AF692202

Encapsulation Nanotechnologies

Scrivener Publishing
100 Cummings Center, Suite 541J
Beverly, MA 01915-6106

Publishers at Scrivener
Martin Scrivener (martin@scrivenerpublishing.com)
Phillip Carmical (pcarmical@scrivenerpublishing.com)

Encapsulation Nanotechnologies

Edited by

Vikas Mittal

Chemical Engineering Department,
The Petroleum Institute,
Abu Dhabi, UAE

Scrivener Publishing

WILEY

Copyright © 2013 by Scrivener Publishing LLC. All rights reserved.

Co-published by John Wiley & Sons, Inc. Hoboken, New Jersey, and Scrivener Publishing LLC, Salem, Massachusetts.
Published simultaneously in Canada.

No part of this publication may be reproduced, stored in a retrieval system, or transmitted in any form or by any means, electronic, mechanical, photocopying, recording, scanning, or otherwise, except as permitted under Section 107 or 108 of the 1976 United States Copyright Act, without either the prior written permission of the Publisher, or authorization through payment of the appropriate per-copy fee to the Copyright Clearance Center, Inc., 222 Rosewood Drive, Danvers, MA 01923, (978) 750-8400, fax (978) 750-4470, or on the web at www.copyright.com. Requests to the Publisher for permission should be addressed to the Permissions Department, John Wiley & Sons, Inc., 111 River Street, Hoboken, NJ 07030, (201) 748-6011, fax (201) 748-6008, or online at http://www.wiley.com/go/permission.

Limit of Liability/Disclaimer of Warranty: While the publisher and author have used their best efforts in preparing this book, they make no representations or warranties with respect to the accuracy or completeness of the contents of this book and specifically disclaim any implied warranties of merchantability or fitness for a particular purpose. No warranty may be created or extended by sales representatives or written sales materials. The advice and strategies contained herein may not be suitable for your situation. You should consult with a professional where appropriate. Neither the publisher nor author shall be liable for any loss of profit or any other commercial damages, including but not limited to special, incidental, consequential, or other damages.

For general information on our other products and services or for technical support, please contact our Customer Care Department within the United States at (800) 762-2974, outside the United States at (317) 572-3993 or fax (317) 572-4002.

Wiley also publishes its books in a variety of electronic formats. Some content that appears in print may not be available in electronic formats. For more information about Wiley products, visit our web site at www.wiley.com.

For more information about Scrivener products please visit www.scrivenerpublishing.com.

Cover design by Russell Richardson

Library of Congress Cataloging-in-Publication Data:

ISBN 978-1-118-34455-2

Printed in the United States of America

10 9 8 7 6 5 4 3 2 1

Contents

Preface

The encapsulation process is prevalent in the evolutionary processes of nature, where nature protects the materials from the environment by engulfing them in a suitable shell. These natural processes are well known and have been applied to numerous processes in the pharmaceutical, food, agricultural, and cosmetics industries. Thus, this allows one to combine the properties of the various components along with the time point of combination, if the release from such capsules can be controlled.

In recent years, owing to the increased understanding of the material properties and behaviors at nanoscale, research in the encapsulation field has also moved to the generation of nanocapsules, nanocontainers, etc. One such example is the generation of self-healing nanocontainers containing corrosion inhibitors which can be used in anti-corrosion coatings. The processes used to generate such capsules have also undergone significant developments. Various technologies based on chemical, physical and physic-chemical synthesis methods have been developed and applied successfully to generate encapsulated materials.

Owing to the high potential of the developed technologies and products in a large number of commercial processes, it is of significance to compile the recent technological advancements in a comprehensive volume. This volume not only introduces the subject of encapsulation to readers new to the field, but also serves as a reference for experts working in this area.

Chapter 1 details the copper encapsulation of carbon nanotubes. Since copper is a good electrical and thermal conductor and has a low binding energy to carbon, its encapsulation into CNTs would lead to many interesting practical applications. Chapter 2 describes the intercalation of ionically conductive polymers into the layers of molybdic acid. The resulting intercalation compounds were characterized by powder X-ray diffraction (XRD), thermogravimetric analysis (TGA), Fourier-transform infrared spectroscopy (FTIR), and ac impedance spectroscopy. Chapter 3 discusses various aspects of the application of fluid-bed technology for the coating and encapsulation processes. Particular attention has been paid to the principles of the fluidization technique, the miscellaneous fluid-bed coating processes and various coaters configurations with special emphasis on fine powder coating, dry coating and encapsulation. Chapter 4 demonstrates the use of the electrospinning technique for encapsulation. The electrospinning technique, consisting of the application of an electrical voltage to a polymeric solution to generate fiber or capsule-like morphologies, has tremendous potential for the development of encapsulation structures of interest in a number of areas such as biomedicine, food technology, bioremediation, energy storage, etc. Chapter 5 details the concept of microencapsulation by interfacial polymerization. Interfacial polymerization, including polycondensation, polyaddition, *in situ* polymerization as well as other heterophase polymerization processes, is defined by the formation of the capsules shell at or on a droplet or particles by polymerization of reactive monomers. Chapter 6 summarizes the main contributions from the literature for the preparation of a specific example of such hybrid materials, core-shell particles composed of an inner silica core and a poly(methyl methacrylate) outer shell. Chapter 7 provides an overview of recent progress in encapsulation technologies for organic thin-film transistors (OTFTs). General mechanisms of environment-induced degradation to OTFTs is reviewed, along with a discussion on the general requirements of encapsulation. Chapter 8 demonstrates that the derivatives of a hyperbranched polymer (mainly hyperbranched polyethylenimine (PEI)) can encapsulate a variety of guest species, and the encapsulating system shows a rather high guest selectivity, in which a specific interaction is absent or very weak. Chapter 9 presents a description of the initiated chemical vapor deposition (iCVD) process, concentrating on aspects like molecular weight of the deposited polymer, which is important for stability, and deposition rate. Both aspects, molecular weight and deposition rate, are essential for large-scale application in hybrid gas barriers. Chapter 10 provides an overview of the current status of polymer capsule technology, with a specific focus on preparation methods and their areas of application. The preparation of polymer capsules and their general features for applications are addressed. Chapter 11 demonstrates the potentialities of encapsulated ionic liquids (IL) within porous moieties in the proton exchange membranes field.

One approach relies on the IL immobilization in large pore zeolites, which are further deployed as inorganic fillers to the polymer casting solution. Chapter 12 reviews the encapsulation and co-precipitation processes based on the use of supercritical fluids, i.e., carbon dioxide. These processes are classified according to the role of the carbon dioxide (solvent, antisolvent, solute or reaction medium). The focus is set on the process mechanisms description, as well as the evolution of different techniques for overcoming the challenges set according to the physical properties of the different processed materials.

Vikas MITTAL
Abu Dhabi

List of Contributors

Alvise Benedetti is a professor of physical chemistry at the Department of Molecular Sciences and Nanosystems, Università Ca'Foscari Venezia, Italy. He is the author of more than 120 papers published in international journals. His research has focused on physical-chemical studies, mostly from a structural point of view, of amorphous, partially crystalline and polycrystalline systems containing nanostructured phases both in surface and/or in bulk systems.

Rabin Bissessur received his PhD from Michigan State University in 1994, and is currently professor of chemistry at the University of Prince Edward Island. His research interests include the development of nanocomposites for lithium rechargeable batteries and carbon capture. He has co-authored 38 refereed articles, and 4 book chapters.

María José Cocero founded the High Pressure Process Group at the University of Valladolid (Spain) in 1998. Since then, she has published more than 200 papers on natural bioactive compounds extraction and formulation, supercritical water oxidation for the treatment of highly contaminated wastewater and biorefinary applications, among other topics.

Douglas C. Dahn received his PhD from the University of British Columbia in 1985, and is currently associate professor of physics at the University of Prince Edward Island. He has co-authored 22 refereed articles and two patents on topics including scanning probe microscopy and condensed matter and materials physics.

Adela Eguizábal received her diploma in chemical engineering in 2008 and the MSc degree in chemical engineering in 2010 from the University of Zaragoza, Spain. She is currently a research associate in the Department of Chemical and Environmental Engineering and also works in the Nanoscience Institute of Aragon (INA). Her research interests are focused on composites based on microporous materials, high temperature PEMFCs and polymer based microsystems prepared by soft litography for preconcentration and reaction applications.

Maria José Fabra is a post-doctoral researcher at the Novel Materials and Nanotechnology Group of IATA-CSIC. She has published thirty papers, one book and eight book chapters. The main research interests are the development of new biodegradable packaging materials and the encapsulation of functional and bioactive compounds.

Isidora Freris is a post-doctoral researcher at the Department of Molecular Sciences and Nanosystems, Università Ca'Foscari Venezia, Italy. She obtained her PhD in chemistry from Monash University, Australia in 2007. Her current research is focused on the development of nanostructured hybrid materials, particularly organic-inorganic core-shell hybrids and luminescent materials via sol-gel processing. She has co-authored 9 scientific publications.

Yu Fu received his doctorate degree in materials science and engineering from the National Taiwan University in 2011 and is now general manager of Yu Crystal Encapsulation Co.

Blakney Hopkins worked on an honours project under the supervision of Professor Rabin Bissessur. She graduated with a BSc (Honors) degree in chemistry in 2010 from the University of Prince Edward Island.

José M. Lagaron, PhD, is Founder and Group Leader of the Novel Materials and Nanotechnology Group of the IATA-CSIC (Valencia, Spain) and is part-time professor of materials science at the Universitat Jaume I. He has published more than one hundred peer-reviewed papers and has fourteen patent applications in nanotechnology applied to polymers.

Amparo López-Rubio PhD, is a research scientist and project leader in the encapsulation area within the Novel Materials and Nanotechnology Group of the Institute of Agrochemistry and Food Technology (IATA) of the Spanish Council for Scientific Research (CSIC). She has published more than forty five papers in peer-reviewed international journals on the subjects of food technology, nanotechnology, packaging and biopackaging.

Ángel **Martín** is a senior researcher at the University of Valladolid (Spain). During his PhD and postdoctoral visits to the universities of Delft (The Netherlands) and Bochum (Germany), he specialized in the development of new materials by supercritical fluids techniques for a wide portfolio of applications, from energy to pharmaceutics.

Boateng Onwona-Agyeman received his PhD from Saga University in Japan. He is currently a senior lecturer at the Department of Materials Science and Engineering, University of Ghana. His current research includes the development of nanoporous structured materials and thin films for solar cell applications and has 30 publications in peer-reviewed journals.

Jong Myung Park is currently a professor in the fields of polymer materials and coatings in the Graduate Institute of Ferrous Technology at Pohang University of Science and Technology (POSTECH), Korea. He received his PhD in polymer science and engineering from Lehigh University, U.S.A. in 1990. He has more than 25 years of industrial R&D experience in the fields of organic coatings and corrosion protection/surface treatments and holds more than 90 patents and published more than 50 scientific papers. His research interests include (1) polymer synthesis and characterization, (2) morphology control for polymeric and hybrid particles, (3) functional coatings for corrosion control/self-healing and (4) functional nano-materials for bio- and energy-related areas.

Rocío Pérez-Masiá has an Msc in food science and engineering and is a PhD student in the Novel Materials and Nanotechnology group at IATA-CSIC. She is focused in the development of new materials through the electrospinning technology for active packaging applications and has coauthored 4 publications in the field of food packaging.

María Pilar Pina received her diploma in chemistry in 1994 and her PhD in chemistry in 1998 from the University of Zaragoza, Spain. She is currently associate professor with tenure at the Chemical Engineering and Environmental Department at the University of Zaragoza and active member of the Nanoscience Institute of Aragon (INA). Her research activities are mainly focused on microfabrication using zeolite membranes as structural layers for reaction, separation and sensing applications; development of polymer based microsystems by soft lithography and modified with nanostructured materials; and chemical sensors for gas detection at trace level.

Jatindra Kumar Rath Manager Utrecht University lab at HTC, Eindhoven, Netherlands, has over 25 years of experience in thin films silicon solar cells and has published more than 250 papers. His main research interests are transient and dusty plasmas in PECVD, nanocrystalline silicon and quantum dots, multijunction and heterojunction solar cells and solar cells on nano-textured surfaces and plastics.

Soraya Rodríguez-Rojo is assistant lecturer at the University of Valladolid, Spain where she earned her doctorate in chemical engineering (2008) on the hydrodynamics of supercritical fluidized bed for microparticle coating. During her two post-doctoral research fellowships (ETH-Zurich, Switzerland, and ITQB-IBET, Portugal), she has specialized in the formulation of nutraceutical compounds.

Fabien Salaün is a professor assistant at ENSAIT/GEMTEX, France. His research interests focus on polymer synthesis, encapsulation, and functional coatings for textile applications. His obtained his PhD in 2004 from the University of Lille 1, France. He has published more than 20 articles in refereed journals and 3 book sections in these research fields.

Toshifumi Satoh received his PhD from Hokkaido University in 1996. He subsequently joined the faculty of this university and was promoted to a professor in 2013. He has 177 publications to his credit, including research papers, reviews, and book chapters. His current fields of interest are branched polymers and unimolecular micelles

Ruud Schropp received his PhD in science from the University of Groningen in 1987. After that he worked in R&D at Glasstech Solar, Inc. in Colorado, USA on solar cells. In 1989 he joined Utrecht University and in 2000, he was appointed Full Professor in "Physics of Devices". In 2012 he joined the Energy Research Center of the Netherlands (ECN), while continuing professorship in thin film photovoltaics at Eindhoven University of Technology.

Diederick Spee studied physics at Utrecht University where he completed his master thesis on back contacted HIT solar cells in 2009. Currently, he is completing his PhD research on the hot wire chemical vapor deposition of flexible thin film organic/inorganic multilayer moisture barriers.

Yong Sun received his PhD from Kyushu Institute of Technology in Japan. He is currently an associate professor at the Department of Applied Science for Integrated System Engineering, Kyushu Institute of Technology. His research area includes the electromagnetic and acoustic properties of nano-materials and semiconductors.

Roman Grzegorz Szafran is an assistant professor at the Wroclaw University of Technology, Faculty of Chemistry, Department of Chemical Engineering, Poland. He is a specialist in the field of chemical engineering, fluid-bed and spout-fluid bed systems, coating, CFD modeling and microengineering. He is the author of 44 publications and 9 patent applications.

Feng-Yu Tsai received his doctorate degree in materials science from the University of Rochester in 2002 and is an associate professor of materials science and engineering at the National Taiwan University. His research interests include atomic and molecular layer deposition, nanotechnologies, and organic and flexible electronics including light-emitting diodes, organic photovoltaics, and thin-film transistors. Dr. Tsai has more than 50 publications and patents in related fields.

Decheng Wan received his PhD from Fudan University in 1999. He joined the faculty of Tongji University in 2006 and was promoted to a professor in 2011. He has (co)authored 68 research papers, reviews, and book chapters. His research interest is macromolecular synthesis and supramolecular chemistry.

1

Copper Encapsulation of Multi-Walled Carbon Nanotubes

Yong Sun[1] and Boateng Onwona-Agyeman[2]

[1]*Dept. of Applied Science for Integrated System Engineering, Kyushu Institute of Technology, Tobata-ku, Kitakyushu-city, Japan*
[2]*Graduate School of Bioresource and Bioenvironmental Sciences, Department of Agro-environmental Sciences, Kyushu University, Hakozaki, Higashi-ku, Fukuoka-city, Japan*

Abstract
Properties of hollow carbon nanotubes (CNTs) could be modified by introducing foreign materials into the interior. Different materials used to fill CNTs include water molecules, DNA segments, metals and many others. Among CNTs filled with different materials, metal-filled CNTs show great potential in numerous applications, such as data storage nanotechnology, due to their small size. In addition, the carbon sheets of CNTs provide an effective layer against oxidation and therefore ensure long-term stability of the encapsulated metals. Since copper is a good electrical and thermal conductor and has a low binding energy to carbon, its encapsulation into CNTs would lead to many interesting practical applications. Typically, CNTs filled with Cu are useful for the fabrication of ultra-low resistance nanoscale electronic devices. Recently, bamboo-like tapered CNTs with only copper located at the tip region were also found to be useful for tube spot welding using current-induced Joule heating. The Cu impregnation in the hollow inner region of CNTs can be attained *in situ* during the CNT growth by incorporating metals or metal precursors along with the carbon source. The other fabrication method is to fill copper into the prepared CNTs by various means, such as electrodeposition, wet chemistry, capillary suction and plasma irradiation.

Vikas Mittal (ed.) Encapsulation Nanotechnologies, (1–40) © 2013 Scrivener Publishing LLC

In this chapter we will introduce three general copper encapsulation methods; electric arc discharge, chemical vapor deposition and laser ablation. The mechanism of the encapsulation will also be discussed.

Keywords: Multi-walled carbon nanotube, copper, encapsulation, electric arc discharge, chemical vapor deposition, laser ablation, vapor-liquid-solid model, tip growth, root growth

1.1 Introduction

Since its discovery in the 1990s [1–4], carbon nanotubes (CNTs), including single-wall carbon nanotube (SWNT) and multi-wall carbon nanotubes (MWCNTs), have attracted great industrial and academic interest. Due to their superior mechanical, thermal, electrical and optical properties, CNTs are expected to replace many classic components in the near future [5–7]. It has also been practically shown that they possess extremely good mechanical properties and remarkable electrical transport properties, therefore enabling their potential use in nanoelectronic devices, energy storage, field emission displays, chemical and biological sensors and other technological fields [8, 9]. Since CNTs possess hollow cylindrical structures they could be used as containers of atoms and small molecules [10–12], and also can be used for hydrogen storage [13].

Different materials used to fill CNTs include water molecules [14], DNA segments [15], metals [16, 17] and many others [18, 19]. Among CNTs filled with different materials, metal-filled CNTs show great potential in numerous applications, such as data storage nanotechnology, due to their small size. In addition, the carbon sheets of CNTs provide an effective layer against oxidation and therefore ensure long-term stability of the encapsulated metals. One such example is the filling of iron in CNTs demonstrated by Borowiak-Palen *et al.* [19]. The encapsulation of iron in CNTs is suitable for use as magnetic field sensors due to the ferromagnetic behavior of the system at room temperatures. Also, CNTs filled with ferromagnetic fillers can be used in controlling the heating of tumor tissues [20].

Since copper is a good electrical and thermal conductor and has a low binding energy to carbon, its encapsulation into CNTs would lead to many interesting practical applications. Recently, bamboo-like tapered CNTs with only copper located at the tip region were found to be useful for tube spot welding using current-induced Joule heating inside a transmission electron microscope (TEM) [21].

1.2 Preparation of Copper Encapsulated CNTs

Modification of CNTs provides an effective strategy to expand, improve or change their properties and functions giving way to many promising applications [22–24]. Cu impregnation in the hollow inner region of CNTs can be attained *in situ* during the CNT growth by incorporating metals or metal precursors along with the carbon source. Among the metals, copper shows the highest thermal and electrical conductivity apart from silver, and exhibits a low binding energy towards carbon about 0.1 eV [25]. Therefore copper-filled CNTs show potential applications as mentioned above. Various studies have been conducted in the filling of different materials into CNTs [26–29]. For the preparation of copper-filled CNTs we will discuss three general methods; electric arc discharge, chemical vapor deposition (CVD) and laser ablation.

1.2.1 Arc Discharge

The arc discharge method is a common and easy way of producing CNTs. It is a technique that produces a complex mixture of components and sometimes requires further purification to separate the CNTs from the soot and other residual materials. The method creates CNTs through arc vaporization of two carbon rods placed end to end, separated by a small gap, for example, 1 mm in a chamber filled with an inert gas at low pressure. A direct current (DC) of 50–100A, driven by a potential difference creates a high temperature discharge between the carbon rod electrodes. The discharge vaporizes the surface of one of the carbon electrodes and forms a deposit of materials on the surface of the other electrode. The evaporated carbon atoms coagulate to form carbon nanoparticles including fullerenes. A part of the evaporated carbon is deposited on the adjacent cathode (at lower temperature) and MWCNTs grow there.

A. Setlur and coworkers [30] have prepared large quantities of CNTs filled with pure copper by using hydrogen arc. In their method, the interaction of small copper clusters with polycyclic aromatic hydrocarbons (PAH) was shown to form CNTs and encapsulated copper nanowires. The DC arc chamber used in this method was filled with hydrogen to the operating pressure range of several hundred Torr. Two graphite rods of approximately 10 mm in diameter were used as electrodes. A 6 mm diameter hole is made 20 mm deep into the anode and a copper rod is inserted. The arc was generated by a DC supply (100 A, 200 V) and its stability maintained by adjusting the electrode spacing. Materials produced by the arcs were examined by TEM. The authors observed the following; 1. the deposits produced by the hydrogen arcs with the copper composite anodes differ greatly from arcs operated with pure graphite anodes, 2. the rod used as the cathode is covered with a leafy growth. For the 100 and 500 Torr cases, the leaves appear to have small copper particles deposited on them, indicating that the temperature around the deposited rod is less than 1083°C, the melting point of copper. For 500 Torr case, the leaves have a rubbery texture while at 100 Torr the leaves are generally harder. The leaves produced in 500 Torr of hydrogen contain carbon nanotubes, many of which are filled with copper. For the 100 Torr, the leaves produced are less and consist of graphitic sheets and copper particles. From these observations, the authors proposed that the PAH molecules produced by the arc interact with copper clusters to form nuclei for nanotube growth. Once the interaction occurs between the PAH molecules and the copper clusters, growth proceeds by the addition of atoms, chains and rings. Figure 1.1a is a low magnification image of a portion of the soot produced at 500 Torr of hydrogen, consisting of long hollow carbon nanotubes. Figure 1.1b shows a copper rich region of the soot, which has copper-filled nanotubes, copper nanocrystals and larger copper crystals. It is estimated that, in these regions about 80–90%

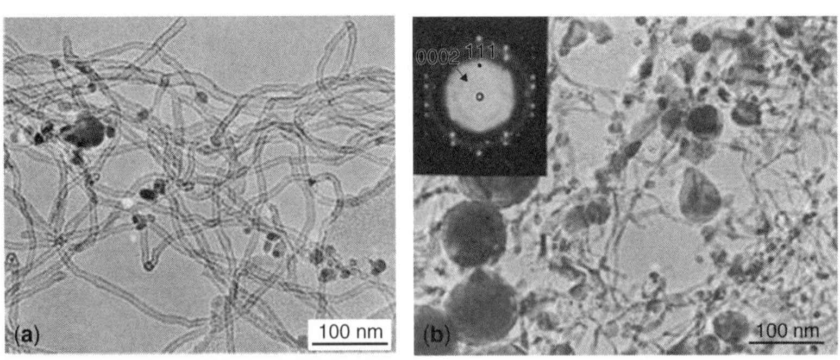

Figure 1.1 TEM images of the soot formed in 500 Torr of hydrogen with a copper composite anode. (a) Long hollow nanotubes. (b) A copper rich region of the soot, the inset is SAED pattern with (111) twin of the copper encapsulation and the (0002) graphite layer.

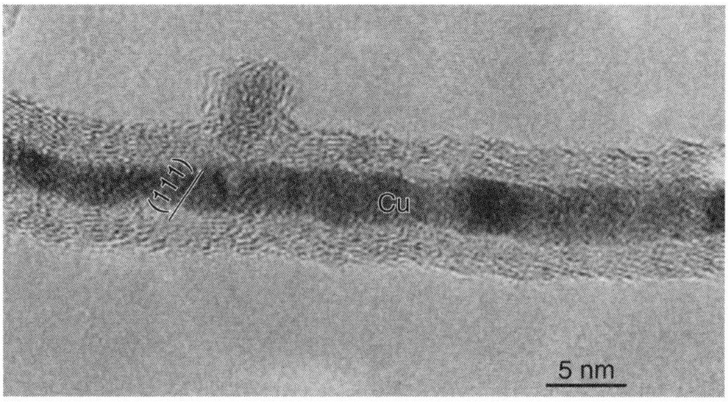

Figure 1.2 HRTEM image of a copper-filled nanotube with a diameter of about 10 nm.

of the nanotubes are completely filled with copper. The selected area electron diffraction (SAED) pattern (inset) shows the presence of crystalline copper (111) and graphitic layers. Figure 1.2 shows a high resolution transmission electron micrograph (HRTEM) of the filled nanotube. The copper in the nanotubes is polycrystalline with twins occurring in some tubes. It was estimated through TEM observations that 20–30% of the nanotubes were filled with copper. To explain the observation of both filled and unfilled nanotubes, the authors proposed the following model as shown schematically in Figure 1.3. Small copper clusters produced by the arc must either coagulate with other copper clusters or interact with PAH molecules as shown in Figures 1.3(a), (b) and (c) to reduce their energy. The authors proposed that in these experiments, the PAH molecules produced by the arc resembling small graphitic sheets interact with copper clusters similarly to graphite to form nuclei for nanotube growth in Figure 1.3(c). It is evident from their results that copper and PAH molecules interact to form nuclei for nanotube growth. In a copper rich region, Figure 1.1(b), there is copper available to fill the nanotubes as seen in Figure 1.3(d). In a copper poor region, Figure 1.1(a), there is not enough copper to fill the nanotubes as they grow, resulting in the empty nanotubes shown in Figure 1.3(e).

Z. Wang and coworkers [31] have also reported a simple arc-discharge method for *in situ* synthesis of copper-filled CNTs with coal as carbon precursor. The experiment was carried out in a DC arc discharge reactor in an argon gas ambient. A high purity

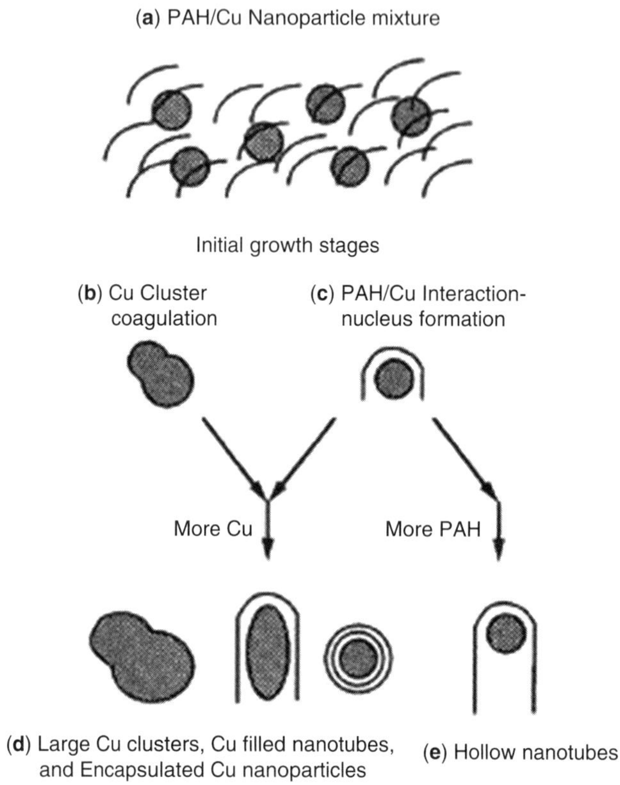

Figure 1.3 Schematic diagram of Cu/PAH interactions and nanotube growth. (a) PAH/Cu from hydrogen arc. (b) Coagulation of copper clusters to reduce surface energy. (c) Interaction of copper clusters with PAH molecules, which forms the nucleus for nanotube growth. (d) A copper rich region of the leaves containing large copper clusters, copper-filled nanotubes, and copper-encapsulated nanoparticles. (e) A region of the leaves or soot that contains hollow nanotubes.

graphite tube filled with a mixture of coal (anthracite) and CuO powder, particle size less than 150 μm, was used as the anode while the cathode was made of high purity graphite rod. The weight ratio of CuO to coal in the mixture was 1:9. The arc discharge was carried out with a direct current of 70 A and voltage of 20 V in argon ambient at 80–90 kPa. After the discharge, the deposits on the cathode were collected and examined using TEM. Figure 1.4(a) shows a low magnification TEM image of the as-prepared sample showing the complete synthesis of copper encapsulated CNTs of several tens micrometers long. They also observed that in some CNTs, there were several distorted defects such as kinks and curls in which the

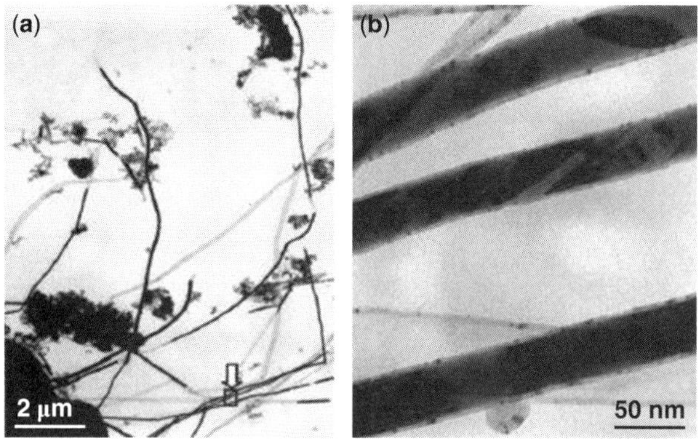

Figure 1.4 TEM images of Cu-filled CNTs prepared with coal as carbon source: (a) image of super-long Cu nanowires; (b) an image of three Cu-filled CNTs from (a), indicated by white arrow.

distance between the defects varies from hundreds of nanometers to several micrometers. The HRTEM image in Figure 1.4(b) shows that the CNTs are completely filled with copper with a diameter of about 30–80 nm and the aspect ratio of the copper filled CNTs is about 200–360. Repeated experiments indicated that on average more than 40–50% of the as-prepared CNTs are filled with copper as can be seen in Figure 1.5. The SAED patterns of the distorted nanowires are shown in the insets of Figures 1.5(b) and (d). The observed diffractions consist of regular arrays of sharp spots together with short arc due to the (002) diffraction of hexagonal graphite indicating the presence of well-developed monocrystalline structure in the copper nanowires. These diffraction patterns are in good agreement with typical diffraction pattern of a face-centered cubic (fcc) copper along the (011) zone axis. They also showed a HRTEM image of a 30 nm diameter copper-filled CNT in Figure 1.6 in which monocrystals have been observed in long-range order as well as the outside coating consisting of well-oriented graphite layers (about 20 layers with a separation of about 0.34 nm). They concluded that these results show that the encapsulated material inside the CNTs was pure copper consisting of several long monocrystals. A one-step synthesis by J. Ding and colleagues [32] was used to prepare pure copper nanowire in carbon nanotubes with different structures by DC arc discharge. The as-prepared

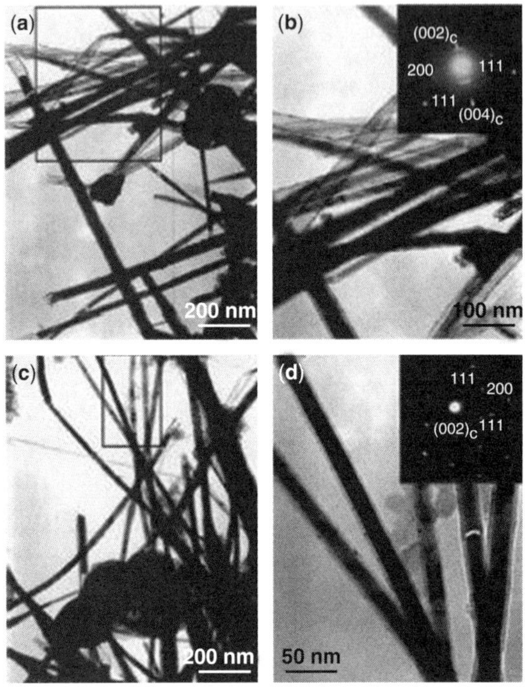

Figure 1.5 TEM images of the Cu-filled CNTs. (a) and (c): Magnified images and (b) and (d): SAED patterns showing CNTs filled with Cu nanowires.

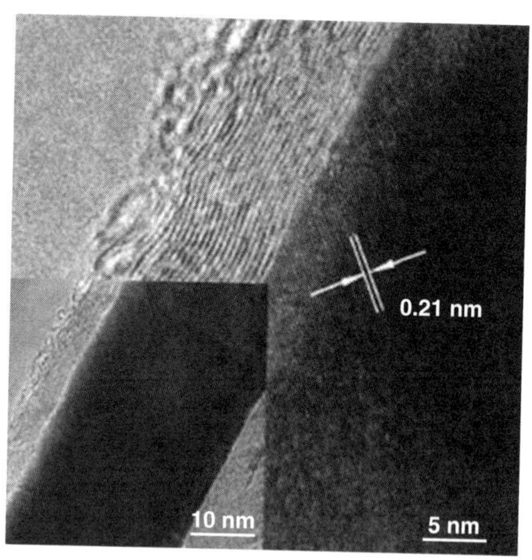

Figure 1.6 HRTEM image of one Cu-filled carbon nanotube.

copper encapsulated CNTs (Cu@CNTs) exhibited three different structures, including well-filled Cu@CNT nanocables, symmetrically trifurcate Cu@CNT nanocables and twice capsulated Cu@CNT nanocables. The DC arc discharge system they used consisted of anode-cathode assembly installed in a stainless steel cylindrical chamber capped at both ends. The cathode was a highly pure graphite rod and the anode 65 mm long with outer and inner diameters of 10 and 6 mm before arcing respectively. The anode, being hollow was packed with metal copper powders. The experiment was carried out in a helium/hydrogen ambient (volume ratio: 1:1) at total pressure of 400 Torr, and the arc discharge was created by a current of 120 A. The gap between the cathode and anode was kept at 2 mm by fixing the consumed anode and advancing the cathode manually. The crystal structures of the deposited powder were studied using X-ray diffraction (XRD), and the microstructure and surface morphology were characterized by scanning electron microscope (SEM) and HRTEM. Figure 1.7 shows XRD pattern of the samples with peaks corresponding to graphite, copper carbide and copper respectively. No diffraction peaks corresponding to

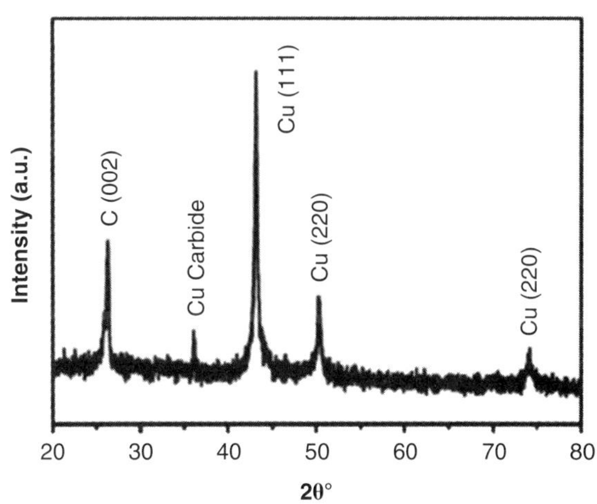

Figure 1.7 XRD pattern of the sample.

other phases can be observed. They observed that the diffraction signals were from CNTs, small amounts of copper carbide and copper clusters. In order to study the microstructure and morphology of the samples of the encapsulated copper, TEM images were taken. Figure 1.8(a) shows the CNTs nanostructures consisting of unfilled, partially-filled and well-filled nanotubes marked with U, P and W respectively. It indicates that over 85% of CNTs can be filled with copper and the CNTs walls will still remain intact. The inset

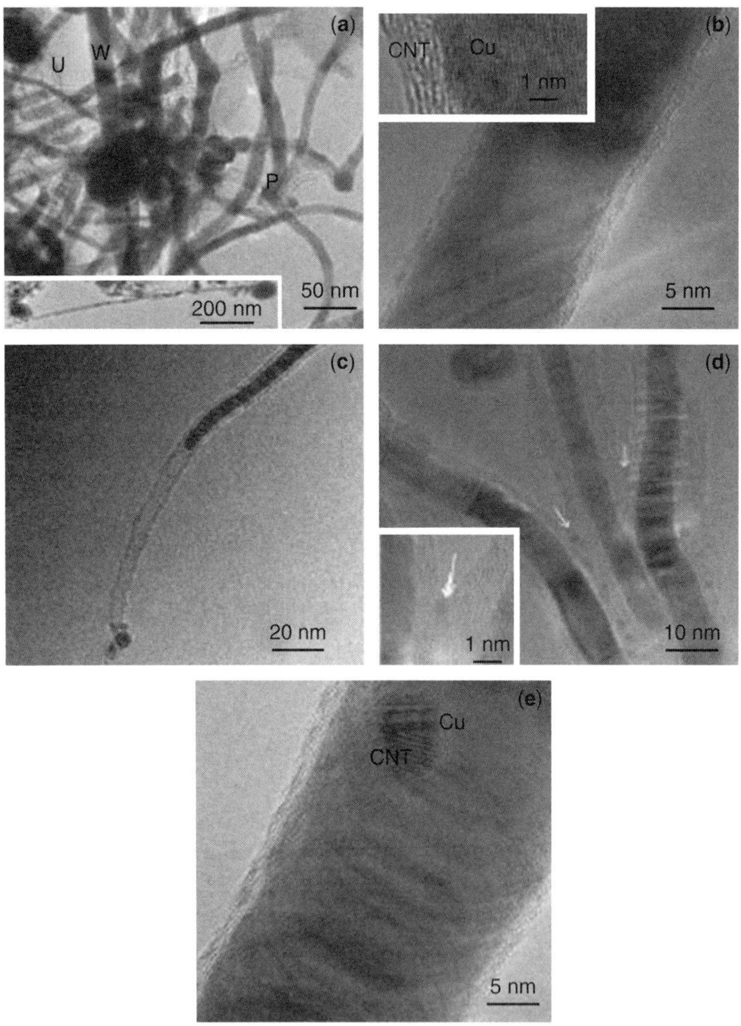

Figure 1.8 (a) TEM image of the sample, (b) HRTEM image of single Cu@CNT, (c) image of terminal single Cu@CNT, (d) a trifurcate Cu@CNT, (e) HRTEM image of twice encapsulated Cu@CNT.

of Figure 1.8(a) shows that well-filled CNTs can be as long as over one micrometer. A HRTEM image of a single Cu@CNT is shown in Figure 1.8(b) indicating well-filled CNTs with oriented graphite layers and encapsulated copper crystals inside the MWCNTs. The inset shows the d-spacing of the graphite layers (about 6 layers) and the encapsulated copper crystals with (111) atomic plane. Figure 1.8(c) shows a terminal morphology of an individual Cu@CNT. The hollow structure of the CNT, the tube's wall and the copper nanowire level inside can be seen. Also, the filled section of the Cu@CNT has a larger diameter compared with the hollow one. They attributed this to the continuous incorporation of the copper clusters into the MWCNTs during growth. Figure 1.8(d) reveals a trifurcate Cu@CNT nanocable and well-filled copper nanocables. The inset of Figure 1.8(d) indicates non-crystal copper nanoparticles embedded into the branched spot, which may be due to the formation of interfacial copper carbide that favors infiltration of liquid copper nanoparticles into CNTs and resides at defect sites. Figure 1.8(e) shows that copper nanocrystalline grains encapsulated in CNTs are found to exist inside copper CNT nanocables, implying that the growth process of copper CNT nanocables is very delicate. Copper carbide will possibly be formed at interface between the twice encapsulated CNTs [33]. The authors explained the growth mechanism of the copper encapsulated CNT by using the vapor-liquid-solid (VLS) model [34]. As shown in Figure 1.9, first the carbon atoms that are evaporated from graphite or decomposed from carbon-rich gases (hydrocarbons resulting from interaction of carbon and hydrogen buffer gas during arc discharge) dissolve into liquid copper clusters as shown in Figure 1.9(a). Copper then

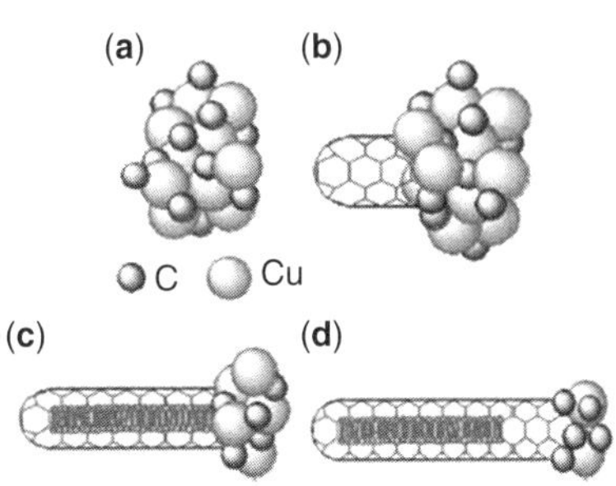

Figure 1.9 Schematic diagram of the growth mechanism of Cu@CNT: (a) carbon atom diffusion within the molten copper particles, (b) initial growth of the MWCNTs, (c) part of copper clusters is pulled into the MWCNTs, and (d) formation of partially-filled Cu@CNTs.

catalyzes the decomposition of the carbon precursor and leads to the supersaturated carbon precipitation to grow the CNTs shown in Figure 1.9(b). Later, part of the liquid copper is sucked into the hollow of the CNT shown in Figure 1.9(c). The authors attributed this sucking to capillary attraction, and also the low solubility of copper with carbon is responsible for the outer walls of CNTs being free from copper clusters.

Copper encapsulated nanoparticles were synthesized by a modified arc plasma method using methane as carbon source by C. Hao *et al.* [35]. In the arc reactor, two electrodes for the DC arc discharge were fixed with a 5 mm gap between them. The upper electrode was tungsten and the lower electrode (anode) was graphite crucible packed with copper metal rod. The chamber was filled with helium and methane gas with a pressure of 100 kPa after it was vacuumed to Pa. The discharge current was 80 A and the arc plasma was ignited using a high frequency initiator in the chamber. The copper rods were melted and evaporated by the generated high temperature. The evaporated copper and carbon were deposited on the inner walls of the chamber. The morphologies and size of encapsulated copper particles were determined by SEM and HRTEM. Also, the phase and crystal structure of the particles were characterized by XRD. Figure 1.10 shows the XRD patterns of pure copper

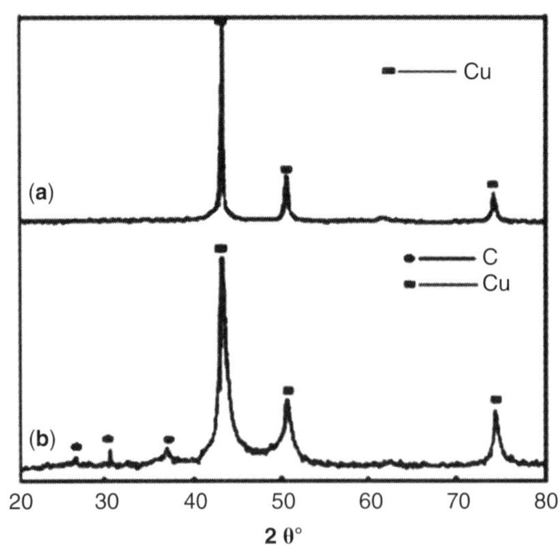

Figure 1.10 XRD patterns of (A) pure copper nanoparticles and (B) copper encapsulated carbon nanoparticles.

nanoparticles (helium/methane =1:2) and copper encapsulated nanoparticles respectively. In Figure 1.10(a) it can be seen that the position of peaks for pure copper nanoparticles is consistent with the reflection lines of fcc copper. In addition to the copper peaks, three peaks due to carbon were also observed in the XRD pattern of the copper encapsulated nanoparticles as shown in Figure 1.10(b). To identify the existence of core-shell structure, SEM and HRTEM images were observed. Figure 1.11(a) shows a typical SEM image of the copper encapsulated nanoparticles and Figure 1.11(b) shows the TEM image. Figure 1.11(c) shows the HRTEM micrograph of copper encapsulated nanoparticles. The authors observed that the

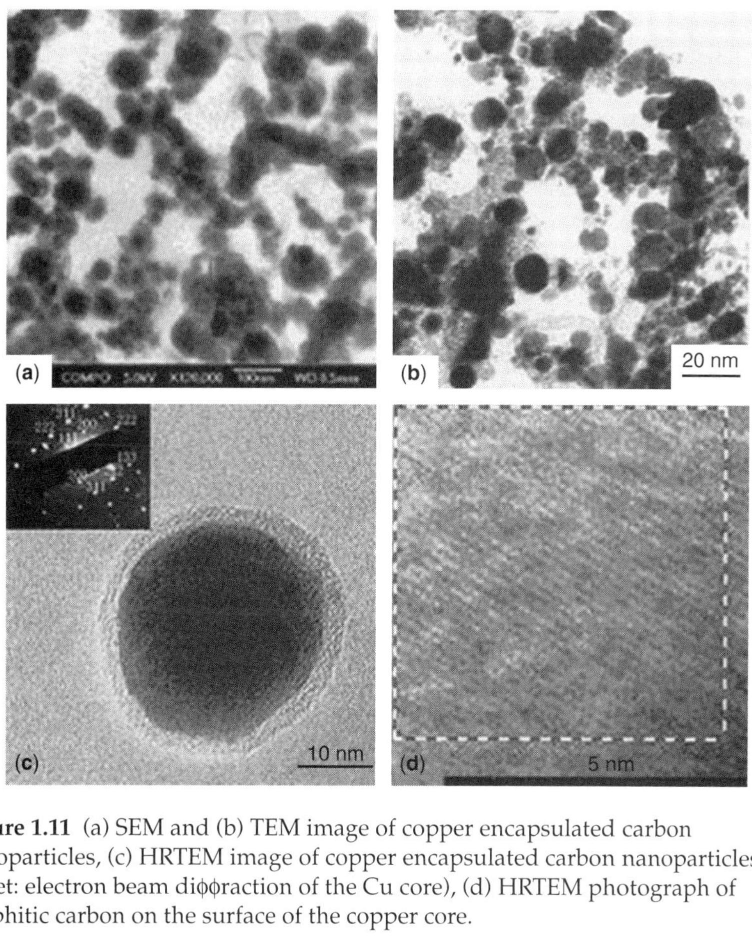

Figure 1.11 (a) SEM and (b) TEM image of copper encapsulated carbon nanoparticles, (c) HRTEM image of copper encapsulated carbon nanoparticles (inset: electron beam diϕϕraction of the Cu core), (d) HRTEM photograph of graphitic carbon on the surface of the copper core.

copper nanoparticles were covered with 3–5 nm carbon layers. The SAED shown in the inset of Figure 1.11(c) indicates that the core is composed of fcc copper. The diameter of the core-shell copper/carbon nanoparticles was about 30 nm. Figure 1.11(d) shows a HRTEM image of the carbon shell. It can be observed that the shells outside the core are not amorphous but ordered graphitic carbon. The interlayer spacing of these graphitic planes is about 0.34 nm. The authors observed that as temperature was increased, the decomposition of hydrocarbons occurred resulting in the formation of copper and carbon vapor. The carbon then dissolves in the copper particles reducing the vapor energy of the copper. The final formation of the product was determined by the cooling rate and the solubility of carbon in copper. The authors also observed the formation of copper nanoparticles under helium and hydrogen atmosphere as shown in the image in Figure 1.12(a). The copper particles were spherical in shape and the average particle size is about 40 nm. Under helium and methane ambient, copper encapsulated CNTs were produced and it was noted that a change in the volume ratio of helium/methane affects the morphologies and size of the copper encapsulated particles. When the ratio of helium/methane is 1, part of the copper nanoparticles clinched to each other as shown in Figure 1.12(b) and the average size is about 40–50 nm. When the ratio is decreased to 1/2, the particle size becomes smaller as can be seen in Figure 1.11(b). The authors also observed that compared

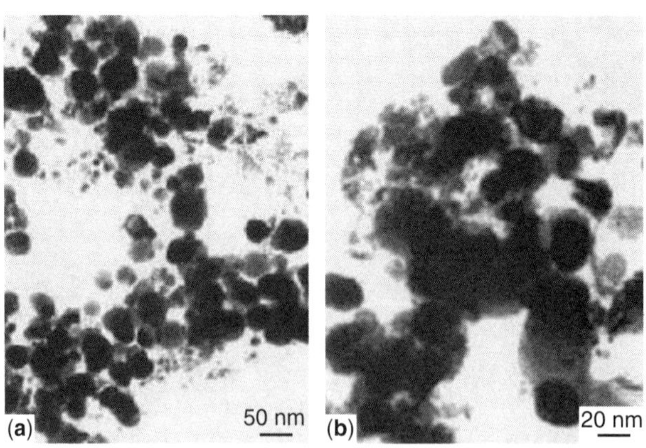

Figure 1.12 (a) TEM micrograph of copper nanoparticles VHe/VH2 = 1:1, (b) TEM micrograph of copper encapsulated carbon nanoparticles VHe/VCH4= 1:1.

with pure copper nanoparticles, the size of the copper encapsulated nanoparticles is evenly distributed. They attributed this to the presence of the carbon shells which limits the growth of the particles and inhibits aggregation of copper particles.

1.2.2 Chemical Vapor Deposition

Chemical vapor deposition of hydrocarbons over metal catalyst is a classic method that has been used to produce various carbon materials such as carbon fiber, diamond-like carbon and recently graphene. Large amounts of CNTs can be formed by CVD of acetylene over metals supported on silica, zeolite or alumina. Currently, the formation of CNTs directly on the metal plate by CVD has attracted much attention because the metal plate can act as the substrate and a catalyst for the growth of the CNTs at the same time. An advantage of the method is that infiltration of unwanted materials into the CNTs can be avoided.

From their experiment, J. Lin *et al.* [36] found that CNTs could be produced in high yield by catalytic decomposition of methane using a copper catalyst, especially when $CuSO_4$ was used with γ-alumina as the support material. The preparation of the CNTs was carried out using a fixed bed quartz tube reactor. The $CuSO_4/Al_2O_3$ catalyst was prepared by impregnating the γ-alumina with an aqueous solution of $CuSO_4.5H_2O$. The catalyst was then loaded into the reactor and treated with helium gas at different temperatures (600–1100°C) after which a mixture of methane/helium in a ration 3/1 was allowed to flow into the reactor at required temperatures for the synthesis of the CNTs. Figure 1.13 shows the catalytic activity of 5 wt.% copper sulfate/alumina at different temperatures for the synthesis of CNTs. From the graph, the growing of CNTs starts at about 600°C and reaches a maximum at about 800°C, and then drops to zero when grown in temperatures that exceed 1000°C. Figure 1.14 shows the SEM and TEM images of CNTs at 800°C for 1 hour on copper nitrate/alumina and copper sulfate/alumina catalysts. The authors observed that the formation rate of CNTs on copper catalyst drops to a barely detectable level when copper nitrate was used as the copper precursor instead of copper sulfate, and also, the CNTs appeared to be the fish-bone type of carbon nanotube shown in Figure 1.14(b). The TEM image in Figure 1.14(c) suggests that the growth of

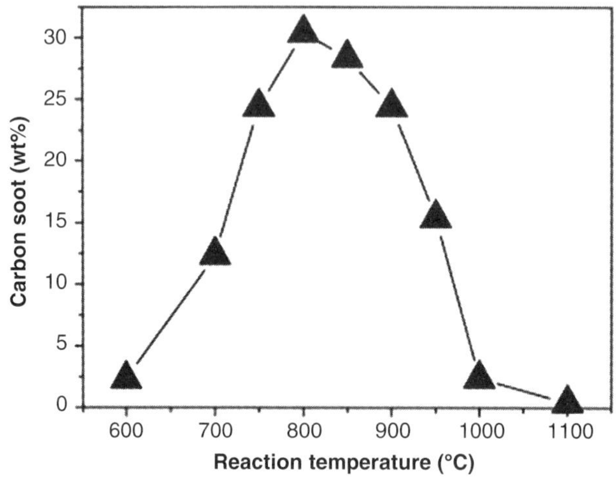

Figure 1.13 Relation between the catalytic activity of 5% Cu SO_4/Al_2O_3 and temperature during the synthesis of carbon soot in CH_4/He (3/1).

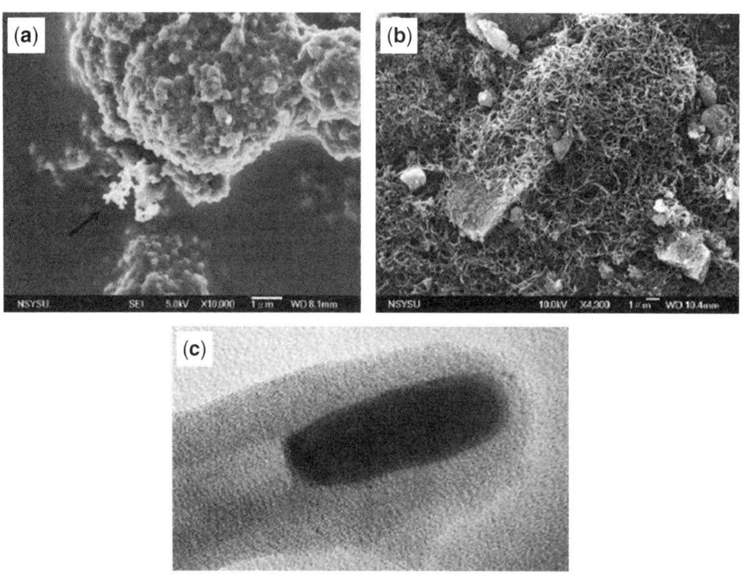

Figure 1.14 SEM images of CNTs on (a) 5% $Cu(NO_3)_2/Al_2O_3$, (b) 5% Cu SO_4 / Al_2O_3, and (c) HRTEM image of CNTs on 5% $CuSO_4/Al_2O_3$.

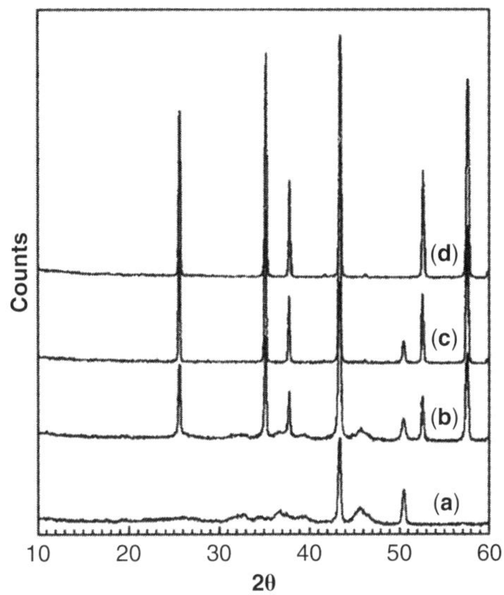

Figure 1.15 XRD patterns of 5% $CuSO_4$/ Al_2O_3 pre-treated at (a) 800°C, (b) 1000°C, (c) 1100°C in He for 2 hr, and (d) α-Al_2O_3.

CNTs on copper catalyst is consistent with a typical tip-growth mechanism where carbon diffusion is followed by precipitation at the rear of the metal particles to form the body of the CNTs. The authors then treated the copper/sulfate catalyst with a stream of helium gas at temperatures between 800 and 1100°C for 2 hours and analyzed the structure by XRD. As shown in Figure 1.15 a broad gamma alumina diffraction pattern is observed at 800°C. An alpha alumina diffraction pattern develops gradually when the temperatures are higher than 800°C, and gamma alumina diffraction pattern fades away completely when temperatures are higher than 1000°C. From the XRD data, the authors postulated that the behavior of copper for catalyzing the CNT synthesis may correlate with the interactions between the copper and gamma alumina. It is well known that copper and gamma alumina forms a mixed oxide with a spinel-type structure. However, high temperature treatment converts the gamma alumina to alpha alumina and destroys the active spinel structure. Therefore a decrease of catalytic activity for the CNT synthesis is observed.

J. Zhu *et al.* [37] have studied the synthesis of bamboo-like CNTs on copper foil by the CVD using ethanol. They investigated the effects of temperature (700–1000°C) on the growth of the CNTs, as well as the structural and morphology of the resultant CNTs. In their experiment, a 50 μm thick pure copper foil was placed on an alumina tube and inserted into a horizontal tube furnace. The system was sealed and evacuated to 10^{-2} Torr before admitting Ar gas and raising the temperature. When the target temperature was attained, the Ar gas was redirected into an ethanol bath before entering the system. After a certain time, the system was allowed to cool down and the copper foil was collected and its surface analyzed. They observed that the size and yield of the CNTs increased with temperature, those prepared at 700°C had a copper droplet tip and those at 800–900°C had a copper nanoparticle inside. On the other hand, an amorphous carbon film consisting of porous and non-porous layer was deposited on the copper foil and CNTs were grown from this layer. They therefore concluded that a carbon film first is deposited on the surface of the copper foil while the surface layer of the copper foil partially melted and migrated across the carbon film where the CNTs formed. Figure 1.16(a) is an SEM image of the cross section of a film of the sample prepared at 900°C for 30 minutes. A high magnification image is also shown in the inset of the Figure. The film consists of two layers (A and B). The thickness of the top layer was about 50 nm (A layer) while the bottom layer was about 760 nm. From its large thickness, the authors concluded that the thick carbon film was not graphene. The EDS results indicated that this black film was a carbon film with about 3.5 at.% of copper shown in Figure 1.16(e). On the surface of the carbon film, clusters of nanostructures were found. The nanostructures were curled with a smooth geometry as shown in the SEM image in Figure 1.16(b). They were extracted and examined by TEM and were confirmed to be CNTs in Figure 1.16(f). The diameter and length of the CNTs were determined to be about 130 nm and several microns respectively. In the TEM images shown in Figure 1.16(c) some particles with a size of about 12 nm (indicated by the dark arrows) were found inside the CNTs near the tips. The particles were not copper oxide as no oxygen signal was found. These CNTs were further examined by HRTEM as shown in Figure 1.16(d) and these CNTs had a bamboo-like structure with complete knots. The authors also studied the structure of the CNTs and their copper catalyst prepared at different temperatures. Figure 1.17 shows the

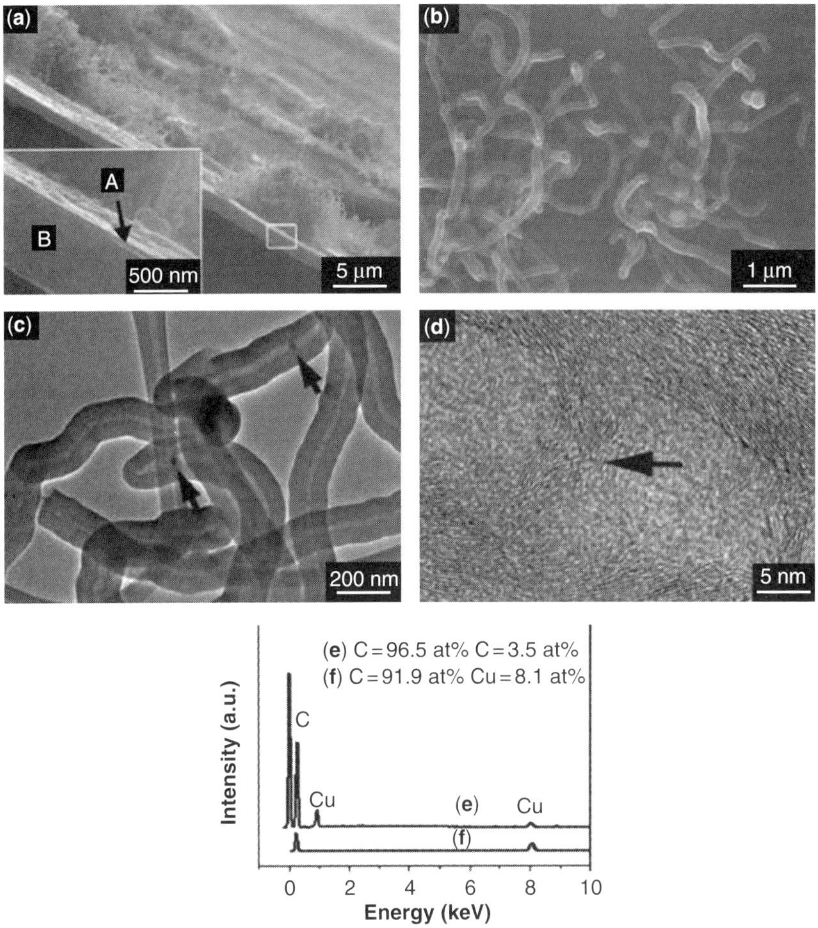

Figure 1.16 (a) SEM image of the CNTs/carbon film of the sample prepared at 900°C for 30 min and magnified image of the carbon film (inset). (b) SEM and (c) TEM images of the CNTs from the same sample. (d) HRTEM image of the CNT. EDS spectra: (e) and (f) from arrowed regions in (a) and (c), respectively.

TEM images of the CNTs collected from samples prepared at 700, 800 and 1000°C for 30 minutes. Their diameter increased from 40 to 210 nm when temperature was increased from 700 to 1000°C, while their length extended from about 500 nm to 2–3 μm. These results and others are listed in Table 1.1. The CNTs prepared at 700°C were short and straight as seen in Figure 1.17(a), but those at higher temperatures were long and curly as shown in Figures 1.17(b) and (c). All the CNTs appeared multi-walled with a bamboo-like structure.

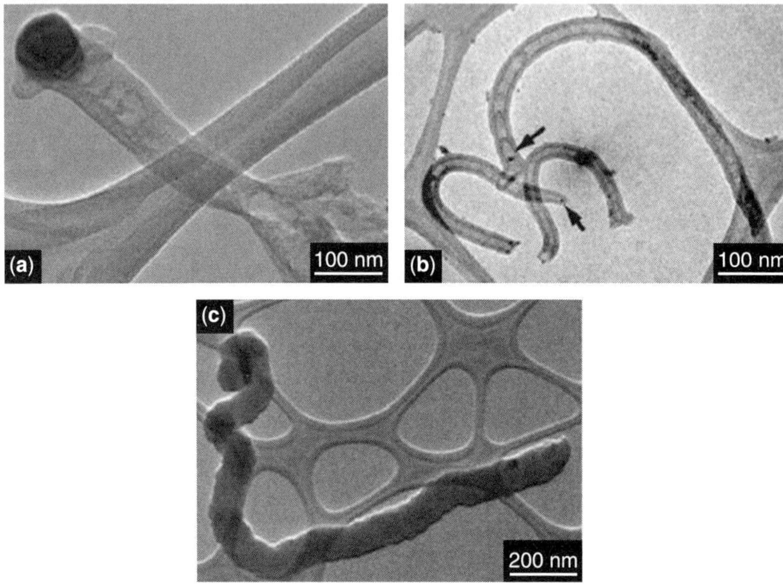

Figure 1.17 TEM images of samples prepared for 30 min at (a) 700, (b) 800, and (c) 1000°C.

Table 1.1 Diameters and lengths of the CNTs, and the I(D)/I(G) ratios of the samples prepared at different temperatures for 30 min.

Samples	**700°C**	**800°C**	**900°C**	**1000°C**
Outer diameter (nm)	73	83	130	175
Inner diameter (nm)	35	28	19	13
Length (μm)	0.5	1	2.5	2
I(D)/I(G)	0.81	0.87	0.82	0.80

Copper droplet tips were found in CNTs prepared at 700°C as shown in Figure 1.17(a). The authors suggested that their growth followed the VLS model [34].

Copper nanoparticles were found inside the CNTs prepared at 800 and 900°C near their tips as indicated by the dark arrows in Figures 1.17(b) and 1.16(c). The copper particle found in the sample prepared at 700°C was about 100 nm in size in Figure 1.17(a) located at the tip of the CNT. Those found inside the CNT tip prepared at 800 and 900°C were about 12 nm, and no copper particles were found at the tips or inside CNTs Table 1.1 Diameters and lengths of the CNTs, and the I(D)/I(G) ratios of the samples prepared at different temperatures for 30 min.

prepared at 1000°C. The authors observed the decrease and disappearance of the copper particles with increasing temperature, and suggested that the copper atoms would be more likely to be mobile and form smaller particles when the temperature is close to its melting point of 1083°C. The HRTEM images of the graphite layers in the walls of the CNTs prepared at 900°C indicated that they were well oriented as shown in Figure 1.16(d), but the CNTs prepared at other temperatures showed low graphitization. Therefore, 900°C was chosen as the optimum temperature for preparing samples with high yield, small diameter and high graphitization. The authors illustrated the growth of the CNTs in their work using schematic diagrams in Figure 1.18. When incoming ethanol vapor is in contact with hot copper foil shown in Figure 1.18(a), carbon from the decomposed ethanol was deposited on the surface of the copper foil to form a film as shown in Figure 1.18(b). With increasing duration, the carbon film became thicker and copper was found to diffuse into the carbon film and parts of the copper nanoparticles accumulated on the upper surface as shown in Figure 1.18(c), leaving pits in the substrate. The copper particles on the surface of the

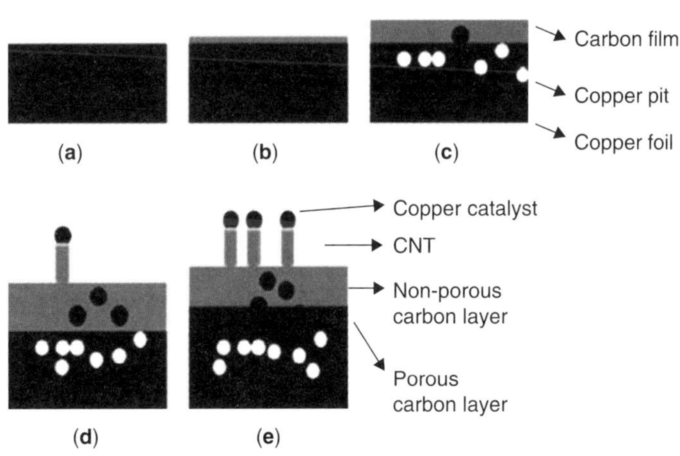

Figure 1.18 Schematic diagrams to illustrate the formation of the CNTs on the copper foil.

carbon film acted as the catalyst for the growth of the CNTs via the tip mode VLS process as indicated in Figure 1.18(d). At the same time, the bottom surface of the carbon film interacted with the copper foil and became porous as shown in Figure 1.18(e).

Q. Zhang and colleagues [38] have prepared carbon nanotubes with totally hollow channels and totally filled copper nanowires using methane decomposition on copper microgrid as a catalyst at 1173 K. The aim of their work is to develop a method to prepare CNTs with totally hollow channels and to *in situ* fill copper into the nanotubes. They reported that by using this method, the filling ratio of the copper can be up to 50% of the totally hollow channels of the CNTs. They also reported that the encapsulated copper species can form continuous single crystalline copper nanowires (8–10 μm) by tailoring the copper catalyst and the composition of feed gas. In their method, nanometer-sized copper species were placed on a microgrid, usually used as the sample carrier for the HRTEM observation. The microgrid with the nanosized copper was inserted into a horizontal quartz tube reactor. Then, a mixture of hydrogen, methane and argon with flow rates of 100, 100 and 400 ml/min, respectively was fed into the reactor and decomposed to synthesize the CNTs at 1173 K at atmospheric pressure. The products were directly deposited on the microgrid. After 30 minutes, the power was switched off and the reactor was cooled to the ambient condition. The carbon-based product on the microgrid was directly characterized by HRTEM. As shown in Figure 1.19(a), the relatively low magnification TEM image shows that there are large amounts of CNTs growing along the edge of the microgrid. Most of the CNTs are straight and 6–10 μm long as in Figures 1.19(b) and (c), indicating their relatively uniform growth rate from the microgrid. There are about 70% CNTs with tips free of metal catalyst and 30% CNTs with large metal particles at the tip as shown in Figures 1.19(b) and (d). Also most CNTs have a larger tip as compared with its diameter (Figure 1.20) which the authors could not explain. Regardless of their different growth modes, most CNTs are totally hollow or are totally filled by copper as in Figures 1.19(c)(d) and Figure 1.21. The authors compared the CNTs grown on pure copper catalyst and then on iron-copper catalyst. Grown on the iron-copper catalyst by the intentional addition of iron to the copper catalyst, the CNTs obtained were bamboo-like with nearly no hollow channels as shown in Figure 1.22(a). The EDS characterization indicated the iron in the iron-copper alloy catalyst has an atomic ratio of 1.3% as shown in Figure 1.22(b), and catalyst responsible for the filling of

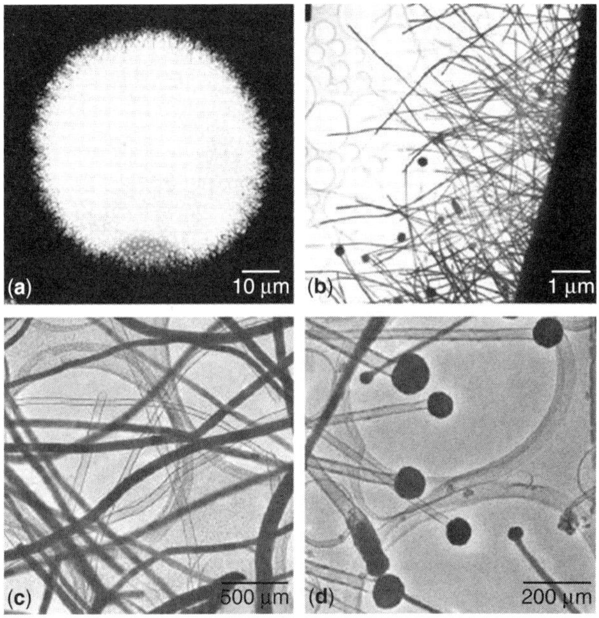

Figure 1.19 (a) TEM image of CNTs on the edge of microgrid; (b) TEM image of 70% CNTs following base growth mode; (c) image of the relatively straight CNTs filled or unfilled with copper in (b); (d) TEM image of CNTs with totally hollow core and large copper tips.

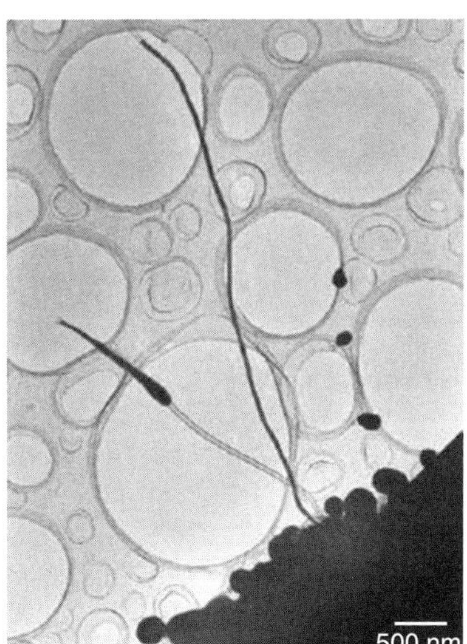

Figure 1.20 Image of sintered copper nanoparticles on the microgrid and the CNTs following the tip growth mode or base growth mode.

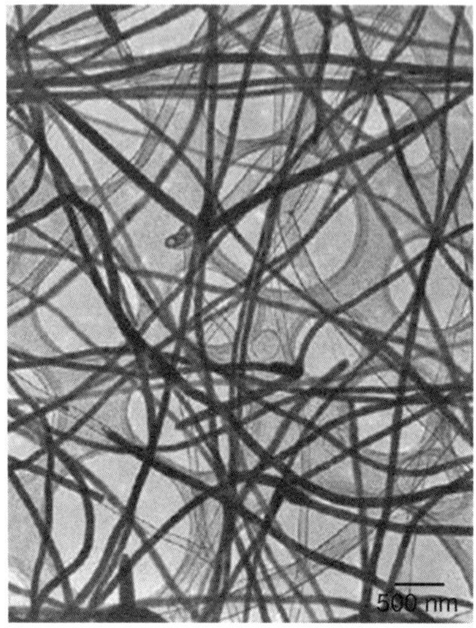

Figure 1.21 TEM image of large amount of Cu@ CNTs and CNTs with hollow channel, without amorphous carbon on the outer wall.

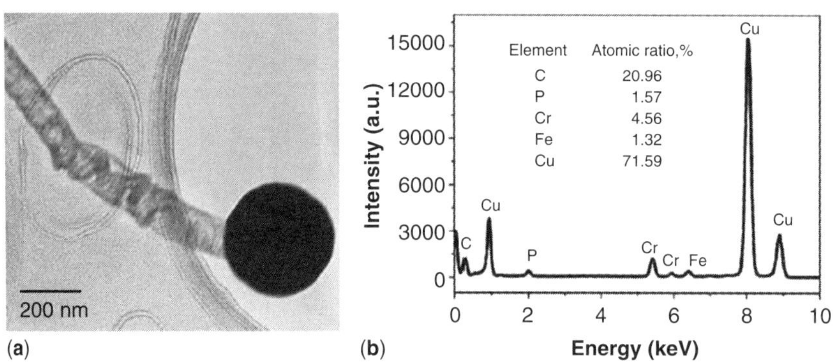

Figure 1.22 (a) TEM image of bamboo-like CNTs prepared from copper catalyst containing 3% iron; (b) EDS pattern of copper-iron nanoparticles in (a).

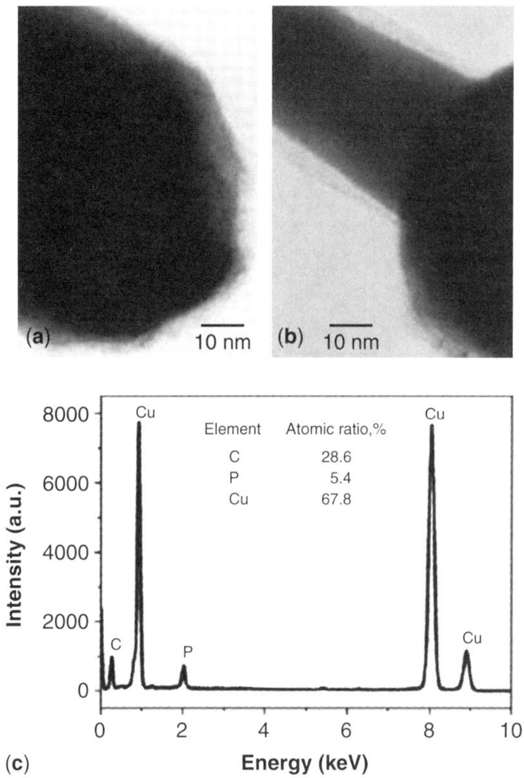

Figure 1.23 (a) Copper nanoparticle for the growth of CNTs in tip growth mode, with thin carbon layer smaller than 2 nm; (b) the thin carbon layer formed at the carbon-copper interface; (c) EDS of the copper tip with high purity in (b).

CNTs with hollow channel is pure copper as seen in Figure 1.23. The authors argued that the pure state of the copper is important for controlling the carbon supply rate as compared with iron, cobalt and nickel. Also, copper has a weak interaction with carbon and it is difficult to form copper carbide. Therefore, the bulk phase of the particles must maintain a pure metallic state and not be in a carbide state as shown in the HRTEM image (Figure 1.24) and confirmed by the low atomic ratio of copper to carbon in the CNT tip by EDS (Figure 1.23[c]). The authors also investigated the presence of hydrogen in the feed gas on the formation of CNTs with totally hollow channels. They found out that, it is necessary to add hydrogen into the feed gas to increase the purity of copper catalyst for the analysis of desirable CNTs with totally hollow channels.

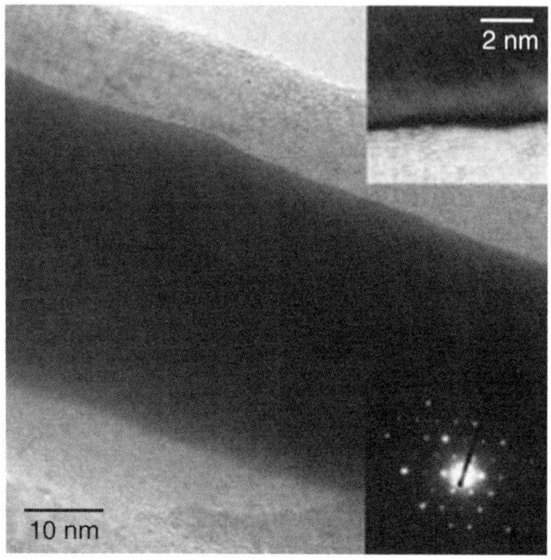

Figure 1.24 HRTEM image of the nanotubes filled with copper. The upper insert shows the detailed copper lattice and carbon layer; the lower insert is the SAED pattern of the single crystalline copper nanowires with fcc structure.

Carbon nanotubes filled with copper nanoneedles at the tips have been synthesized using alkali-element doped copper catalyst by a simple thermal CVD method by X. Tao *et al.* [39]. XRD revealed that the copper nanoneedles have perfect fcc structure. SAED indicates that these copper nanoneedles are single crystalline with fine quality. In their method, the catalyst was prepared by combustion of a certain amount of high-quality $Cu(NO_3)_2 3H_2O$, KNO_3, $Mg(NO_3)_2 3H_2O$ which were dissolved in a minimum amount of water to yield a molar ratio of K/Cu/Mg = 0.06/1/2. The solution was transferred into a quartz boat and placed in a furnace at 500°C where it was ignited and fired for about 10 minutes. The boat was then allowed to cool to room temperature and the resultant foamy materials ground to a fine powder. A one-step process was then used to obtain the carbon nanomaterials as follows; the catalyst was introduced into a furnace with a quartz tube heated to 700°C and to expel air, a flow of nitrogen at 600 ml/min was maintained for 4 minutes. After this, a mixture of $C_2H_2/NH_3/N_2$ = 100:300:200 at a flow rate of 600 ml/min was introduced into the furnace. The furnace was cooled to room temperature under nitrogen flow, and for analysis some products were collected and treated with 50 ml HNO_3 (1M) at 70°C for 2 hours and kept in acidic solution overnight at room temperature. A black, soot-like product was obtained after filtering and washing, which was

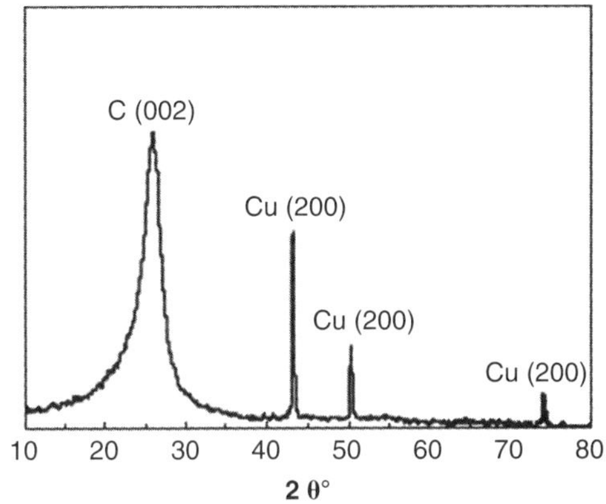

Figure 1.25 XRD pattern of the sample purified by acid treatment.

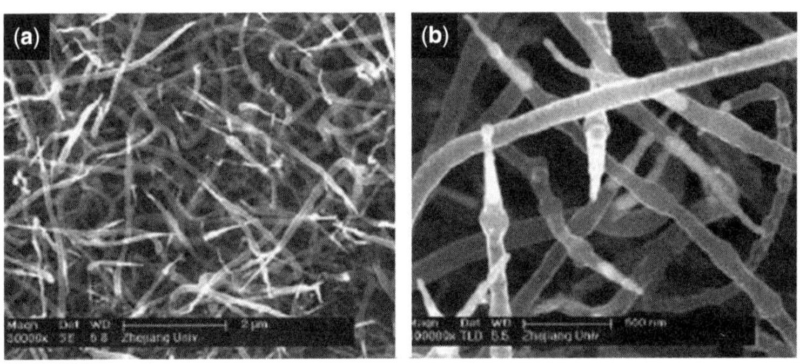

Figure 1.26 (a) FE-SEM images of Cu nanoneedles; (b) filled CNTs at the tips.

then characterized by FE-SEM, XRD and TEM. The acid-treated sample was characterized by XRD as shown in Figure 1.25. The XRD pattern shows that graphite carbon is the dominant feature and a large amount of copper is also detected in the sample. No other diffraction peaks, for example, CuO, Cu_2O and $Cu(NO_3)_2$, were found indicating that copper particles were encapsulated inside the carbon shells. Figure 1.26(a) shows a low-magnification FE-SEM image of dense CNTs without acid treatment. These CNTs are up to 5 μm long with outer diameters in a range of 40–80 nm. A high-magnification FE-SEM image shown in Figure 1.26(b) shows that all the CNTs have tips filled with metal nanoneedles. Further observation shows that it is difficult to find CNT without copper

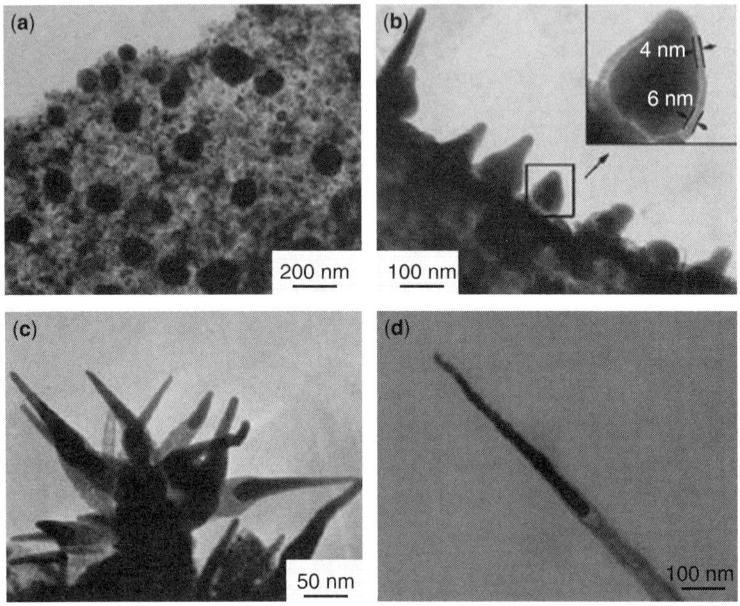

Figure 1.27 TEM images of the samples with different growth time: (a) 1 min, (b) 2 min, (c) 5 min, and (d) 30 min. The inset in (b) is the magnified image of the rectangular region.

filling, indicating the ratio of copper filling is very high. Figure 1.27 shows the TEM images of as-grown products reacted for different time periods. Figure 1.27(d) shows a typical copper-filled CNT synthesized for 30 minutes. The authors concluded that copper nanoneedles become thinner and longer with increasing reaction time, and also, the catalyst for the growth of CNTs should be in a molten state. Typical HRTEM images reveal that copper nanoneedles are encapsulated in graphite walls which are usually 4–6 nm thick shown in Figure 1.28(a), and the inset of Figure 1.28(a) is the corresponding SAED pattern of copper nanoneedles along the [112] zone axis showing that the copper nanoneedles is single crystalline. A magnified HRTEM image of Figure 1.28(b) reveals that the interlayer spacing of the CNT is about 0.34 nm, consistent with the (002) plane of graphite. The EDS spectrum reveals the presence of copper and carbon as shown in Figure 1.29 which indicates that copper plays the role of catalyst in the CNT formation. Based on these results, the authors explained the formation mechanism of copper-nanoneedles-filled CNTs schematically in Figure 1.30. The decomposition of acetylene on the surface of potassium-doped copper nanoparticle resulted in the formation of bimolecular hydrogen and carbon atoms as shown in Figure 1.30(a). Due to the stress between the graphite layer and the copper particle, the copper particles are transformed into nanocones in Figure 1.30(b). During the growth of the carbon walls, some carbon species accumulated at the bottom of copper can form the compartment graphite layers in Figure 1.30(c). If the carbon species are supplied with a steady-state manner, the compartment layers will appear periodically as shown in Figure 1.30(d).

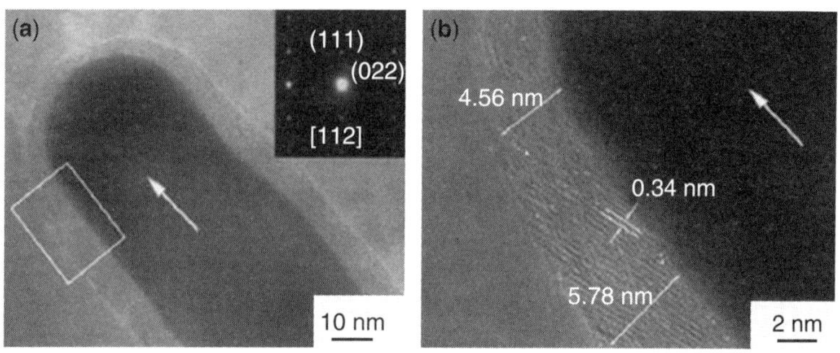

Figure 1.28 (a) HRTEM image and the corresponding SAED pattern (inset) of a Cu@CNT after acid treatment. (b) The magnified image of the rectangular region in (a). The big arrows indicate the growth direction of the CNTs.

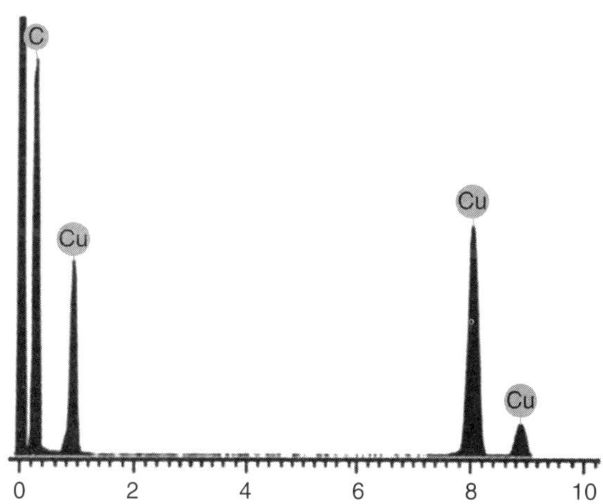

Figure 1.29 Typical EDS spectrum of Cu-filled CNTs after acid treatment.

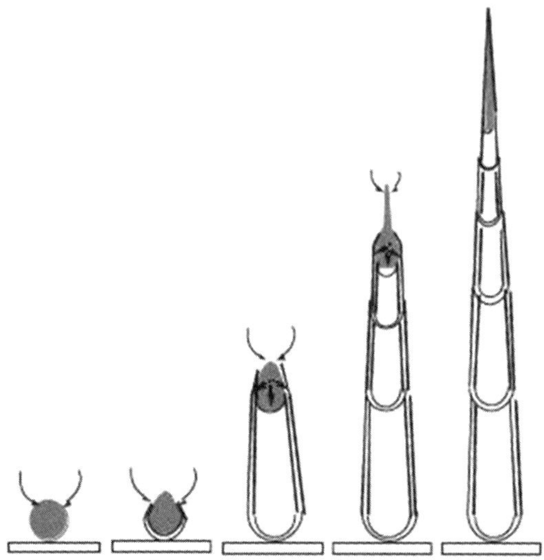

Figure 1.30 Schematic diagrams of the growth of a Cu-nanoneedle-filled CNT.

1.2.3 Laser Ablation

The laser ablation method involves the ablation of a carbon target containing a small amount of catalyst materials such as copper, nickel and cobalt with intense laser pulses. During the CNT preparation, a flow of inert gas is passed through the growth chamber to collect the grown CNTs. Carbon nanotubes filled completely with polycrystalline copper were synthesized by laser vaporization of copper and graphite under high-pressure argon gas ambient by F. Kokai and coworkers [40]. The authors noted that depending on the argon gas pressure (100–900 kPa) and the copper content (1–40 at.%) in graphite targets for laser vaporization, various products with different morphologies were observed by SEM and TEM. In their work, copper powder (100 μm grain size) was mixed with graphite powder (4 μm grain size) with the copper content ranging from 1–40 at.%. The mixed powder was pressed into copper/graphite pellets (10-mm diameter, 2-mm thickness). A continuous wave Nd:YAG laser (500 W peak power) was used for the vaporization of copper/graphite pellet targets at room temperature. The laser beam was focused on the target through a quartz window in a stainless-steel chamber filled with argon gas at pressures ranging from 100 to 900 kPa. Figure 1.31 shows typical SEM images of

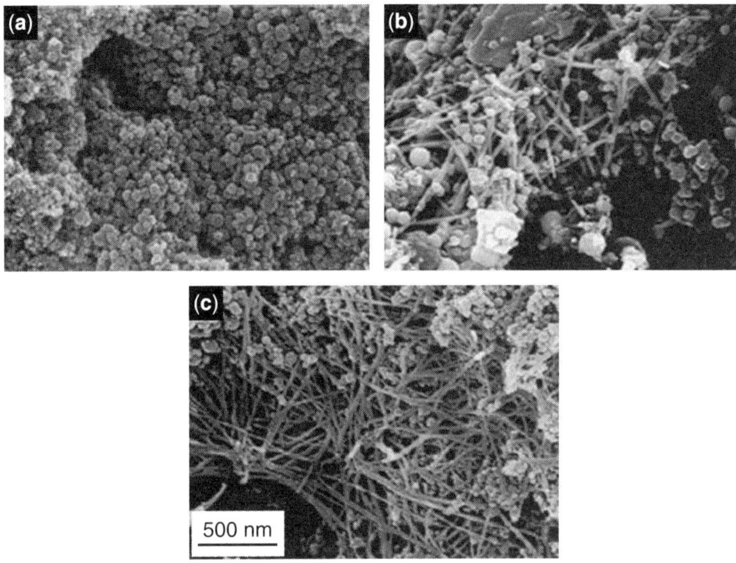

Figure 1.31 SEM images of the deposits produced at Ar gas pressures of (a) 100, (b) 500, and (c) 900 kPa.

the deposits obtained at argon gas pressures of 100, 500 and 900 kPa. Sphere-like particles with diameters of 30–130 nm were dominant at the lower pressure region of argon (100–300 kPa). When they increased the argon gas pressure to 900 kPa, the particle size was increased and the deposits were found to contain straight one-dimensional structures in addition to the sphere-like particles as shown in Figures 1.31(b) and (c). TEM observations indicated the sphere-like particles obtained at lower argon gas pressures were composed of amorphous carbon (AC) and single-wall carbon nanohorn (SWNH) particles. Figures 1.32(a) and (b) are typical TEM images of AC and SWNH particles revealing diameters of 80–150 nm including copper-filled CNTs. Figure 1.32(c) shows a TEM image observed near a core copper particle of a SWNH particle. Figure 1.33 is a typical TEM image of deposits obtained at an argon pressure of 900 kPa, consisting of 1D structures and sphere-like particles. Figures 1.34(a), (b) and (c) are examples of HRTEM images of the 1D structures consisting of copper nanowires with diameters of 18–20 nm surrounded by one, two or three graphitic layers. No unfilled or intermittently-filled CNTs were observed and all grown CNTs were found to contain copper from their roots to their tips in TEM observations of more than 300 copper-filled

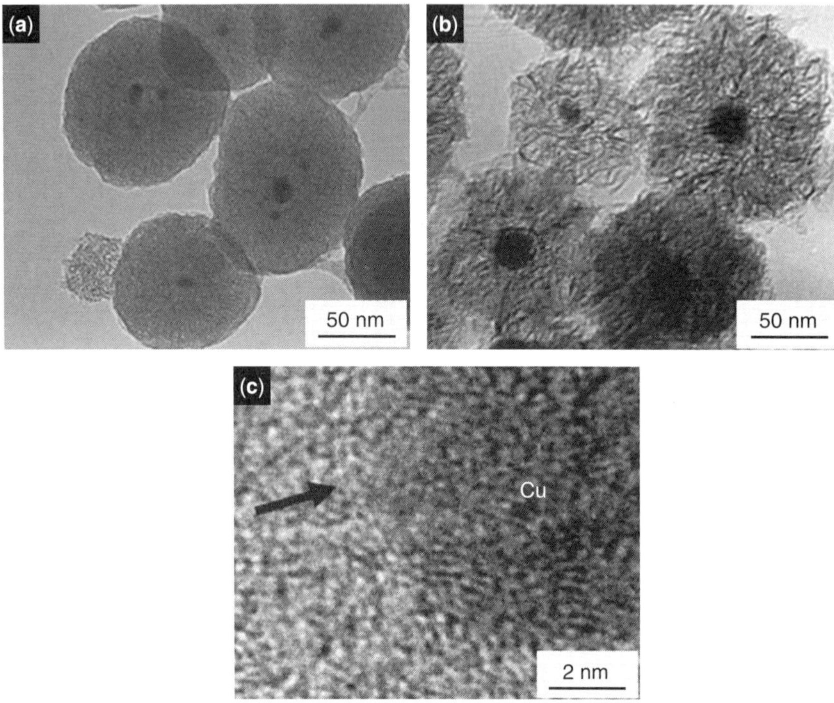

Figure 1.32 TEM images of (a) AC and (b) SWNH particles including Cu@CNC. (c) TEM image observed near the core Cu particle in a SWNH particle.

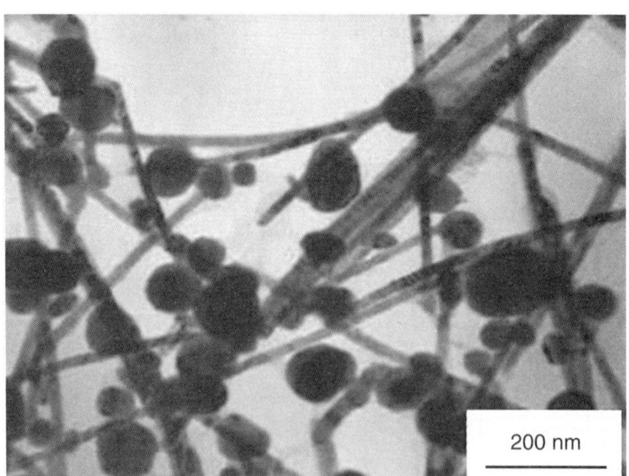

Figure 1.33 TEM image of a deposit obtained at Ar gas pressure of 900 kPa.

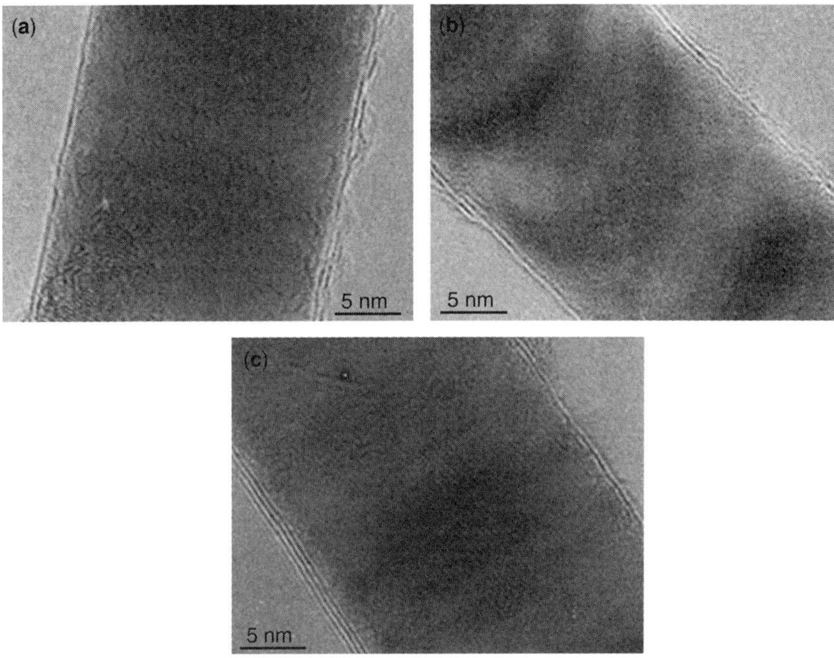

Figure 1.34 TEM images of 1D structures with (a) one, (b) two, and (c) three graphitic layers.

CNTs. A HRTEM image focusing on the part of a copper nanowire and its corresponding SAED is shown in Figure 1.35. Reflections assigned to the graphite (002) plane and the copper (111), (200) and (220) planes were also observed in the SAED pattern. These characteristics indicate that the encapsulated copper nanowire forms a polycrystal with an fcc structure. To understand the growth mechanism, the authors examined by TEM the ends of the copper-filled CNTs possessing sphere-like particles as shown in Figure 1.36(a). Graphitic layers similar to those covering copper were also examined by TEM as shown in Figure 1.36(b). The authors stressed that the presence of the sphere-like particles indicates the contribution of molten particles in forming the Cu@CNTs. But the mechanism of growth of Cu@CNTs by laser vaporization cannot be the same as CNT formation which occurs through the well-known vapor-liquid-solid mechanism, because their products do not contain CNTs. Also, hydrogen was not used in their experiment (laser vaporization method), although its contribution has been suggested in earlier experiments on the growth of the Cu@CNTs [30, 31].

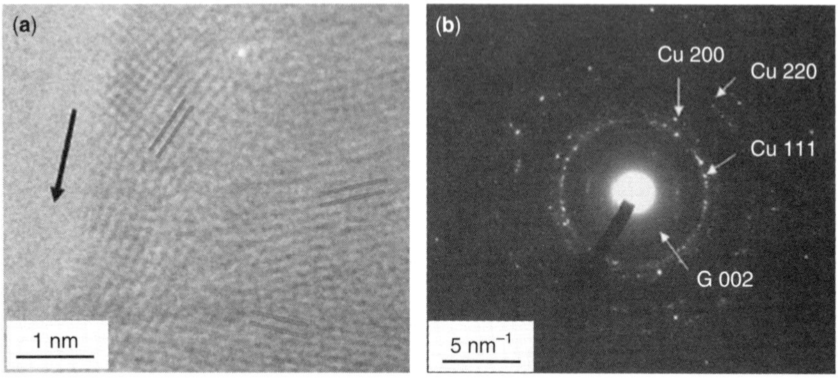

Figure 1.35 (a) TEM image focusing on the part of a Cu nanowire, and (b) its corresponding SAED pattern. Arrow indicates the growth direction and the distance between the parallel fringes is close to the space of Cu (111) planes.

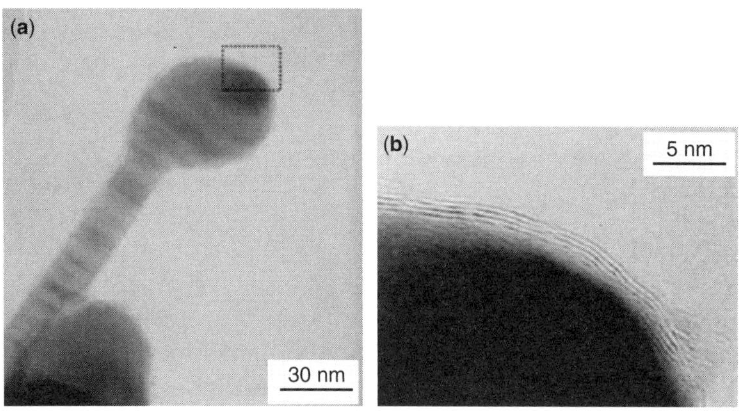

Figure 1.36 (a) TEM image of Cu@CNT with a spherical particle at its tip, and (b) another TEM image of the outer region of the sphere-like particle (rectangular area in (a)).

The authors proposed that collisions between carbon and copper species would be enhanced in a space confined by high-pressure (900 kPa) argon gas. The induced interaction between the carbon and copper gives rise to the formation of molten copper-carbon particles with carbon-rich composition at elevated temperature, even though carbon interaction with copper at normal atmospheric pressure is known to be weak and the carbon solubility is very low [41]. They also stated that molten carbon-copper composite particles with certain small sizes seem to play a crucial role in the formation of the Cu@CNTs.

Y. Sun and his colleagues [42] reported that the resistivity of multi-walled carbon nanotube networks can be changed by filling copper into the nanotubes as well as by preparing the CNT networks with various densities. They found out that the resistivity can be controlled to be lower than the c-axis resistivity of graphite, and also has a low coefficient of about over the temperature range of 20–500 K. In their work, laser vaporization of a carbon target containing copper was carried out in an argon atmosphere at a pressure of 500 kPa. A continuous wave Nd:YAG laser was used to vaporize the copper/carbon target at room temperature. The Cu@CNT powders were then characterized by XRD, SEM and TEM. The powders were pressed into pellets at room temperature and in a vacuum at pressures of 50, 76, 128 and 191 MPa for 30 minutes. Resistivity of the pellets was measured by means of a four–probe technique using a resistance tester. A typical SEM image of a copper CNT pellet is shown in Figure 1.37(a). They suggested from

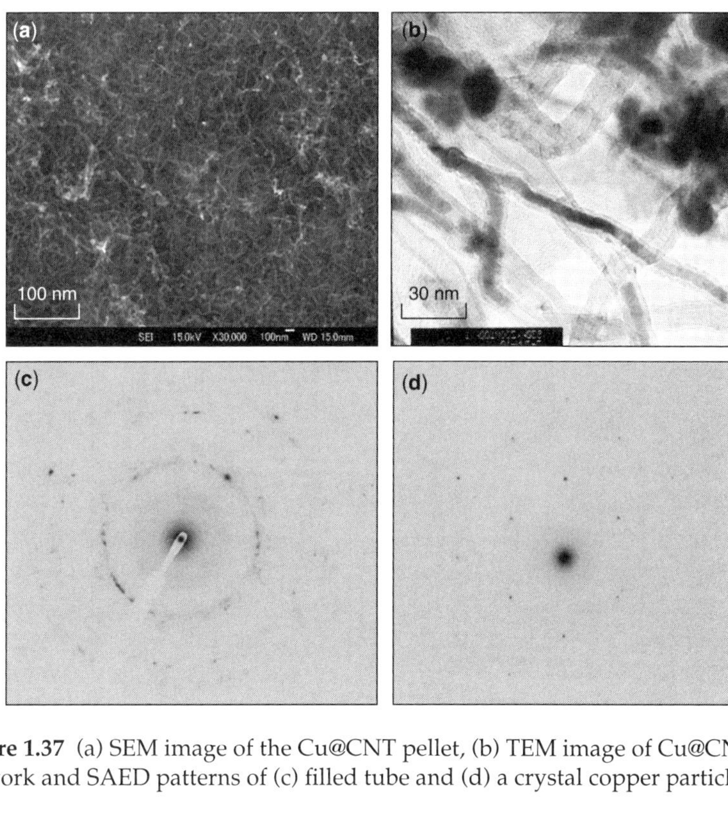

Figure 1.37 (a) SEM image of the Cu@CNT pellet, (b) TEM image of Cu@CNT network and SAED patterns of (c) filled tube and (d) a crystal copper particle.

the SEM image that the resistance of the network will be determined by the total resistance of the inter- and intra-tubes, whereas in the filling of copper only the resistance of the intra-tube changes. Figure1.37(b) is a TEM image of the network showing filled and hollow tubes with an average diameter of 20 nm. Using the electron beam diffraction, they showed that the hollow tube has the graphite structure, the filled tube is copper in CNT and the large particles are copper crystals. The electron beam diffraction pattern is shown in Figures1.37(c) and (d). The diffraction shows graphite (200) plane as well as (111), (200), (220) and (311) planes of fcc copper. The authors also measured the XRD of the Cu@CNT pellet. Figures 1.38(a) and (b) show the patterns of the Cu@CNT pellet exposed to air for one and nine weeks. Diffractions are from graphite (200) and from (111), (200) and (220) planes of fcc copper as well as peak from Cu_2O (111). They found that from the intensity ratios of the Cu_2O (111) to the Cu (111) were 0.10 and 0.18 for the exposure times of one and nine weeks, meaning that the single crystal copper particles in the network are bare or are covered by a defective graphite layer. The temperature dependences of the resistivities of the copper-filled and pristine CNT pellets prepared under pressure of 128 MPa are shown in Figure 1.39. The upper and bottom curves in the Figure are for pellets with carbon/copper ratios of 0.73 and 0.57. The resistivity of the Cu@CNT network decreases with increasing the copper yield filled into the tubes. They observed

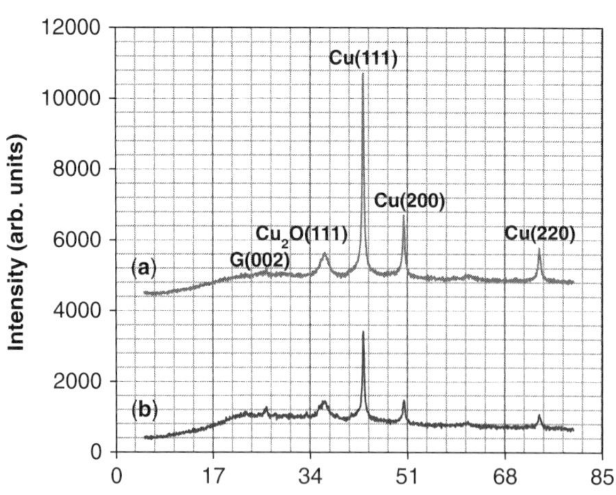

Figure 1.38 XRD patterns of the Cu@CNT powders exposed to air for (a) one week, and (b) nine weeks.

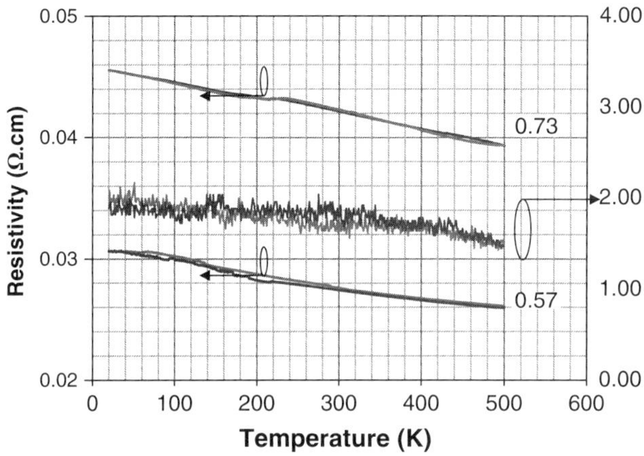

Figure 1.39 Temperature dependent resistivities of the Cu-filled and pristine CNT pellets prepared by applying pressure of 128 MPa during heating and cooling processes. The upper and bottom curves are related to the pellets with the C/Cu ratios of 0.73 and 0.57.

that the resistivity is almost inversely proportional to the temperature over the range of 20–500 K. They finally concluded that: The resistivities of the copper/CNT network at 300 K are 0.042 and 0.028 Ωcm for the carbon/copper ratio of 0.73 and 0.57. The values are lower than the resistivity of MWCNT film (1 Ωcm) at 300 K and also lower than the c-axis resistivity (0.1 Ωcm) of highly oriented pyrolytic graphite (HOPG) at 300 K. The measured temperature coefficient of the copper/MWCNT networks has smaller value of over the temperature range of 20–500 K. This is due to the fact that the MWCNT has a negative temperature coefficient indicating that the copper filling can decrease the intra-tube resistivity of the Cu@ CNT network.

References

1. S. Ijima. *Nature* 354 (1991) p. 56.
2. X. Gong, J. Liu, S. Baskran, R.D. Voise, and J.S. Young. *Chem. Mater.* 12 (2000) p. 1049.
3. P. Calvert. *Nature* 399 (1999) p. 210.
4. M.S.P. Shaffer, A.H. Windle. *Adv. Mater.* 11 (1999) p. 937.
5. J.W. Ding, X.H. Yan, and J.X. Cao. *Phys. Rev. B* 66 (2002) p. 073401.

6. O. Gulseren, T. Yildirim, and S. Ciraci. *Phys. Rev. B* 68 (2003) p. 115419.
7. A.H. Nevidomskyy, G. Csanyi, and M.C. Payne. *Phys. Rev. Lett.* 91 (2003) p. 105502.
8. R. Saito, G. Dresselhaus, and M.S. Dresslhaus. *Physical Properties of Carbon nanotubes*, Imperial College Press, London, 1998.
9. M.S. Dresselhaus, G. Dresselhaus, and P.C. Eklund. *Science of Fullerenes and Carbon Nanotubes*, Academic Press, New York, 1996.
10. J. Zhao, A. Buldun, J. Han, and J.P. Lu. *Nanotechnology* 13 (2002) p. 195.
11. M.R. Pederson, and J.Q. Broughton. *Phys. Rev. Lett.* 69 (1992) p. 2689.
12. V.V. Ivanovskaya, C. Köhler, and G. Seifert. *Phys. Rev. B* 75 (2007) p. 075410.
13. A. Quintel. In *Electronic Properties of Novel Materials- Molecular Nanostructures*, Edited by H. Kuzmany, J. Fink, M. Mehring and S. Roth, AIP Conf. Proc., Vol. 544, (AIP, NEW York, 2000).
14. I. Hanasaki, A. Nakatani. *Nanotechnology* 17 (2006) p. 2794.
15. M.C.G. Lim, Q.X. Pei, Z.W. Zhong. *Physica A: Statistical Mechanics and its Applications* 387 (2008) p. 3111.
16. A. Chu, J. Cook, R.J.R. Heesom, J.L. Hutchison, M.L.H. Green, J. Sloan. *Chemistry of Materials* 8 (1996) p. 2751.
17. Z.X. Zhang, Z.Y. Pan, Q. Wei, Z.J. Li, L.K. Zang, Y.X. Wang. *International Journal of Modern Physics B* 17 (2003) p. 4667.
18. X. Fan, J.E. Barclay, W. Peng, Y. Li, X. Li, G. Zhang, D.J. Evans, F. Zhang. *Nanotechnology* 19 (2008) p. 165702.
19. E. Borowiak-Palen, E. Mendozaa, A. Bachmatuk, M.H. Rummeli, T. Gemming, J. Nogues, V. Skumryev. R.J. Kalenczuk, T. Pichler, S.R.P. Silva. *Chem. Phys. Lett.* 421 (2006) p. 129.
20. S. Costa, E. Borowiak-Palen, A. Bachmatiuk, M.H. Rümmeli, T. Gemming, R.J. Kalenczuk. *Physica Status Solidi (b)* 244 (2007) p. 4315.
21. L.X. Dong, X.Y. Tao, L. Zhang, X.B. Zhang, B.J. Nelson. *Nano Lett.* 7 (2007) p. 58.
22. Y. Lin, A.M. Rao, B. Sadanadam, E.A. Kenik, Y.P. Sun. *J. Phys. Chem. B* 106 (2002) p. 1294.
23. S.C. Tsang, Y.K. Chen, P.J.F. Harris, M.L.H. Green. *Nature* 372 (1994) p. 159.
24. S. Banerjee, and S.S. Wong. *Nano Lett.* 2 (2002) p. 195.
25. S. Seraphin, D. Zhou, and J. Jiao. *J. Appl. Phys.* 80 (1996) p. 2097.
26. F.W. Sun, H. Li, K.M. Liew. *Carbon* 48 (2010) p. 1586.
27. W. Han, P. Redlich, F. Ernst, M. Ruhle. *Appl. Phys. Lett.* 75 (1999) p. 1875.
28. M. Monthioux. *Carbon* 40 (2002) p. 1809.
29. R. Fan, R. Karnik, M. Yue, D. Lei, A. Majumdar, and P. Yang. *Nano Letters* 5 (2005) p. 1633.
30. A.A. Setlur, J.M. Lauerhaas, J.Y. Dai, and R.P.H. Chang. *Appl. Phys. Lett.* 69 (1996) p. 345.
31. Z. Wang, Z. Zhao, and J. Qiu. *Carbon* 44 (2006) p. 1845.
32. J. Ding, X. Yan, B.K. Tay, and Q. Xue. *J. Phys. Chem. Solids* 72 (2011) p. 1519.
33. H.Q. Li, A. Misra, Y.T. Zhu, Z.J. Horita, C.C. Koch, and T.G. Holesinger. *Mater. Sci. Eng. A* 523 (2009) p. 60.
34. J. Gavillet, J. Thibault, O. Stephan, H. Amara, A. Loiseau, C. Bichara, J.P. Gaspard, and F. Ducastelle. *J. Nanosci. Nanotechnol.* 4 (2004) p. 346.
35. C. Hao, F. Xiao, and Z. Cui. *J. Nanoparticle Research* 10 (2008) p. 47.
36. J. Lin, C. Chen, H. Ma, C. Hsu, and H. Chen. *Carbon* 45 (2007) p. 203.

37. J. Zhu, J. Jia, F. Kwong, and D.H.L. Ng. *Carbon* 50 (2012) p. 2504.
38. Q. Zhang, W.Z. Qian, H. Yu, F. Wei, and Q. Wen. *Appl. Phys. A* 86 (2007) p. 265.
39. X. Tao, X. Zhang, J. Cheng, Z. Luo, S. Zhou, and F. Liu. *Diamond & Related Materials* 15 (2006) p. 1271.
40. F. Kokai, T. Shimizu, K. Adachi, A. Koshio, and Y. Takahashi. *Appl. Phys. A* 97 (2009) p. 55.
41. T.B. Massalski, H. Okamoto. P.R. Subramanian, and L. Kaeprzak. *Binary Alloy Phase Diagrams*, (Am. Soc. Metals, Metal Park, 1990) p. 839.
42. Y. Sun, B. Onwona-Agyeman, and T. Miyasato. *Materials Lett.* 65 (2011) p. 3187.

2

Novel Nanocomposites: Intercalation of Ionically Conductive Polymers into Molybdic Acid

Rabin Bissessur#, Blakney Hopkins[1] and Douglas C. Dahn[2]

Department of Chemistry, University of Prince Edward Island, Charlottetown, PE, Canada
[2]Department of Physics, University of Prince Edward Island Charlottetown, PE, Canada

Abstract
Technological improvements continue to force the need for smaller, more powerful batteries. The lithium ion battery is the current battery of choice because lithium is the lightest metal and the lithium ion yields the highest energy for its mass. Research surrounding new cathode and electrolyte materials is currently being conducted.

In this work, the intercalation of ionically conductive polymers into the layers of molybdic acid was explored. The resulting intercalation compounds were characterized by powder X-ray diffraction (XRD), thermogravimetric analysis (TGA), Fourier-transform infrared spectroscopy (FTIR), and ac impedance spectroscopy.

Keywords: Ionically conductive polymers, molybdic acid, intercalation

2.1 Introduction

2.1.1 Battery Technology

Electronic devices continue to benefit from new technological breakthroughs that improve their quality, intricacy, and appearance. While the size of these devices is trending downward, their energy

Dedicated to Radha Bissessur (1923–2013)

Vikas Mittal (ed.) Encapsulation Nanotechnologies, (41–70) © 2013 Scrivener Publishing LLC

demands are rising. This creates a need for smaller and more powerful batteries to complement modern technological advancements. The current battery of choice is the lithium ion battery which allows a high energy output. Lithium is the lightest metal and yields the highest energy for its mass [1].

Current lithium ion batteries utilize layered compounds for both the anode and the cathode materials, which allows for the reversible intercalation of lithium ions [2–5]. Lithium ions are intercalated between the layers of the cathode material after being removed from the anode during the discharge process. Electrons will flow from the anode, through the external load, to the cathode to balance the charge from the lithium ions. The flow of lithium ions and electrons is reversed during the charge process meaning the lithium ion battery is a secondary type battery also known as a rechargeable battery. Figure 2.1 illustrates the charge/discharge mechanism of the lithium ion battery.

Research into the lithium ion battery is being conducted around the world and focuses on improvements to the cathode, the anode and the electrolyte.

The cathode is the site of reduction during the discharge process (Figure 2.1). In order to be a suitable candidate for the layered cathode material, the substance should be stable, environmentally friendly and of low cost. The material must be able to undergo oxidation-reduction reactions and must be capable of undergoing reversible intercalation of lithium ions. The reaction with lithium should be fast with a high free energy change [6]. Layered materials such as $LiTiS_2$, $LiVSe_2$, $LiCoO_2$, $LiNiO_2$, and $LiNi_yMn_yCo_{1-2y}O_2$ have all been used as cathode materials [6]. Many ratios exist for

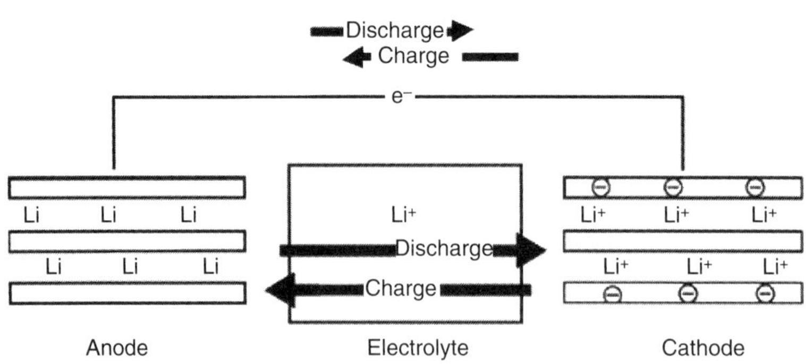

Figure 2.1 Charge and discharge mechanism of a typical lithium ion battery.

the $LiNi_yMn_yCo_{1-2y}O_2$ layered compound, however recent research shows that the $LiNi_{0.33}Mn_{0.33}Co_{0.33}O_2$ system (y = 0.33) demonstrates the best performance in battery applications [7].

The anode is the site of oxidation in the discharge process (see Figure 2.1). It is the source of lithium ions and electrons. Anode materials are limited compared to the range of cathode materials that are available. Previously, lithium metal was used as the anode material [8]. This was problematic because of the extreme reactivity of lithium. There were thermal runaway issues where the temperature would reach the melting point of the anode during discharge, causing explosive and flammable gases to be produced [8]. Since then, the use of lithiated graphite has evolved as the standard anode material. Graphite has a high efficiency, a low cost, and a high abundance [9]. These properties make the improvement of anode materials a challenging and ambitious undertaking.

The electrolyte functions as an electrical isolator between the anode and the cathode (Figure 2.1). This isolation forces the electrons to flow external to the cell and is therefore a key factor in the performance of the overall system. The electrolyte must also facilitate the flow of ions from the anode to the cathode in order to maintain charge balance. These factors dictate that the properties of the electrolyte material include high ionic conductivity and very high electronic resistance [10, 11]. Our current research is focused on the synthesis and characterization of nanocomposites that can potentially be utilized as electrolyte materials.

2.1.2 The Polymer Electrolyte

The use of polymers as electrolytic materials is an active area of research. Polymeric materials in general are much easier to contain than liquids which makes polymer electrolytes more appealing to smaller volume battery packages [12]. The polymers chosen in our research are electronically insulating and have reasonably good ionic conduction when complexed with inorganic salts, in particular those of lithium, thus making them prospective candidates as electrolytes for lithium ion batteries.

The commercial viability of polymer electrolytes is limited by the required criteria for mass production of batteries containing these substances [5]. These include low toxicity, low cost, resistance to mechanical, thermal, and electrochemical decomposition between -20°C and 60°C. In addition, as previously mentioned, the

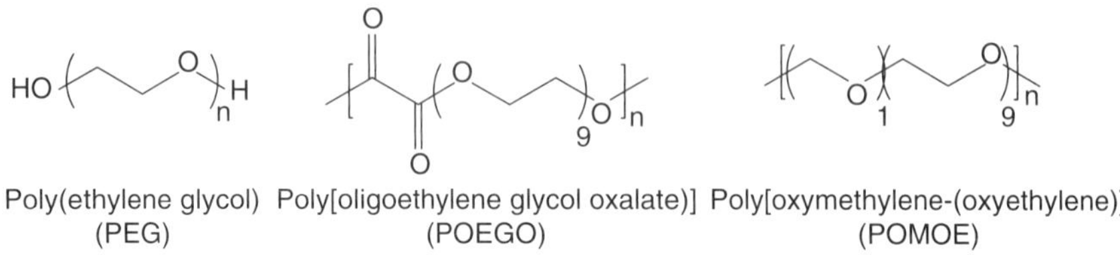

Figure 2.2 Ionically conductive polymers.

polymer must be electronically insulating and ionically conducting [5]. Batteries containing polymer electrolytes could offer easier packaging, lower cost of manufacturing, and higher energy density [13].

Figure 2.2 depicts the structure of the polymers that were used in this work. Among this series of polymers, poly(ethylene glycol) has been studied most extensively as an electrolyte material. It is semi-crystalline, with reduced mechanical freedom in the crystallized segment of the polymer where ion-transport is hindered [14, 15]. To circumvent this problem the use of PEG-derivatives such as poly[oligo(ethyleneglycol)-oxalate] [16], poly[oxymethylene-(oxyethylene)] [17], and poly[bis-(methoxyethoxyethoxy)phosphazene] [18], which are completely amorphous, has been proposed. However, these amorphous polymers are mechanically unstable which creates leaking problem when assembled in a battery [19]. Several methods have been employed as attempts to increase the mechanical and dimensional stability of these polymer electrolytes. One such method is the addition of fine ceramic powders to the polymer [12]. Another method is the insertion of the polymer into layered structures that can minimize the tendency of the polymer to crystallize while adding to the mechanical stability [20–24].

In order to be a feasible electrolyte, an observed conductivity of 10^{-3} S/cm or higher at 25°C must be observed [25]. For PEG-based systems the conductivity has generally been on the order of 10^{-6} S/cm [1]. To achieve these conductivity values, lithium salts are added. The polymer acts as a solvent system for lithium salts [14], with lithium ions coordinating to the electron rich sites of the polymer. Lithium trifluoromethanesulfonate as depicted in Figure 2.3 is an ideal salt for complexation with the polymer as a result of its low crystal energy. While the lithium ion is small enough to travel freely throughout the polymeric matrix, the bulky trifluoromethanesulfonate anion does not [14].

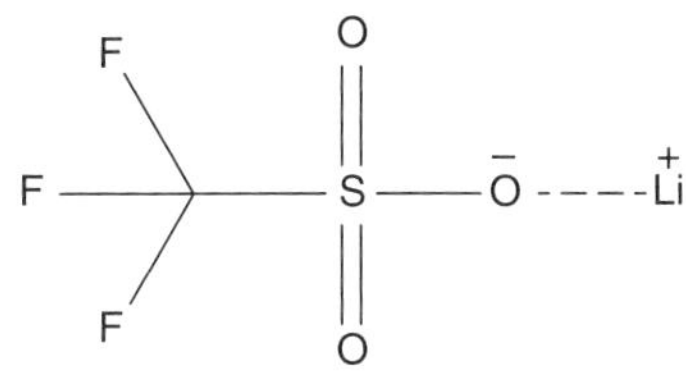

Figure 2.3 Lithium trifluoromethanesulfonate.

2.1.3 Intercalation Chemistry

Intercalation is the reversible insertion of a guest species into a host material. In most cases the host is a layered material and the guest is inserted between the layers. In our research, an exfoliation/restacking process is used. During the exfoliation step the layers are separated in solution. At this point a guest species is introduced. The guest species is then inserted between the layers upon restacking. This process is illustrated in Figure 2.4. Even though the exfoliation/restacking process is not reversible, the product is often referred to as an intercalated material, since it consists of a guest species between the layers of a host. The region between the layers is referred to as the interlayer gap or gallery space. The layer spacing or lamellar spacing is the distance from the center of one host layer to the center of the next. The layers in the host material are held together by weak van der Waals forces.

Although two dimensional (2D) layered hosts are used in our work, three dimensional (3D), and one dimensional (1D) host structures can also be used in intercalation chemistry [26]. 3D frameworks have vacancies extending in three dimensions. Included in the category of 3D structures are ReO_3 and Mo_6S_8 [27–30]. 2D frameworks have vacancies extending in two dimensions. Examples of 2D layered structures include $Li_xNi_{1-y}Co_yO_2$, TiS_2, FeOCl, $VOPO_4$, and $MgPS_3$ [31–40]. 1D structures are typically chain hosts and are similar to tubes with free space in one dimension [26]. Examples include TiS_3 and $RuBr_3$ [34, 39].

1D frameworks tend to be fragile and unstable as a result of the bond angles and high internal energies within the systems [26]. 3D frameworks tend to be rigid due to the extension of the framework in three dimensions [26]. 2D frameworks are more stable than their 1D analogues, and much more flexible than their 3D analogues. As a result there are many more applications for 2D

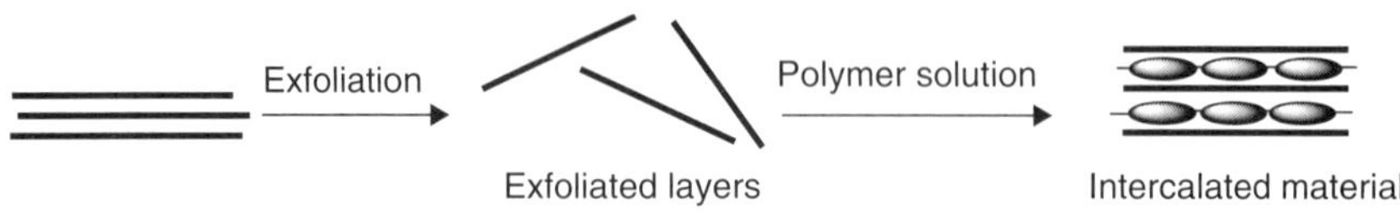

Figure 2.4 Mechanism of layered structure exfoliation/restacking with polymer addition.

layered structures, and many guest species can be inserted in the gallery spaces [40, 41] This research examines the chemical properties of potential electrolyte materials that utilize 2D structures based on molybdenum.

2.1.4 MoO_3 and MoO_3 Derivatives

Molybdenum trioxide (MoO_3) has an orthorhombic crystal structure. An MoO_3 layer is composed of molybdenum atoms with distorted octahedral geometry (as MoO_6) which is illustrated in Figure 2.5. The layer is formed by shared crosslinking oxygen atoms [42].

MoO_3 was an early candidate for layered cathode material as a result of an observed lithium loading of 1.5 lithium ions per molybdenum. Further research into this area was abandoned when the reactions could not reach a satisfactory rate [43–45].

Molybdic acid ($MoO_3{\cdot}nH_2O$) is a hydrated form of MoO_3. Two forms of molybdic acid are known, namely the monohydrated form ($MoO_3{\cdot}H_2O$), and the dihydrated form ($MoO_3{\cdot}2H_2O$) [42]. The structures of these compounds are similar to pure MoO_3 with water molecules between the MoO_3 layers. The solid-state structure of the monohydrated compound includes octahedral $MoO_5(H_2O)$, where 4 vertices are shared. The dihydrated form consists of the bound water molecule along with another coordinated water molecule inside the lamellar space of the layer [42].

Recent research surrounding molybdic acid has involved the intercalation of dithiocarbamate for applications in oxidation catalysis [46]. Another area of research involving molybdic acid was focused on the synthesis of MoO_3 nanostructures. The syntheses of MoO_3 nanorods, nanodisks, and nanoscrolls have been achieved through the intercalation of amines with varying alkyl chain lengths [47].

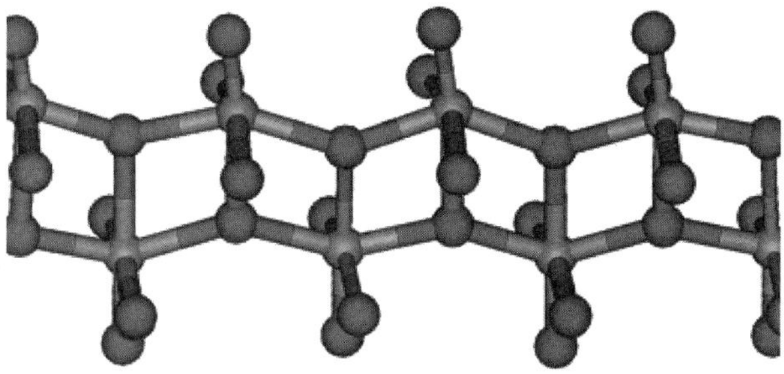

Figure 2.5 An illustration of one MoO_3 layer [42]. Blue represents molybdenum, pink represents oxygen.

2.2 Experimental

2.2.1 Materials

This research dealt with three polymers: poly[ethylene glycol] (PEG), poly[oligoethylene glycol oxalate] (POEGO) and poly[oxymethyleneoxyethylene] (POMOE). PEG (Mw 10000) was purchased from Sigma-Aldrich, and was used as received. POEGO [16] and POMOE [17] were synthesized as described in the literature. Molybdic acid and lithium trifluoromethanesulfonate were purchased from Sigma-Aldrich and were used without modification.

2.2.2 Synthesis of POEGO

PEG 400 (5.04 g, 0.0142 mol) was added to a 100 mL round-bottom flask containing oxalic acid dihydrate (1.59 g, 0.0126 mol). Benzene (35 mL) was then added. The reaction mixture was allowed to reflux, open to air for 5 days. The excess benzene and water were then removed under reduced pressure. The product was then heated in a vacuum oven at 120 °C until a clear viscous product was obtained. The identity of the synthesized polymer was confirmed by ^1H NMR spectroscopy. ^1H NMR ($CDCl_3$): δ= 5.98 (-COO**H**, singlet); 4.40 (-C(O)-C(O)-O-$\mathbf{CH_2}$-, triplet); 3.76 (-C-(O)-C(O)-O-$CH_2\mathbf{CH_2}$-, triplet); 3.62 ((-C-(O)-C(O)-O-CH_2-CH_2-(O$\mathbf{CH_2CH_2}$)$_{n-2}$-O-, triplet).

2.2.3 Synthesis of POMOE

Potassium hydroxide powder (12.5 g, 0.229 mol) was introduced into a three-neck flask connected to a mechanical stirrer under nitrogen purge from a Schlenk line. Dichloromethane (50 mL, 0.589 mol) was syringed into the reaction vessel. Polyethylene glycol 400 (PEG 400) (12.5 mL, 0.0353 mol) was added slowly by means of a dropping funnel to the reaction mixture. The reaction vessel was protected from direct light with aluminum foil. After three days, the excess potassium hydroxide was washed off the thick rubbery product. The thick rubbery product was dissolved in water (500 mL) and purified via dialysis for several days. After dialysis, the solution was filtered to remove any suspended particles, and was then freeze-dried. A clear colorless rubbery mass of the polymer was obtained. The identity of the synthesized polymer was confirmed by ^{1}H NMR spectroscopy. ^{1}H NMR ($CDCl_3$): δ= 3.71 (-O(CH_2CH_2)$_9$-(O**CH_2**)-, triplet); 3.65 (-O(**CH_2CH_2**)$_9$-(OCH_2)-, triplet).

2.3 Intercalation into Molybdic Acid

2.3.1 Intercalation of PEG into Molybdic Acid

Molybdic acid (50 mg) was dissolved in 35 mL of deionized water. One equivalent of PEG was dissolved separately in 10 mL of deionized water. The PEG solution was then slowly added to the aqueous solution of molybdic acid. The reaction mixture was stirred for 2 days and then cast onto a glass substrate. The procedure was repeated using two and four equivalents of PEG.

2.3.2 Intercalation of POEGO into Molybdic Acid

Molybdic acid (50 mg) was dissolved in 35 mL of deionized water. POEGO (0.2 equivalent) was dissolved separately in 10 mL of deionized water. The POEGO solution was then slowly added to the aqueous solution of molybdic acid. The reaction mixture was stirred for 4 days, and then cast onto a glass substrate.

2.3.3 Intercalation of POMOE into Molybdic Acid

Molybdic acid (50 mg) was dissolved in 35 mL of deionized water. POMOE (0.55 equivalent) was dissolved separately in 10 mL of deionized water. The POMOE solution was then slowly added to the aqueous solution of molybdic acid. The reaction mixture was stirred for 4 days prior to casting onto a glass plate.

2.4 Preparation of Polymer-Lithium Complexes

2.4.1 Preparation of POEGO/LiOTf Complexes

POEGO was complexed with lithium trifluoromethanesulfonate (LiOTf) using the literature procedure [9]. A 1:1.7 ratio of lithium (Li) to etheric oxygens ([EO]) was chosen. Freeze-dried POEGO (2.4764 g, 5.7 mmol) was transferred into a vial. The vial was then brought inside a dry box where LiOTf (0.5270 g, 3.4 mmol) was added. The vial was capped and removed from the dry box. The reaction mixture was placed inside a vacuum oven at 90°C overnight. The mixture was lightly stirred periodically to ensure complete complexation.

2.4.2 Preparation of POMOE/LiOTf Complexes

POMOE was complexed with lithium trifluoromethanesulfonate (LiOTf) using the literature procedure [9] for the complexation of POEGO. A 1:1.7 ratio of lithium (Li) to etheric oxygens ([EO]) was chosen. Freeze-dried POMOE (2.2056 g, 5.6 mmol) was transferred into a vial. The vial was then brought inside the inert atmosphere of a dry box where LiOTf (0.5052 g, 3.2 mmol) was added. The vial was capped and removed from the dry box. The reaction mixture was placed inside a vacuum oven at 90°C overnight. The mixture was lightly stirred periodically to ensure complete complexation.

2.4.3 Preparation of PEG/LiOTf Complexes

PEG was complexed with lithium trifluoromethanesulfonate (LiOTf). A 1:16 Li/[EO] ratio was chosen as this is the accepted value for optimizing ionic conductivity [16]. PEG (0.2964 g, 6.7 mmol) along with LiOTf (0.0656 g, 0.42 mmol) were dissolved in 10 mL of deionized water. The mixture was allowed to stir overnight and then freeze-dried.

2.4.4 Intercalation of Polymer/LiOTf into Molybdic Acid Compounds

The polymer salt complexes were intercalated into molybdic acid using the same procedure as described in Section 2.3.

2.5 Instrumentation

2.5.1 Powder X-ray Diffraction

Powder X-ray Diffraction (XRD) analyses were performed on a Bruker AXS D8 Advance Diffractometer. The instrument was equipped with a graphite monochromator, variable divergence and anti-scattering slits, and a scintillation detector. Cu(Kα) radiation (λ = 1.542 Å) was used for the measurements. The samples were run in air, under ambient conditions, from 2–60° (2θ).

2.5.2 Thermogravimetric Analysis

Thermogravimetric analyses (TGA) were performed using a TGA Q500 from TA Instruments. Analyses were performed in air with a sample purge rate of 60.00 mL/min. A heating rate of 10.00°C/min was used on all samples.

2.5.3 Fourier Transform Infrared Spectroscopy

Fourier transform infrared spectroscopy (FTIR) analyses were performed using the Bruker Equinox 55 FT-IR instrument with resolution of 0.5 cm^{-1}. All samples were run as pressed KBr pellets.

2.5.4 Nuclear Magnetic Resonance Spectroscopy

^1H – NMR was performed on a Bruker 300 MHz NMR. All samples were prepared in $CDCl_3$ or D_2O.

2.5.5 AC Impedance Spectroscopy

AC impedance measurements were performed by using a Solarton 1250 frequency response analyzer, over the frequency range 10kHz to 0.01 Hz, and at temperatures ranging from 310 K to 240 K. The procedure is described in more detail in reference [48]. Samples were run as thin films cast between two stainless steel electrodes fitted on a glass slide. The samples were run under vacuum (<10 mTorr), and the samples were placed in the vacuum chamber at least one day prior to running the analyses.

2.6 Results and Discussion

2.6.1 Molybdic Acid

The pristine molybdic acid was characterized with several techniques. First and foremost, powder X-ray diffraction (Figure 2.6) was used to determine the interlayer spacing of the material as well as its crystallite size. The interlayer spacing of the material was found to be 10.1 Å, which is 3.1 Å larger in comparison with layered MoO_3, suggesting that molybdic acid consists of a monolayer of water molecules bound to the molybdenum atoms. The presence

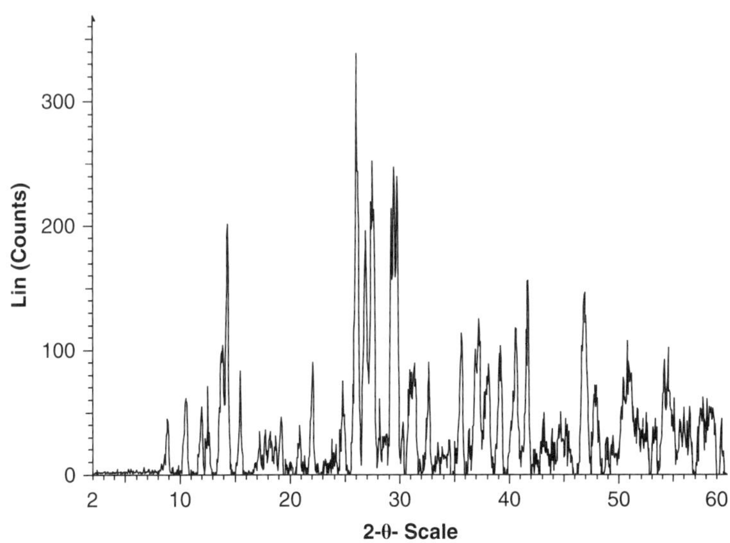

Figure 2.6 X-ray diffractogram of pristine molybdic acid.

of water molecules was confirmed by thermogravimetric analysis (*vide infra*). The average crystallite size of the molybdic acid was also determined from its powder pattern by making use of the Scherrer Equation shown below. The average crystallite size was found to be 34 Å.

The Scherrer Equation is, $D_{hkl} = \frac{K\lambda 57.3}{\beta \cos\theta}$, D_{hkl} = average crystallite size (Å), λ is the wavelength of the Cu (Kα) radiation used (λ=1.542 Å), β = peak width at half-height (2θ) and θ = position of the peak in degrees. The constant 57.3, is the conversion factor from radians to degrees. K is a constant depending on the shape of the crystallites. The crystallite shape of these materials is not known, but because we are primarily interested in trends, not the actual values, we use K = 0.9 (for spheres) for all samples.

The molybdic acid was also characterized by TGA. Figure 2.7 depicts the thermogram of molybdic acid. The material is stable in air up to 210°C, thereafter losing weight till a temperature of about 300°C is reached. The observed weight loss is attributed to the loss of inter-lamellar water molecules. The thermal decomposition patterns indicate that there is one water molecule per unit of MoO_3, which is consistent with the XRD data. The TGA was run up to 650°C in air, and an XRD pattern was collected on the product obtained at that temperature. The collected product was determined to be MoO_3 as shown in Figure 2.8.

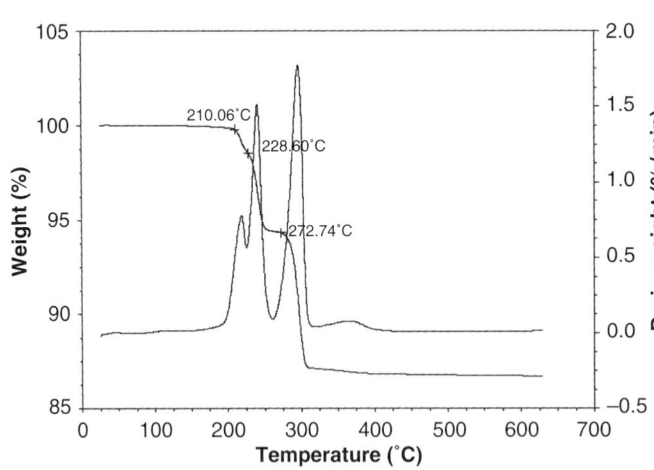

Figure 2.7 Thermogram of pristine molybdic acid.

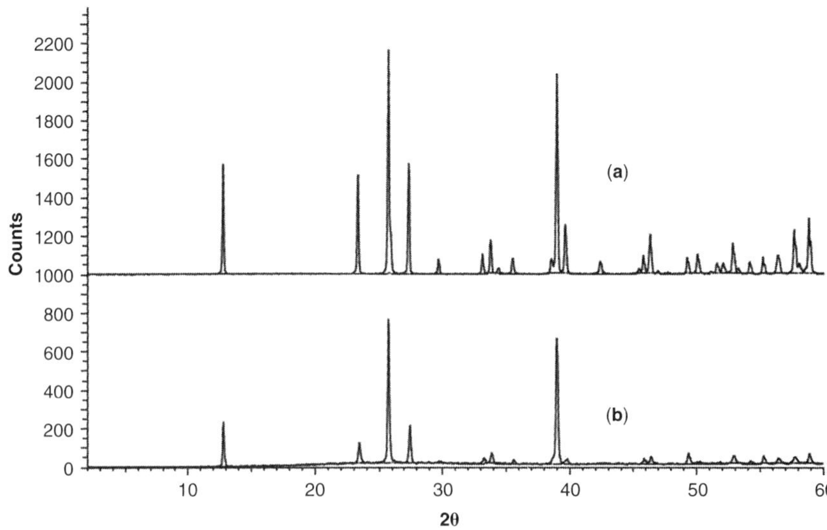

Figure 2.8 Diffractogram of (a) Pristine MoO_3, (b) molybdic acid after TGA in air up to 650°C.

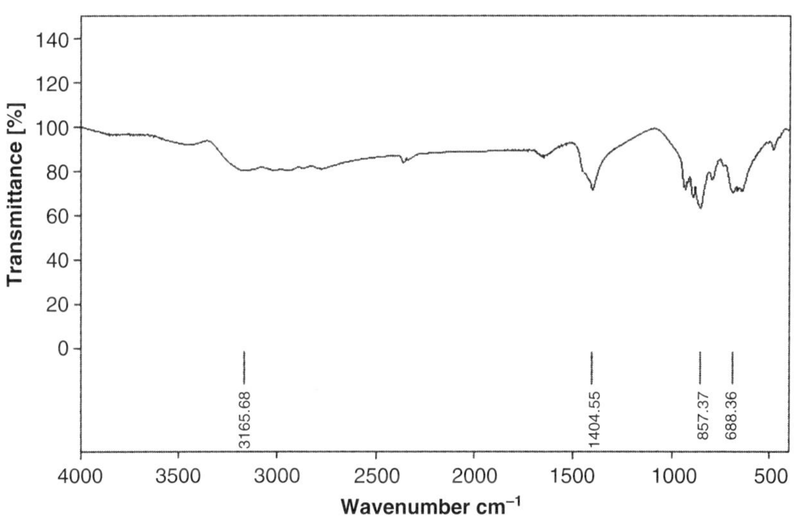

Figure 2.9 Infrared spectrum of pristine molybdic acid.

The molybdic acid was also characterized by FTIR spectroscopy. Figure 2.9 shows the IR spectrum of molybdic acid which reveals the presence of the following vibrations: OH stretching at 3167 cm^{-1} due to the presence of inter-lamellar water molecules, broad OHO bending vibration at 1404 cm^{-1}, and Mo-O vibrations in the fingerprint region: 1000-500 cm^{-1}.

2.6.2 Polymers

PEG, POEGO and POMOE were characterized by techniques such as XRD, TGA and IR.

2.6.2.1 Poly(ethylene glycol)

The X-ray diffractogram of PEG as shown in Figure 2.10 illustrates the semi-crystalline nature of the material, i.e., both the crystalline and amorphous properties of the polymer can be observed. Using Bruker Diffrac.Suite Eva software (version 2.1, 2011), the % crystallinity of PEG was determined to be 51.2 %. The thermogram of PEG as depicted in Figure 2.11 illustrates that the polymer is stable in air up to about 162°C. The Infrared spectrum of POEGO, shown in Figure 2.12, reveals the following main vibrations: C-H asymmetric bend at 2895.57 cm^{-1}, CH_2 symmetric bend at 1344.82 cm^{-1}, and COC stretch at 1101.94 cm^{-1}.

2.6.2.2 Poly[oligo(ethylene glycol)oxalate]

The X-ray diffractogram of POEGO as shown in Figure 2.13 confirms that the polymer is completely amorphous. The thermogram

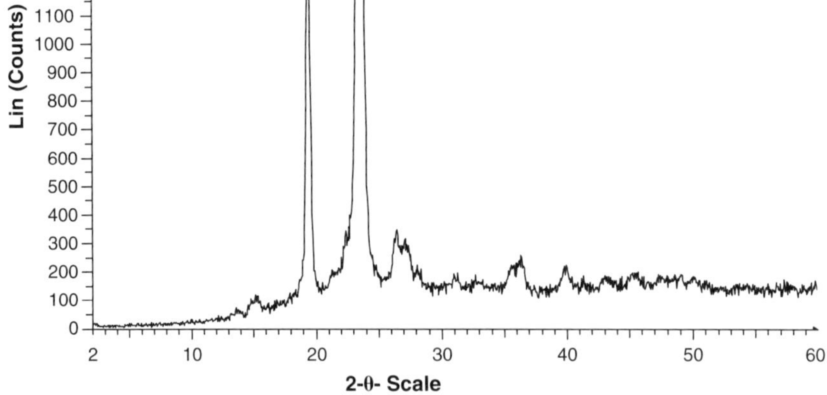

Figure 2.10 Diffractogram of PEG.

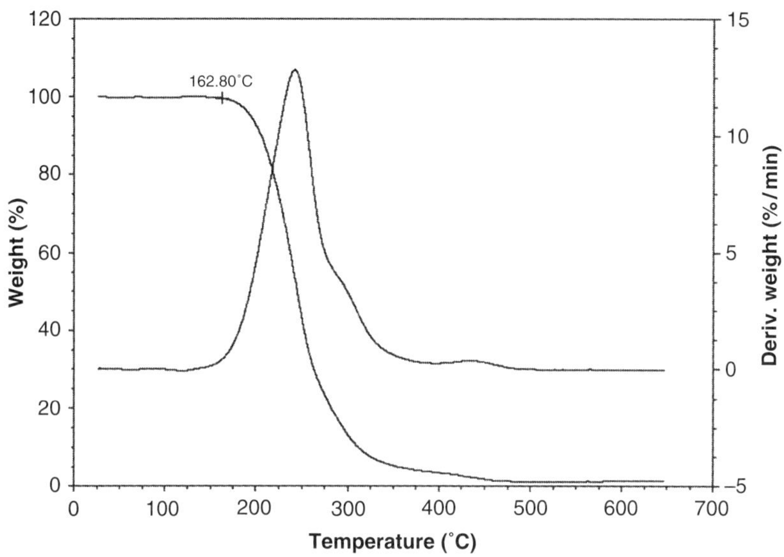

Figure 2.11 Thermogram of PEG.

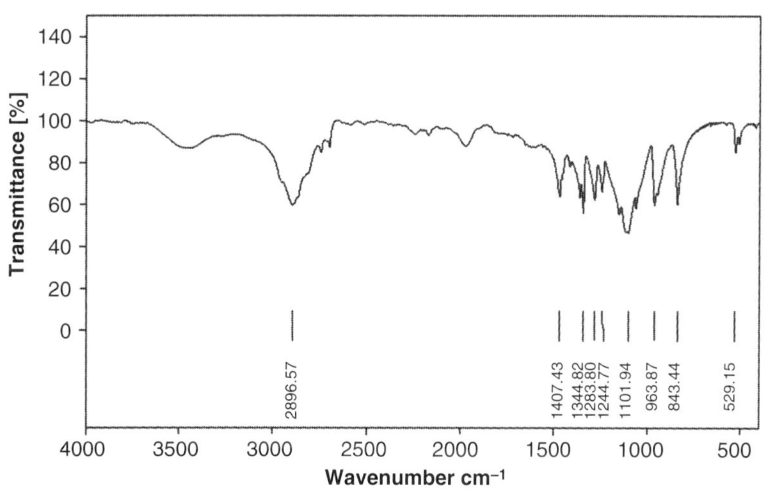

Figure 2.12 Infrared spectrum of PEG.

of POEGO (see Figure 2.14) illustrates that the polymer is stable up to 180°C. The IR spectrum (Figure 2.15) reveals the following major vibrations: *sp*^{3} C-H stretch at 2881.30 cm^{-1}, C=O stretch at 1748.72 cm^{-1}, C-O-C stretch at 1111.17 cm^{-1}, and CH_2 rocking at 953.28 cm^{-1}.

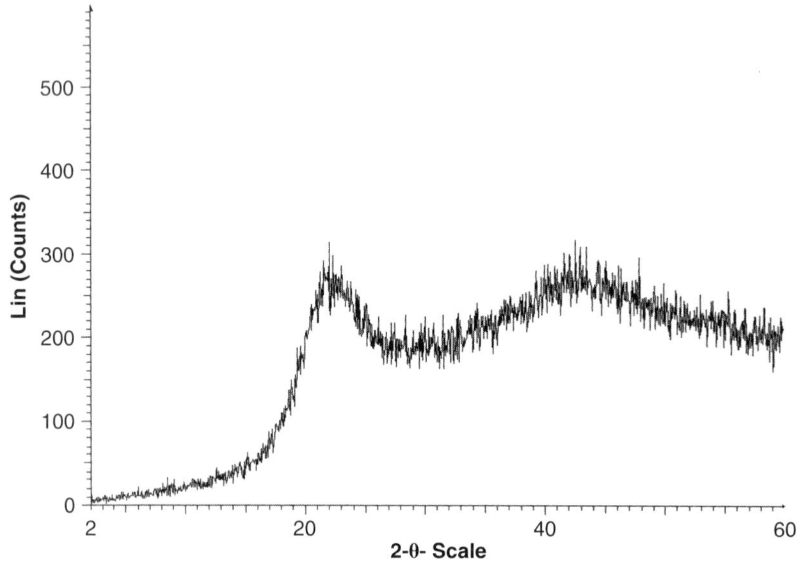

Figure 2.13 Diffractogram of POEGO.

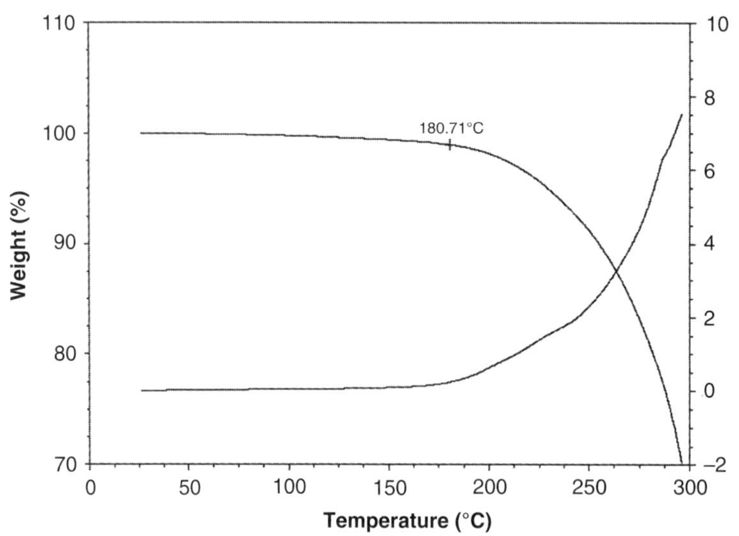

Figure 2.14 Thermogram of PEOGO. Thermal decomposition begins around 180°C.

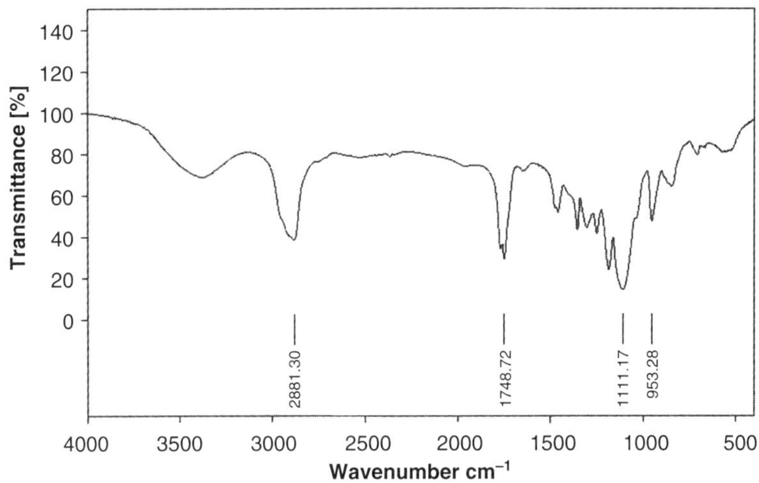

Figure 2.15 Infrared spectrum of POEGO.

2.6.2.3 Poly[oxymethylene-(oxyethylene)]

X-ray diffraction shows that POMOE is completely amorphous (Figure 2.16). TGA shows that the polymer is stable in air up to 170°C (Figure 2.17). The Infrared spectrum of POMOE, shown in Figure 2.18, reveals the following main vibrations: C-H asymmetric bend at 2877.95 cm^{-1}, CH_2 symmetric bend at 1354.87 cm^{-1}, C-O stretch at 1252.45 cm^{-1}, C-O-C stretch at 1110.86 cm^{-1}, and CH_2 rocking at 953.59 cm^{-1}.

2.6.3 Formation of Intercalated Nanocomposites

2.6.3.1 PEG/Molybdic Acid

The X-ray diffraction pattern of the PEG/molybdic acid system as shown in Figure 2.19 demonstrates complete intercalation of the polymer into the layered structure, as no molybdic acid phase could be observed. The interlayer spacing of the nanocomposite is 13.6 Å. Compared to pristine molybdic acid, this corresponds to an interlayer expansion of 3.5 Å, which corresponds to a monolayer of the polymer chain sandwiched between the layers of MoO_3. It is interesting to point out that increasing the ratio of PEG to the molybdic acid does not increase the interlayer spacing value, suggesting that a monolayer of the polymer is preferable, and any excess polymer stays on the surface and edges of the layered compound.

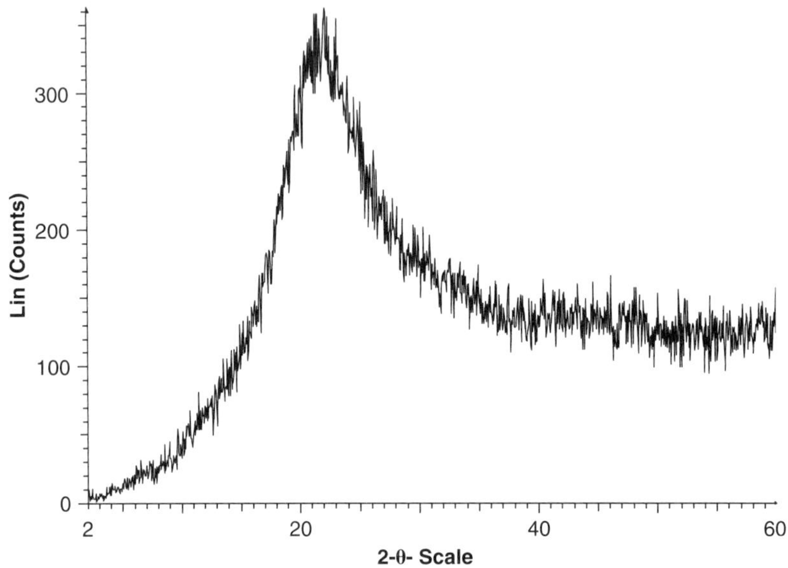

Figure 2.16 Diffractogram of POMOE.

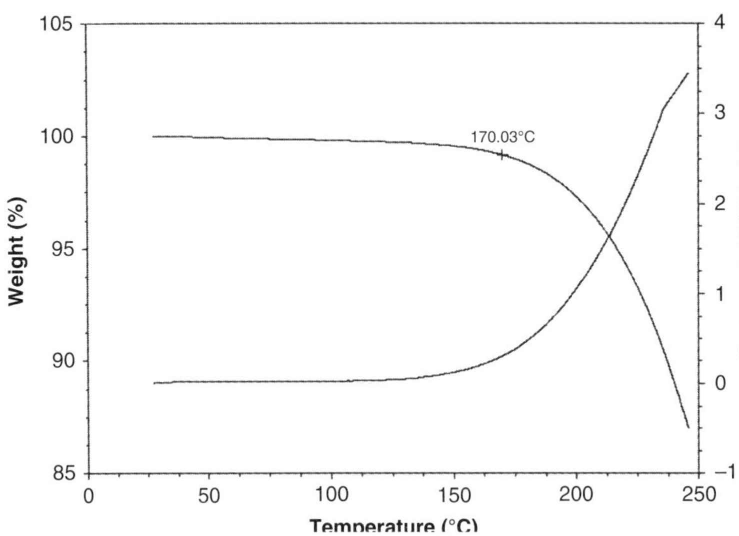

Figure 2.17 Thermogram of POMOE. Thermal decomposition begins around 170°C.

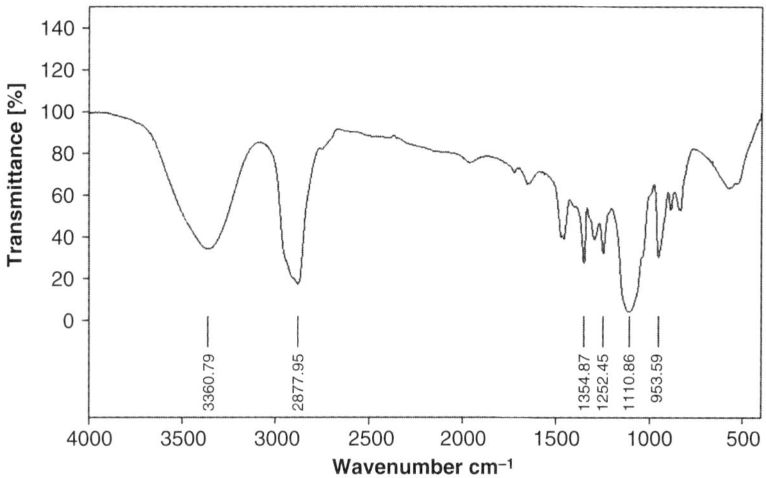

Figure 2.18 Infrared Spectrum of POMOE.

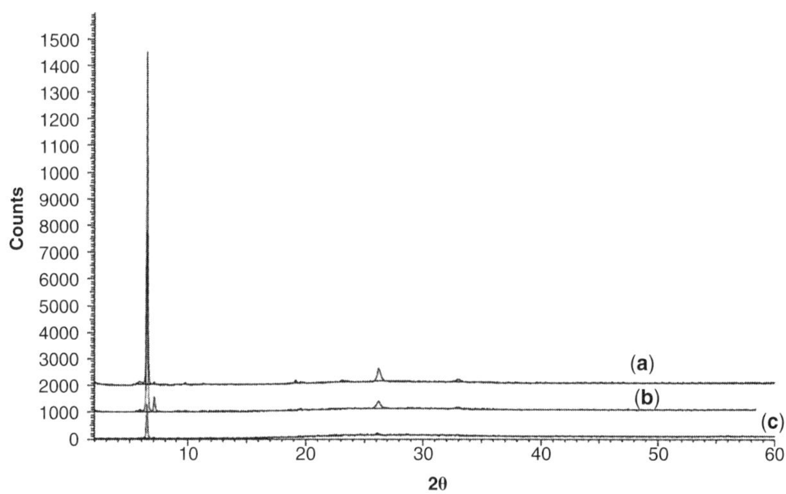

Figure 2.19 Diffractograms of PEG/ molybdic acid system: (a) 1:4 ratio, (b) 1:2 ratio, and (c) 1:1 ratio.

The crystallite size of PEG/molybdic acid system was found to 58 Å, as determined from the powder pattern. This is roughly a two-fold increase over the crystallite size of molybdic acid. This information coupled with the observed sharp peaks in the diffractogram of the PEG/molybdic acid indicates that a system of higher

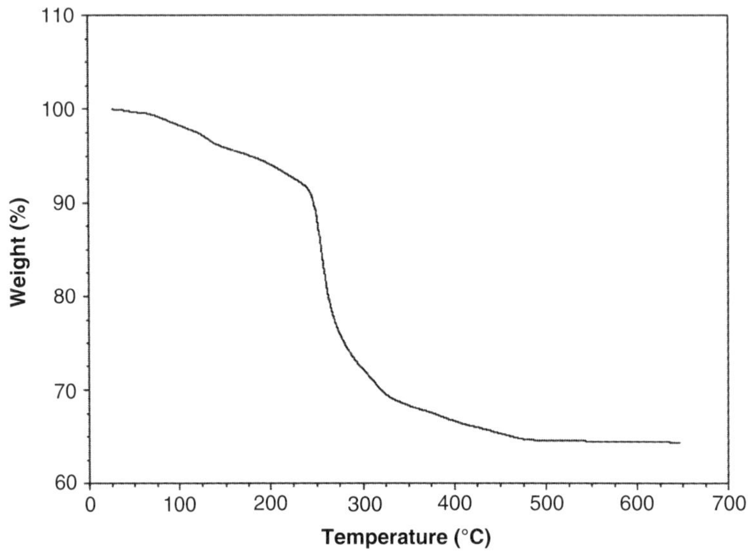

Figure 2.20 Thermogram of PEG/ molybdic acid system.

structural order was obtained upon the intercalation of PEG into molybdic acid.

The thermogram of the PEG/molybdic acid system (Figure 2.20) reveals three weight loss steps. The first weight loss which occurs from the start of the TGA run up to about 162°C, corresponds to the evaporation of co-intercalated water molecules. Since the reaction was performed in an aqueous medium it is reasonable to assume the co-insertion of water molecules. The second weight loss step which occurs in the temperature range 162–200°C is attributed to the loss of externally lying (unintercalated) polymer, and finally the major decomposition starting at 200°C is ascribed to the removal of the inserted PEG. The final phase obtained at 650°C was shown to be MoO_3 from X-ray diffraction. From the TGA, the stoichiometry of the PEG-molybdic acid system was found to be $(H_2O)_{0.54}(PEG_{out})_{0.15}(PEG_{in})_{1.4}MoO_3$, where PEG_{out} corresponds to the externally lying polymer, and PEG_{in} to the intercalated polymer. The ratio of MoO_3 to the total amount of PEG as observed from TGA is 1:1.55. This calculated ratio is in good agreement with the experimental ratio used, which was 1:1.25. It is interesting to note that the decomposition temperature of the externally lying polymer matches that of the bulk polymer, while the intercalated polymer begins to decompose at 200°C, which corresponds to a thermal enhancement of 38°C.

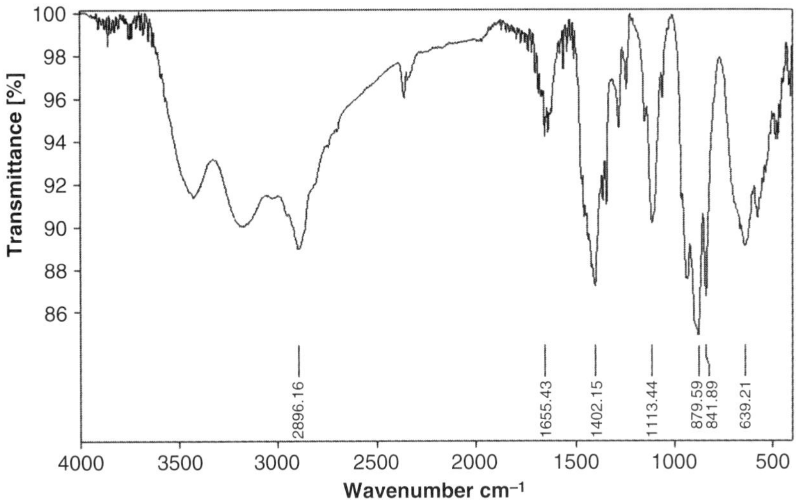

Figure 2.21 Infrared Spectrum of PEG/ molybdic acid system.

The infrared spectrum of the PEG/molybdic acid system (Figure 2.21) reveals vibration peaks of the polymer which are shifted to higher wavenumbers, with the C-H vibration slightly shifted to a lower wavenumber. A shift to lower wavenumber is expected when a polymer is intercalated because it takes less energy to vibrate the bond in a single isolated chain of the polymer compared to the bulk polymer. When the polymer chain is intercalated between the layers of a structured material it is fairly isolated from other polymer chains and as a result will vibrate at a higher wavelength (lower wavenumber) than the pure polymer. A shift to higher wavenumber is also expected when a polymer is intercalated, because when the motility of the polymer is restricted, the bonds become more rigid and therefore require more energy to vibrate. The results are summarized in Table 2.1.

2.6.3.2 POEGO/Molybdic Acid

The X-ray diffraction pattern of the POEGO/molybdic acid system, as shown in Figure 2.22, demonstrates an interlayer spacing value of 15.5 Å. The intercalation of POEGO is complete, similar to that of PEG, as no molybdic acid phase is visible in the XRD. The observed interlayer spacing value of 15.5 Å corresponds to an interlayer expansion of 5.4 Å. An interlayer expansion of this magnitude

Table 2.1 Assignment Table for PEG and PEG/ molybdic acid infrared spectra.

Assignment	PEG	PEG + Molybdic Acid	Shift Wavenumber (cm^{-1})
	Wavenumber (cm^{-1})	Wavenumber (cm^{-1})	
C-H asymmetric Bend	2895.57	2896.16	–0.59
CH_2 symmetric Bend	1344.82	1402.15	+57.33
C-O-C Stretch	1101.94	1113.44	+11.5

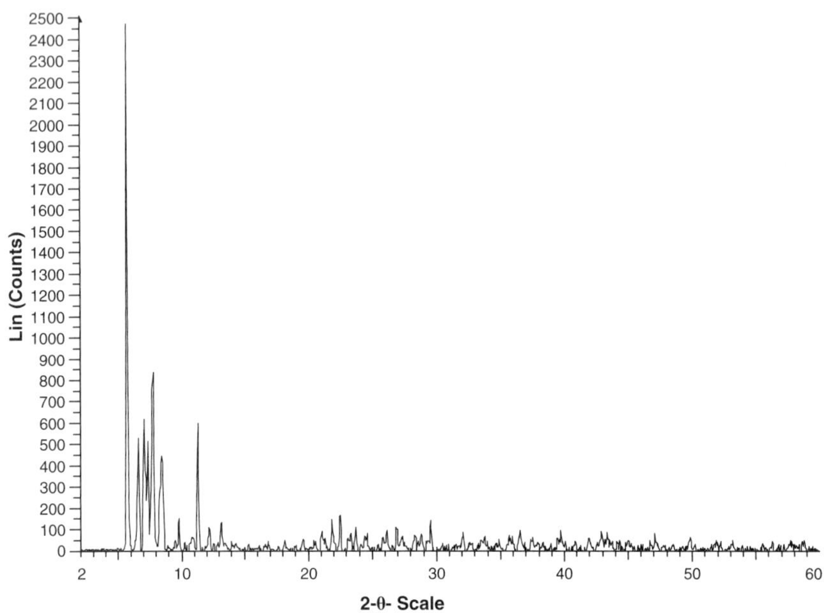

Figure 2.22 Diffractogram of POEGO/molybdic acid system.

indicates that a monolayer of the polymer has been intercalated between the layers of molybdic acid.

From the powder pattern, the crystallite size of the POEGO/molybdic acid system was determined by using the Scherrer Equation, and was found to be 72 Å. This is a two-fold increase in crystallite size when compared to the pristine layered material. This information

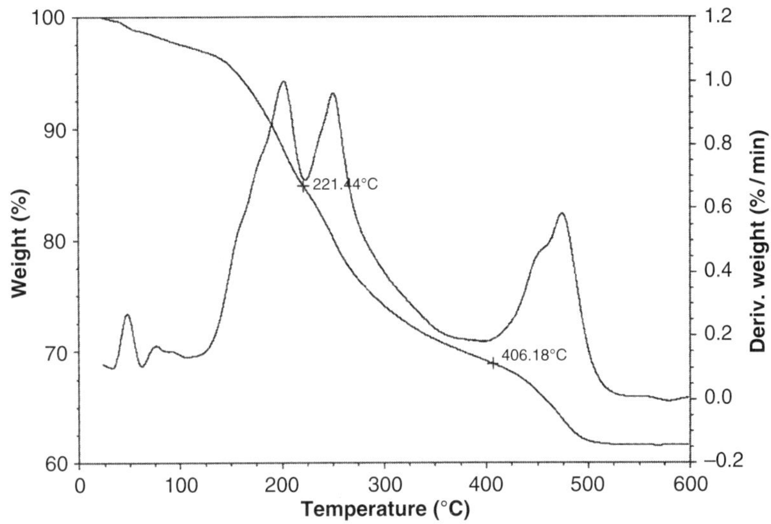

Figure 2.23 Thermogram of POEGO/ molybdic acid system.

coupled with the observed sharp peaks in the diffractogram of the POEGO/molybdic acid indicates a highly ordered system.

Analysis of the thermogram obtained for this system yields the following stoichiometic calculation: $(H_2O)_{2.62}(POEGO_{out})_{0.06}(POEGO_{in})_{0.13}MoO_3$. The ratio of MoO_3 to the total amount of POEGO as observed from TGA is 1:0.19. This ratio is in very good agreement with the experimental ratio used which was 1:0.17. The thermogram shown in Figure 2.23 depicts the external polymer starts to burn off at 190°C, which corresponds very well with the onset decomposition temperature of the bulk polymer. The thermogram in Figure 2.23 also depicts that the internal polymer begins to decompose at around 405°C, and this clearly indicates an increase of over 200°C in thermal stability of the intercalated polymer.

The infrared spectrum of the POEGO/molybdic acid system (Figure 2.24) reveals vibration peaks of the polymer which are shifted to lower wavenumbers when compared to the pure polymer. The shift to lower wavenumbers provides supporting evidence for intercalation. Less energy is required to vibrate the bonds in the polymer when enclosed in the constrained environment of the gallery space of the layered host, where interaction with other polymer chains are minimized compared to the polymer in the bulk state. The IR data are summarized in Table 2.2.

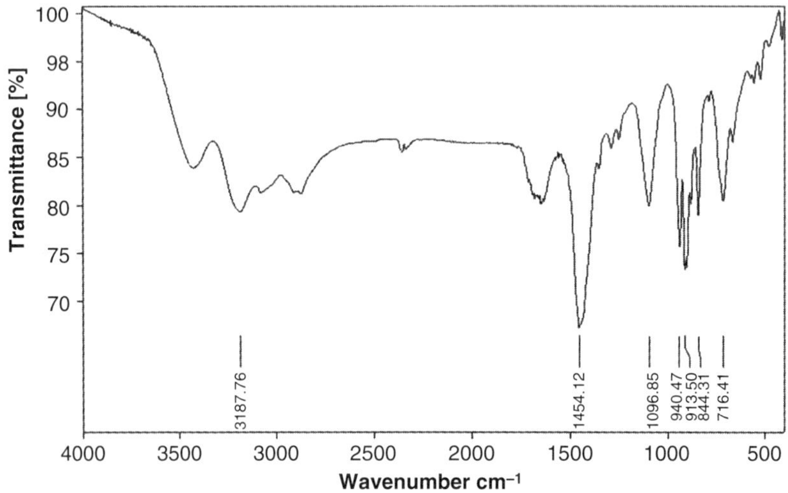

Figure 2.24 Infrared spectrum of POEGO/ molybdic acid system.

Table 2.2 Assignment Table for POEGO and POEGO/ molybdic acid spectra.

Assignment	**POEGO**	**POEGO + Molybdic Acid**	**Shift Wavenumber (cm^{-1})**
	Wavenumber (cm^{-1})	**Wavenumber (cm^{-1})**	
Sp^3 C-H Stretch	2881.30	—	—
C=O Stretch	1748.72	1454.12	–294.60
C-O-C Stretch	1111.17	1096.85	–14.32
CH_2 Rocking	953.28	940.47	–12.81

2.6.3.3 POMOE/Molybdic Acid

The X-ray diffraction pattern of the POMOE/ molybdic acid system as shown in Figure 2.25 demonstrates an interlayer spacing of 15.8 Å. This correlates to an interlayer expansion of 5.7 Å. An interlayer expansion of this magnitude indicates a monolayer arrangement of POMOE in the gallery space of the layered structure.

The crystallite size of the intercalated nanocomposite as determined from its powder patterm was found to be 102 Å . This is a

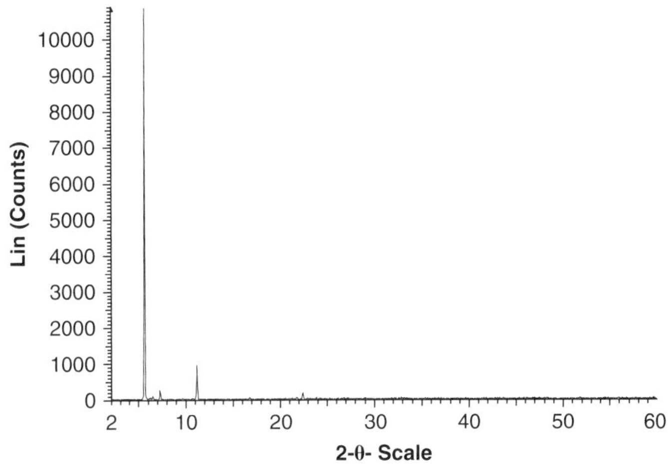

Figure 2.25 Diffractogram of POMOE/ molybdic acid system.

three-fold increase in crystallite size when compared to molybdic acid, suggesting that intercalation of the polymer results in a highly ordered structural framework.

Analysis of the thermogram for this system yields the following stoichiometry: $(H_2O)_{0.62}(POMOE_{out})_{0.40}(POMOE_{in})_{0.12}MoO_3$. The ratio of MoO_3 to the total amount of POMOE as observed from TGA is 1:0.53. This ratio is in very good agreement with the experimental ratio used, which was 1:0.55. The thermogram as shown in Figure 2.26 depicts that the externally lying polymer starts to burn off at 170°C which matches the onset decomposition temperature of the bulk polymer. The thermogram also depicts that the intercalated polymer begins to degrade at around 390°C, which correlates to an increase in thermal stability of over 200°C compared to the pure polymer.

The infrared spectrum of the POMOE/molybdic acid system (Figure 2.27) reveals vibration peaks of the polymer which are shifted to lower wavenumbers, with the C-H vibration shifted to higher wavenumber. These shifts in wavenumbers provide supporting evidence that the polymer is in fact intercalated in the layered host system. The IR data are summarized in Table 2.3.

2.6.4 Ionic Conductivity

Ionic conductivity was apparent in three of the samples (Table 2.4). The ionic conductivity of the samples increases with temperature,

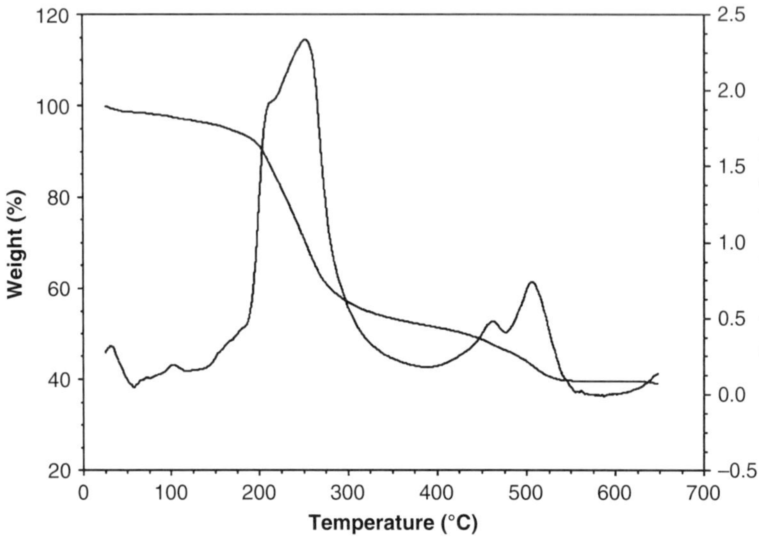

Figure 2.26 Thermogram of POMOE/ molybdic acid system.

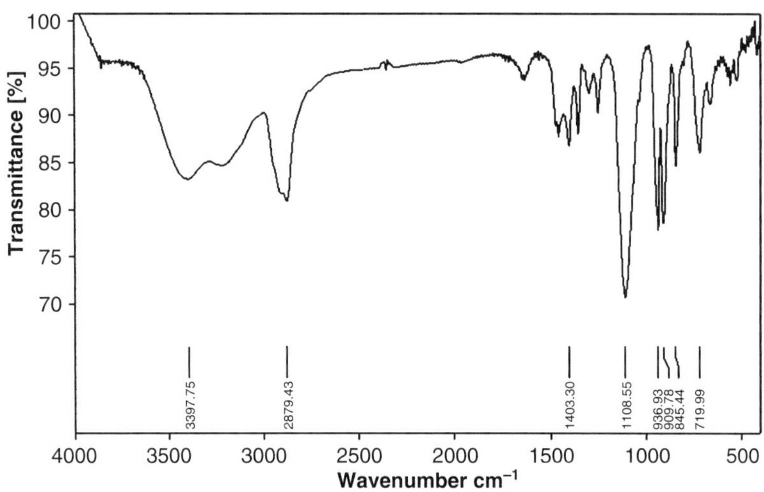

Figure 2.27 Infrared spectrum of POMOE/molybdic acid system.

and is thus thermally activated. Conductivity appears to persist to a lower temperature in Molybdic acid + PEG/LiOTf than in the other samples. (Table 2.4). However, this is due to the fact that this sample had the greatest thickness, so that its resistance was lower and remained within the measureable range to a lower temperature.

Table 2.3 Assignment Table for POMOE and POMOE/ molybdic acid spectra.

Assignment	POMOE	POMOE + Molybdic Acid	Shift Wavenumber (cm^{-1})
	Wavenumber (cm^{-1})	Wavenumber (cm^{-1})	
C-H asymmetric Bend	2877.95	2879.43	+1.48
CH_2 symmetric Bend	1354.87	--	--
C-O Stretch	1252.45	--	--
C-O-C Stretch	1110.86	1108.55	-2.31
CH_2 Rocking	953.59	936.93	-16.66

Table 2.4 Ionic Conductivity Data.

Material	Conductivity (S/cm)			
	280K	290K	300K	310K
Molybdic Acid PEG	**	**	**	**
Molybdic Acid + POEGO	**	**	2×10^{-6}	7×10^{-6}
Molybdic Acid + POMOE	**	**	1×10^{-6}	2×10^{-6}
Molybdic Acid + PEG/LiOTf	**	2×10^{-7}	6×10^{-7}	9×10^{-7}
Molybdic Acid + POEGO/LiOTf	**	**	**	**
Molybdic Acid + POMOE/LiOTf	**	**	**	**
***Conductivity too low to measure*				

A microscope image of the molybdic acid + PEG/LiOTf sample with a field of view of 1.8 mm is depicted in Figure 2.28. In this image the "woven" or granular nature of the sample can be seen. The other samples had similar morphology. If the samples were more uniform, with more points of connectivity between adjacent crystallites, the measured ionic conductivities would in principle be higher. Since variations in sample morphology, connectivity between crystallites, and the amount of external polymer could all affect the measured conductivities, it is difficult to come to any conclusions about the relationship between conductivity and composition. All we can conclude is that some samples are ionic conductors.

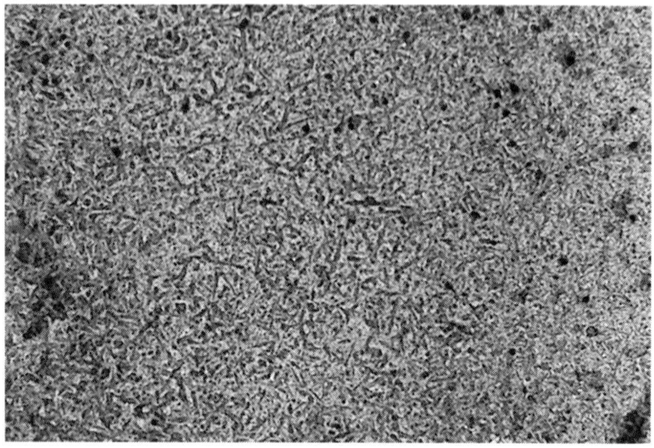

Figure 2.28 Brightfield optical microscope image of molybdic acid +PEG/LiOTf sample. Field of view = 1.8mm

It should also be noted that the thickness of the samples could not be accurately determined, leading to an uncertainty of approximately ±50% in the recorded conductivity values.

2.7 Conclusions

We found that molybdic acid can be readily intercalated with PEG, POMOE and POEGO, by using the exfoliation and re-stacking nature of the layered material. The synthetic methodology used in this research can potentially be extended to other soluble polymers, and molecules. While the conductivity values of the nanocomposites were found to be low (or in some cases too low to be measured), these values can potentially be augmented by increasing the salt content. Hence, these molybdic acid-based nanocomposites have the potential to be used in battery applications.

Acknowledgements

The authors are grateful for financial support from the Natural Sciences and Engineering Research Council (NSERC) of Canada, Canada Foundation for Innovation (CFI), Atlantic Innovation Fund of Canada (AIF), Innovation PEI, and UPEI.

References

1. S.F. Scully. Master's Thesis, University of Prince Edward Island, 2007.
2. M.S. Whittingham. *Science* 1976, 192, 1126.
3. K. Mitzushima, P.C. Jones, P.J. Wiseman, J.B. Goodenough. *Mat. Res. Bull.* 1980, 15, 783.
4. M.M. Thackeray, W.I.F. David, P.G. Bruce, J.B. Goodenough. *Mat. Res. Bull.* 1983, 18, 461.
5. G.A. Nazri, G. Pistoia. *Lithium Batteries: Science and Technology*, Kluwer Academic Publishers: Boston, 2004.
6. M.S. Whittingham. *Chem. Rev.* 2004, 104, 4271.
7. K.B. Kamel, et al. *Ionics* 2008, 14, 89.
8. I. Buchmann. Will lithium-ion batteries power the new millenium? Powerpulse.net Darnell.com Inc., California, 2000.
9. A. J. Proud, R. Bissessur, D. C. Dahn. Polymer Nanocomposite Materials Based on Carbon Nanotubes, In Nanocomposites and Polymers with Analytical Methods, J. Cuppoletti (Ed.). Publisher: Intech Open Access, 2011.
10. D. Linden, T.B. Reddy. *Handbook of Batteries*. 3rd ed. McGraw-Hill: New York, 2002.
11. J.O. Besenhard, ed. *Handbook of Battery Materials*.Wiley-VCH: Weinheim, Germany, 1999.
12. F. Croce, G.B. Appetecchi, L. Persi, B. Scrosati. Nature 1998, 394, 456.
13. F.B. Dias, L. Plomp, J.B.J. Veldhuis. *J. Power Sources* 2000, 88, 169.
14. H.R. Allcock, F.W. Lampe, J.E. Mark. *Contemporary Polymer Chemistry*. 3rd ed. 2003
15. W.H. Meyer. *Adv. Mater.* 1998, 10, 439.
16. W. Xu, J.P. Belieres, C.A. Angell. *Chem. Mater.* 2001, 13, 575.
17. C.V. Nicholas, D.J. Wilson, C. Booth, J.R.M. Giles. *Brit. Pol. J.* 1988, 20, 289.
18. H.R. Allcock, P.E. Austin, T.X. Neenan, J.T. Sisko, P.M. Blonsky, D.F. Shriver. *Macromolecules* 1986, 19, 1508.
19. R. Bissessur, S.F. Scully. *Solid State Ionics* 2007, 178, 877.
20. J. Wu, M.M. Lerner. Chem. Mater. 1993, 5, 835.
21. R. Bissessur, D. Gallant, R. Brüning. *Mater. Chem. Phys.* 2003, 82, 316.
22. R. Bissessur, D. Gallant, R. Brüning. *J. Mater. Sci. Lett.* 2003, 22, 429.
23. R. Bissessur, D. Gallant, R. Brüning. *Solid State Ionics* 2003, 158, 205.
24. R. Bissessur, D. Schipper. *Mater. Lett.* 2008, 62, 1638.
25. M. Riley, P.S. Fedkiw, S.A. Khan. *J. Electrochem. Soc.* 2002, 149, A667.
26. A.V. Powell. *Phys. Chem.* 1993, 90, 177.
27. A.M. Chippindale, P.G. Dickens, A.V. Powell. *Progr. Solid State Chem.* 1991, 21, 133.
28. P.G. Dickens, A.M. Chippindale. *Proton Conductors*. P. Colomban, ed. Cambridge University Press, 1992, 101.
29. R. Schollhorn. *Angew. Chem.* 1980, 19, 983.
30. A.C.W.P. James, J.B. Goodenough, N.J. Clayden. *J. Solid State Chem.* 1988, 77, 356.
31. C. Delmas, I. Saadoune. *Solid State Ionics* 1992, 370, 53.
32. P.G. Dickens, M.F. Pye. *Intercalation Chemistry*. F. Levy, ed., D. Reidel Dordrecht, 1979, 201.
33. M.S. Whittingham. *Progr. Solid State Chem.* 1978, 12, 41.
34. J. Rouxel. *Intercalation Chemistry*. F. Levy, ed., D. Reidel Dordrecht, 1979, 201.

35. J.D. Corbett. *Intercalation Chemistry*. M.S. Whittingham, A.J. Jacobson, eds. Academic Press New York, 1985, 361.
36. A.J. Jacobson, J.W. Johnson, J.F. Brody, J.C. Scanlon, J.T. Lewandowski. *Inorg. Chem*. 1985, 24, 1782.
37. R. Brec. *Solid State Ionics* 1986, 22, 3.
38. P. Fragnaud, R. Brec, E. Prouzet, P. Deniard. *Mater. Res. Bull*. 1993, 28, 337.
39. R. Schollhorn, R. Steffen, K. Wagner. *Angew. Chem*. 1983, 22, 555.
40. D. O'Hare, D.W. Bruce. *Inorganic Materials*. D.W. Bruce, D. O'Hare, eds. Wiley, Chichester, 1992, 4, 165.
41. A.J. Jacobson. *Solid State Chemistry: Compounds*. A.K. Cheetham, P. Day, eds. Clarendon Press, Oxford, 1992, 6, 182.
42. A.F. Wells. *Structural Inorganic Chemistry*. Oxford: Clarendon Press, 1984.
43. M.S. Whittingham. *J. Electrochem. Soc*. 1976, 123, 315.
44. F.W. Dampier. *J. Electrochem. Soc*. 1974, 121, 656.
45. M.S. Whittingham, M.B. Dines. *J. Electrochem. Soc*. 1977, 124, 1387.
46. M. Afsharpour, A. Mahjoub, M.M. Amini. *J. Inorg. Organomet. Polym*. 2008, 18, 472.
47. M.I. Shukoor, H.A. Therese, L. Gorgshvili, G. Glasser, U. Kolb, W. Tremel. *Chem. Mater*. 2006, 18, 2144.
48. E. Monyoncho, R. Bissessur, V. Trenton, D.C. Dahn. *Solid State Ionics* 2012, 227, 1.

3

Fluid-Bed Technology for Encapsulation and Coating Purposes

Roman G. Szafran

Wroclaw University of Technology, Faculty of Chemistry, Department of Chemical Engineering, Wroclaw, Poland

Abstract

This chapter discusses various aspects of the application of fluid-bed technology for coating and encapsulation processes. Particular attention has been paid to the principles of the fluidization technique, the miscellaneous fluid bed-coating processes and various coater configurations, with a special emphasis on fine powder coating, dry coating and encapsulation. Part of the chapter is devoted to fluidized bed chemical, molecular and atomic layer depositions as methods for preparation of functionalized micro- and nanopowders, and presents the classification of powders based on their fluidization behavior, including micro- and nanopowders. As the quality and properties of the coated product strongly depend on the quality of fluidization and are associated with the fluidization regime in which the coater operates, it is important to correctly choose methods, apparatuses and operating conditions to successfully carry out the process. Design, optimization and scale-up of the fluid-bed coating process and apparatus based on classical algebraic equations, dimensionless correlations and numerical simulations are discussed extensively.

Keywords: Encapsulation, coating, fluidization, fluidized bed, scale-up, dry coating, nanopowder, Wurster coater, spouted bed, FBCVD

3.1 Introduction

Fluid-bed coating is one of the various processes that can be applied for granulation, coating and encapsulation in the food, agricultural, pharmaceutical, nuclear, chemical and cosmetics industries. Cosmetics, flavorings, essences, enzymes, proteins, vegetables,

Vikas Mittal (ed.) Encapsulation Nanotechnologies, (71–106) © 2013 Scrivener Publishing LLC

seeds, fertilizers, sweets, nuclear fuel, drugs and pigments are the product of coating and granulation [1, 2].

The objective of the process may vary depending on product form and application. One can obtain tablets, pellets, capsules and granules with specific properties [3]:

a. controlled release of active ingredient (time, quantity) depending on temperature, acidity, pressure, solubility conditions; applicable in medicine to control the biological activity of drugs over a period of time; and for foods during mastication, or to mask odor or bad taste;
b. particular shape, size, or surface texture to facilitate dosage and mixing, to improve flowability or to change the density;
c. extra protection against reactive environment like oxygen, humidity and other constituents during storage or further transformation;
d. enhanced handling and flow of particles with a resistant shell, aimed at avoiding dust and sticking;
e. defined surface properties (catalytic [4] and boiosensing [5, 6]).

It is the specificity of the fluid bed that allows for coating dry solid particles, which leads to forming real capsules—reservoir systems or reservoir systems with multiple layers. Other techniques frequently lead to a matrix with the core material randomly dispersed in a polymer, and may also lead to forming imperfect capsules or granules (e.g., spray drying, durum or pan coating) [1]. The other factors that favor fluid-bed processes (FB) are their high efficiency, scalability and possible operation in a continuous mode that makes FB well suited for a large-scale production of cost-sensitive products, e.g., food or agrochemicals.

Fluidized and conical spouted beds (with and/or without draft tube) have been used mainly for the film coating of particles due to their hydrodynamic properties, such as good particle circulation that bring about high product homogeneity, effective fluid-solid contact (even fine particles) and high rates of heat and mass transfer that lead to shortening of the process duration [7–10]

The groundbreaking discovery in fluid-bed coating was the invention in the early 1950s by Dale E. Wurster [11] at the University of Wisconsin of his spout-fluid bed apparatus for coating tablets

[12–14] which is now extensively used for coating and encapsulation of smaller particles – pellets and capsules [15–17] The Wurster coater is a special variant of a conical spout-fluid bed apparatus with an upfacing nozzle placed at its porous base, and an axially placed draft tube. This construction allows for simultaneous fluidization and spouting with circulation of particles inside the column of the apparatus. Its main use is for the coating and encapsulation of pharmaceuticals for which this is one of the most common methods.

Fluidized beds are also used for granulation, but agglomeration of particles is undesirable in coaters, which are, therefore, designed to minimize it. A number of researchers concentrated their efforts on the improvement of the apparatus performance and product quality by changing construction and operation parameters [18]. A better performance of the apparatus can be obtained by changing bed velocity and circulation rate, and through the elimination of dead zones by means of new gas distributors [19]. To protect nozzles against plugging, special shields are applied or the gas distributor is altered in such a manner as to allow for creating an additional air flow, which blows particles away from the nozzle [20].

As nanoscience has attracted much attention from researchers over the past decades, the possibility of application of the fluid-bed apparatus for encapsulation of micro- and nanoparticles is presently intensively investigated [15]. However, the adhesion of particles caused by Van der Waals forces and electrostatic interactions, as well as their adhesion to the apparatus walls, causes some problems such as the formation of aggregates and nonuniform layers on the surface of particles. The production of microcapsules is growing in importance in new therapies used to fight various types of cancer, like the so-called Neutron Capture Therapy (NCT) [21, 22], and chemoembolization of tumors [16]. Coating of nanosized drug particles with polymers can prevent them from becoming trapped in a mucus barrier, so they can be targeted at specific organs of the body [23], and prevent immune cells from engulfing and eliminating the nanosized drug particles circulating in the blood system [24]. Common techniques utilized for the thin-layer, gas-phase coating of objects are chemical vapor deposition (CVD) [25, 26], atomic layer deposition (ALD), and molecular layer deposition (MLD) [27]. MLD was successfully applied for coating nanoparticles with a polymer film in a fluidized bed reactor. Continuous improvements in the technology of fluid-bed coating of fine particles contribute to the development of personalized medicine of the 21st century.

3.2 Principles of Fluidization

Fluidized beds have many advantages over fixed-bed systems. A very good introduction to the fluidization subject can be found in the book edited by Wen-Chin Yang [28]. Once the solids in the bed are fluidized, the solids inside the bed will behave just like a liquid. Thus the liquid-like behavior of a fluidized bed allows for the solids to be handled like a fluid, which means that continuous feeding and withdrawal become possible. The rigorous mixing in a fluidized bed results in a uniform distribution of temperature in the bed. The fluidized bed can be treated as a stirred-tank reactor with varying solids residence time distribution. Nevertheless, fluidized beds also have some disadvantages. Rigorous solids mixing in the bed produce solid fines through attrition. Operating at high fluidization velocities, fines elutriation and entrainment can become a serious operational problem.

The principle of fluidization is to maintain particles in suspension within the closed space of the apparatus column. Generally, the fluidizing air moves upward, thereby counteracting the gravitational force acting on the bed of solid particles. The phenomenon of fluidization can be characterized by a diagram of a pressure drop across the bed of particles Δp vs. fluidization velocity plot (Figure 3.1). Below the minimum fluidization velocity U_{mf},

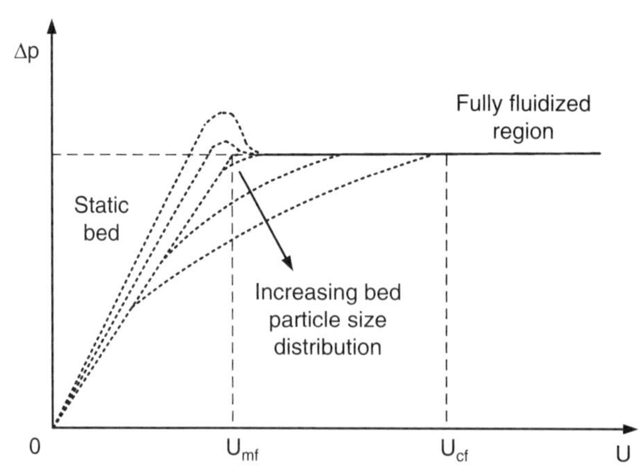

Figure 3.1 Pressure drop vs. fluidization velocity. U_{mf} – minimum fluidization velocity, U_{cf} - complete fluidization velocity. Adapted from [28].

a packed bed of solid particles remains fixed. At the minimum fluidization velocity all the particles are essentially supported by the gas stream. Further increases in gas velocity will not usually cause further increases in pressure drop and will lead to fluidization whose regime depends on gas-solid system properties.

The minimum fluidization velocity U_{mf} is given by Equations (3.1) and (3.2) for particles of diameter $d_p < 100\,\mu m$ and $d_p \geq 100$, respectively.

$$U_{mf} = \frac{\left[\left(\rho_p - \rho_f\right)g\right]^{0.934} d_p^{1.8}}{111\mu^{0.87}\rho_f^{0.066}} \quad d_p < 100\mu m \tag{3.1}$$

$$U_{mf} = \frac{\mu}{\rho_f d_p}\left[\sqrt{1135.7 + 0.0408 Ar} - 33.7\right] \quad d_p \geq 100\mu m \tag{3.2}$$

Where Ar is the Archimedes number given by Eq. (3.9).

Fluidization regimes can be classified into two broad categories: particulate (smooth) and aggregative (bubbling). In particulate (homogeneous) fluidization, solid particles usually disperse relatively uniformly in the fluidizing medium with no readily identifiable bubbles. In the aggregative (heterogeneous) fluidization, there usually occur voids (bubbles) containing no solids. For gas–solid systems, there are five distinguishable regimes of fluidization: fixed bed, particulate fluidization, bubbling fluidization, slugging fluidization, and turbulent fluidization (Figure 3.2).

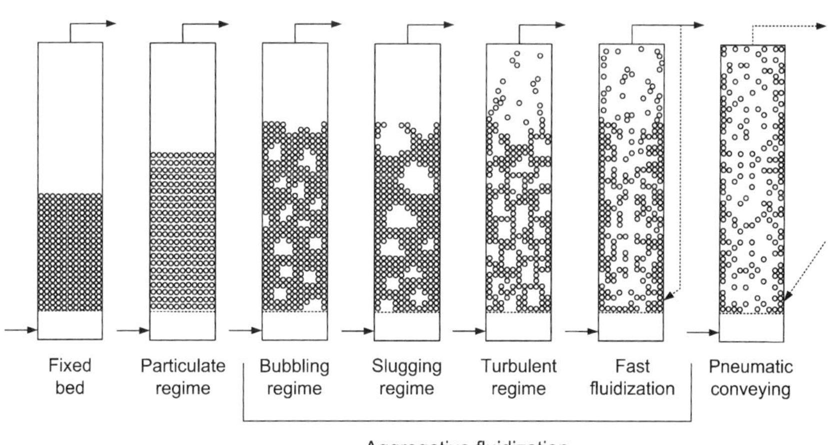

Figure 3.2 Regimes of fluidization. Adapted from [28].

When the operating velocity is higher than the critical (transport) velocity U_{tr}, a significant particle entrainment occurs. Beyond this point, continuing operation of the bed is unlikely to occur without entrained solids being recycled. For Group A and B particles (see Geldart's classification below), the transport velocity U_{tr}, calculated from Eq. (3.3) is slightly larger than the terminal velocity of the individual particles U_{ter}, whereas for Group D particles, the transition velocity equals essentially the terminal velocity of the individual particles, so that transport velocity can be estimated from relations for terminal velocity with reasonable accuracy.

Transport velocity U_{tr} is given by equation:

$$U_{tr} = 1.53 Ar^{0.5} \quad 2 < Ar < 4 \times 10^5 \tag{3.3}$$

The terminal velocity for single particle motion U_{ter} is given by equation:

$$U_{ter} = \sqrt{\frac{4}{3}\frac{d_p\left(\rho_p - \rho_f\right)g}{\rho_f C_D}} \tag{3.4}$$

Drag coefficient C_D is a function of the particle Reynolds number Re_p:

$$\mathrm{Re}_p = \frac{U_p d_p \rho_f}{\mu} \tag{3.5}$$

There are three different regimes distinguishable, depending on the magnitude of the particle's Reynolds number: Stokes, Intermediate and Newton's. Turton and Levenspiel in 1986 [28] proposed a single correlation applicable for the complete range of Reynolds numbers, and considerably simplified the calculation of the single-particle drag coefficient:

$$C_D = \frac{24}{\mathrm{Re}_p}\left(1 + 0.173\,\mathrm{Re}_p^{0.657}\right) + \frac{0.413}{1 + 16.300\,\mathrm{Re}_p^{-1.09}} \tag{3.6}$$

The different regimes for gas–solid fluidization are summarized in Table 3.1.

Table 3.1 Summary description of different regimes of fluidization. Adapted from [28].

Velocity range	Fluidization regime	Fluidization features and appearance
$0 \leq U < U_{mf}$	Fixed bed	Particles are quiescent; gas flows through interstices
$U_{mf} \leq U < U_{mb}$	Particulate regime	Bed expands smoothly and homogeneously with small-scale particle motion; bed surface is well defined
$U_{mb} \leq U < U_{ms}$	Bubbling regime	Gas bubbles form above distributor, coalesce and grow; gas bubbles promote solids mixing during rise to surface and breakthrough
$U_{ms} \leq U < U_{c}$	Slug flow regime	Bubble size approaches bed cross section; bed surface rises and falls with regular frequency with corresponding pressure fluctuation
$U_{c} \leq U < U_{k}$	Transition to turbulent fluidization	Pressure fluctuations decrease gradually until turbulent fluidization regime is reached
$U_{k} \leq U < U_{tr}$	Turbulent regime	Small gas voids and particle clusters and streamers dart to and from; bed surface is diffused and difficult to distinguish
$U > U_{tr}$	Fast fluidization	Particles are transported out of the bed and need to be replaced and recycled; normally has a dense phase region at bottom coexisting with a dilute phase region on top; no bed surface
$U >> U_{tr}$	Pneumatic conveying	Usually a once-through operation; all particles fed are transported out in dilute phase with concentration varying along the column height; no bed surface

Where: U_{mf} is a minimum fluidization velocity, U_{mb} is a minimum bubbling velocity, U_{ms} is a minimum slugging velocity, U_{c} is a critical velocity - a transition velocity between bubbling and transition to turbulent fluidization regimes, U_{k} is a transition velocity to turbulent fluidization regime, U_{tr} is a transport velocity - a transition velocity from the turbulent regime to the fast fluidization regime.

The quality of the coated product depends on the quality of fluidization and is associated with the fluidization regime in which the coater operates. Dense phase fluidization that occurs in bubbling and slug flow regimes facilitates inter-particle collisions, which leads to agglomeration rather than encapsulation. In turn, dilute phase fluidization in turbulent and fast fluidization regimes facilitates encapsulation of fine powders. The regime in which a fluid-bed coater operates depends on its construction, fluidizing medium velocity and the type of fluidized powder. The fluid-bed system is a segregationist system where elutriation and entrainment easily occur. It must be well designed and engineered to avoid these processes and to achieve bed homogeneity in the case of materials with a large size distribution that have a tendency for separation at U_{mf}.

3.3 Classification of Powders

In 1973 Geldart [29] classified the behavior of solids fluidized by gases into four groups characterized by the density difference between the particles and the fluidizing medium ρ_p-ρ_f, and by the mean particle diameter d_p. Geldart's classification has since become the standard to determine the types of gas fluidization. The powder classification diagram for the fluidization by air at ambient conditions was presented by Geldart, as shown in Figure 3.3.

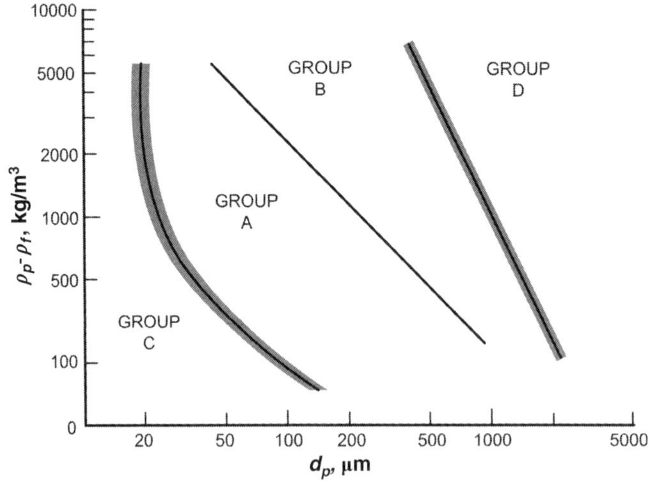

Figure 3.3 Geldart's clasification of powders. Adapted from [28].

Groups of Geldart's classification:

Group A: Bed particles exhibit dense phase expansion after minimum fluidization and before the beginning of bubbling. Gas bubbles appear at the minimum bubbling velocity. Powders of this group are often referred to as "aeratable."

Group B: Gas bubbles appear at the minimum fluidization velocity. Powders of this group are often referred to as "sand-like solids."

Group C: Bed particles are cohesive and difficult to fluidize.

Group D: Stable spouted beds can be easily formed in this group of powders.

The boundaries between groups are expressed numerically as [30]: Between A and B:

$$\left(\rho_s - \rho_f\right)d_p = 225 \tag{3.7}$$

Between B and D:

$$\left(\rho_s - \rho_f\right)d_p^2 = 106 \tag{3.8}$$

Where ρ_s and ρ_f in g/cm^3 are densities of particle and fluidizing medium respectively, d_p in µm is a mean particle diameter in micrometers. Unfortunately, there is no equation proposed for the boundary line between group A and C powders.

3.3.1 Goossen's Classification of Particles by Archimedes Number

Goossen (1998) [31] classified powders on the basis of the Archimedes number:

$$Ar = \frac{\rho_f d_p^3\left(\rho_s - \rho_f\right)g}{\mu^2} \tag{3.9}$$

The proposed classification is of general application, suitable for both liquid fluidization and gas fluidization. The four boundaries he suggested are as follows:

Group C boundary Ar = 0.97
Group A/C boundary Ar = 9.8
Group A/B boundary Ar = 88.5
Group B/D boundary Ar = 176,900

3.3.2 Extended Geldart's Classification for Nanopowders

Many nanopowders form large and compact agglomerates and are very difficult to fluidize because of the large cohesive forces between the particles. Wang *et al.* [32] proposed the classification of the fluidization of nanopowders into "agglomerate particulate fluidization" (APF) and "agglomerate bubbling fluidization" (ABF). APF refers to smooth, liquid-like, bubble-less fluidization. ABF refers to bubbling fluidization with very little bed expansion. Agglomerates with a diameter of 220 μm and an apparent density of 22 kg/m^3 are close to the A/C boundary in the Geldart diagram and sometimes show C-type behavior and at other times show more A-type behavior (homogeneous fluidization). On the other hand, Valverde and Castellanos [33] distinguished two different states of homogeneous fluidization: solid-like fluidization in which the agglomerates are jammed and keeping their place (mostly similar to homogeneous fluidization of Geldart A particles), and liquid-like fluidization in which agglomerates move freely, but no macroscopic bubbles are formed [24]. Using this approach, they defined solid-like to fluid-like to elutriation (SFE) behavior and solid-like to fluid-like to bubbling (SFB) behavior. These two types of behavior would replace the classical Geldart type C behavior with the new type of fluidizable fine and ultrafine powders. The modified Geldart's classification diagram is shown in Figure 3.4. The shaded line represents the boundary between *A* and *C* powders as shown in the original Geldart's diagram.

3.4 Fluidized Bed Coaters

There are many different variations of fluidized beds used in practice. However, for coating and encapsulation, mainly conical fluidized and spouted beds with or without a draft tube (internally

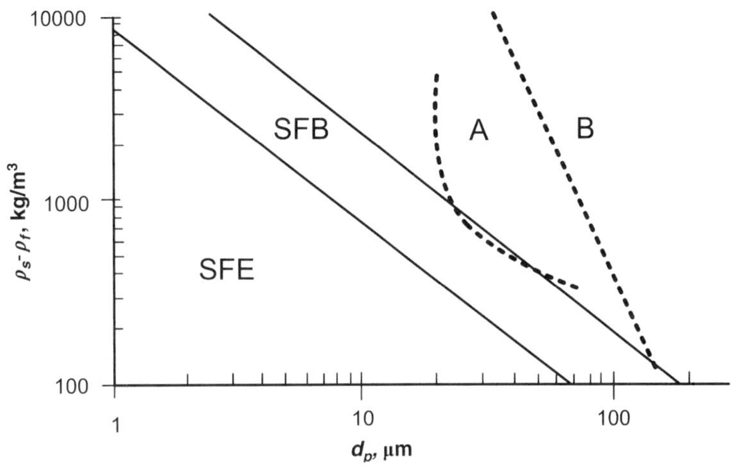

Figure 3.4 Modified Geldart's classification of powders diagram. Solid-to-fluid like to elutriation (SFE) behavior and solid-to-fluid like to bubbling (SFB) behavior. Adapted from [33].

circulating beds) and most of all spout-fluid beds—Wurster-type configurations—are used. In Figure 3.5, different types of fluid-bed coaters are compared.

3.4.1 Top-Spray Fluid Bed Coater

In the top-spray fluid bed coater, the expansion chamber is extended upward conically, which permits uniform deceleration of the air stream, allowing powder to remain fluidized for a longer time (Figure 3.5a). Particles are fluidized in a flow of heated air, which is introduced into the product container via a base plate, and the coating liquid is sprayed into the fluid bed from above against the air flow (countercurrent) by means of a nozzle. At a given fluidization air velocity, a specific range of particle size is determined between the size which is blown off and that which cannot be fluidized [30]. The spray nozzle is placed low in the expansion chamber to reduce distance between the nozzle and coated materials. This reduces the tendency of sprayed droplets to dry. This equipment is used for general coatings by the food, feed and chemical industries to improve the general handling, or for a short-term protection against moisture, oxygen or light [34]. The quality of obtained layers is moderate as neither the particle motion nor the travel distance of droplets from

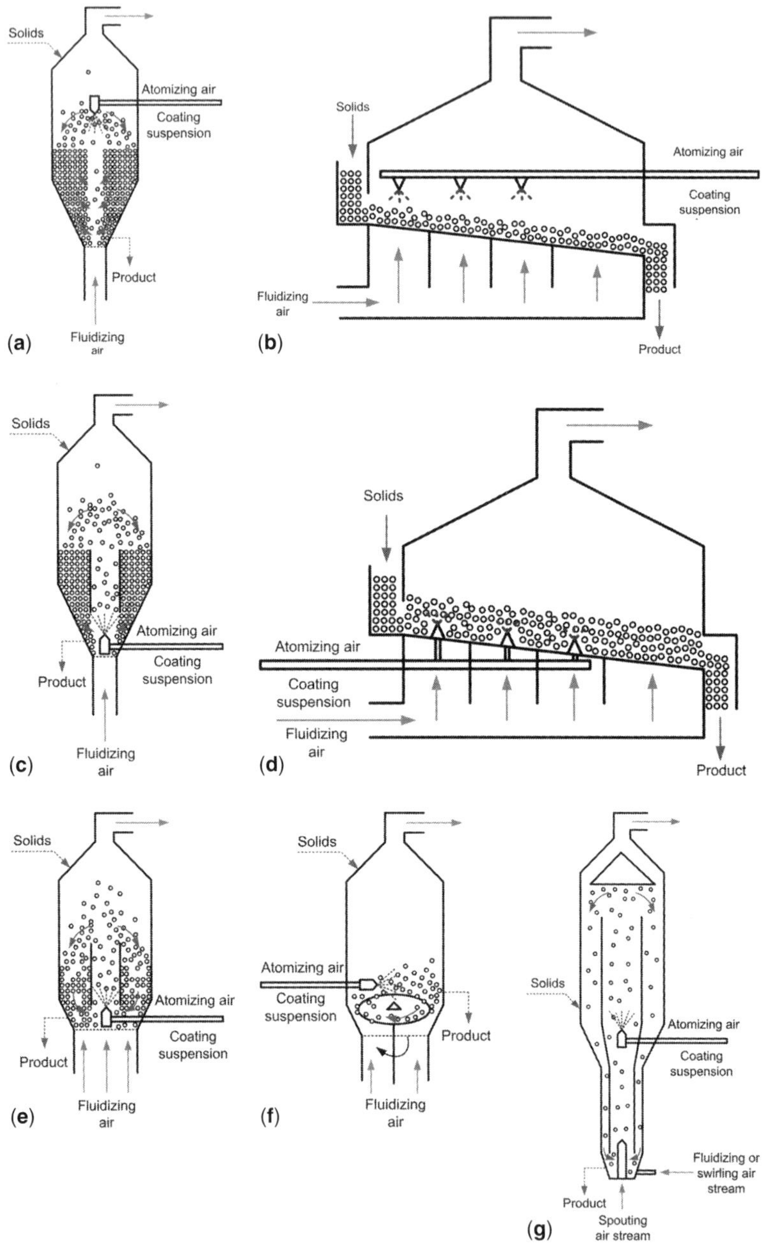

Figure 3.5 Different types of fluid-bed coaters. (A) batch top-spray fluid bed coater, (B) continuous top-spray fluid bed coater, (C) batch conical bottom-spray spouted bed coater, (D) continuous bottom-spray spouted bed coater, (E) batch spout-fluid bed coater (Wurster type), (F) batch rotor (tangential) spray coater, (G) batch fast circulating spout-fluid bed coater.

nozzle to substrate is uniform. However, a perfect film is generally not required for this function. Top-spray coaters can operate in a batch and a continuous mode. Coating in the continuous mode is particularly suitable for protective or color coatings where the product throughput rates are high. In continuous coating the product is fed into one side of the machine and is transported by means of the air flow onwards via the sieve bottom (Figure 3.5b). Depending on the application, the system is subdivided into preheating zones, spray zones, and drying zones. The coated particles are continuously unloaded from the apparatus. As the quality of obtained capsules is not high, the system is typically used for agglomeration and granulation rather than for encapsulation. The capacities of a batch coater are in a range from 2 g up to 1500 kg/batch.

3.4.2 Conical Bottom-Spray Spouted Bed Coater

The equipment is similar to the top-spray coater with a spray nozzle placed at the bottom of the column equipped with a draft tube that facilitates dense bed circulation (Figure 3.5c). The nozzle is placed axially upfacing. The additional air stream is also supplied to the column trough the porous base. Particles fall from the annular zone directly to the draft tube, where particles are entrained in the stream of air flow. Atomized solution (suspension or melt), particles and fluidizing air flow in the same direction, creating a fountain above the outlet of the draft tube. The apparatus has dense moving bed zones (annular) and dilute bed zones (draft tube and fountain), where fast fluidization or pneumatic transport occurs. The coating and layer drying take place in the dilute bed zones where the particle interactions are lower than in a dense or fluidized bed, which reduces particle agglomeration. This configuration has its disadvantages: the access to the pneumatic nozzle is difficult, with its clogging and particles sticking to the nozzle being highly likely.

The configuration is suitable for a large scale manufacture of cost-sensitive products, e.g., food or agrochemicals, that do not need high quality of the formed layer and takes advantage of the continuous mode of operation (Figure 3.5d). In coaters working in a continuous mode, the product is continuously fed into one side of the machine and is transported onwards via the sieve bottom by means of the air flow and then unloaded from the apparatus. The capacities of the batch coater are in a range of between 50 g and 700 kg/batch. The yield of the continuous spouted-bed coater reaches 2–3 metric tons/hour.

3.4.3 Spout-Fluid Bed Coater (Wurster Type)

This type of coater has a combination of the advantages of fluid-bed and spouted-bed coaters, where the liquid is sprayed from the bottom (Figure 3.5e). The bed is circulated as in the spouted-bed coater, but thanks to the wide perforated plate placed at the bottom of the column, the bed also fluidizes in the annular region. The fluidization airflow serves several functions: aerating the annular, enabling pneumatic transport of particles up through the draft tube, and providing drying capacity [2]. Typically, the distributor plate possesses larger holes in the central region and smaller holes in the outer region, favoring gas flow beneath the draft tube (Figure 3.6).

One can distinguish four regions in the apparatus [35, 2]:

a. Upbed region, where particles pass from the annular region through the gap below a draft tube and are pneumatically transported upwards inside it. In this section, particles receive coating from the spray nozzle located at the center of the gas distribution plate. Spray droplets reach the particles surface, then spread, coalesce, and dry to form a film.
b. Deceleration (fountain) region, where after leaving the draft tube particles decelerate and dry, and fall onto the surface of the bed in the annular region.
c. Downbed region, where particles form a dense fluidizing bed. They move slowly downwards to the inlet of the draft tube. If in this region the particles are not sufficiently dry, undesired agglomeration and sticking may occur.
d. Horizontal transport region, where particles move horizontally trough the partition gap below the draft tube. From this region particles enter the upbed region. The partition gap controls the flow of particles and solids circulation rate.

Compared with conventional spouted beds, the configuration of Wurster apparatus allows for the extension of the operation range in particle size from Geldart Group D to Groups A and B. In addition to a better coating performance, the advantages of the Wurster

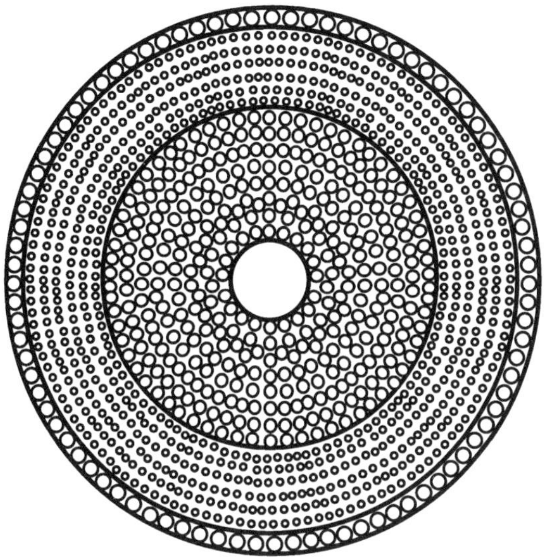

Figure 3.6 Gas distribution plate in the Wurster-type apparatus. Adapted from [19].

coating process include excellent heat and mass transfer within the bed, leading to short batch processing times and the ability to handle particles of a mean diameter of 100 μm [2]. The high rate of particle circulation increases the drying rate and leads to a great homogeneity in the coating quality, with a smooth continuous surface layer development. The drawbacks of this configuration are the nozzle clogging, dead zones in annular region and a further limitation for coating fine particles (< 100 μm) that have a tendency to agglomerate rather than coat, and also to adhere to apparatus walls.

As the Wurster coater provides capsules of high quality, it is used extensively in the pharmaceutical industry for film coating of tablets, pellets, and for encapsulation; in the food industry for coating of food ingredients, and in the production of agrochemicals and fertilizers. The coater configuration enhances operation in a batch mode with a moderate yield and relatively high operating costs, which favors its application in a fine chemicals sector where high operating costs are not the key issue.

3.4.4 Rotor (Tangential) Spray Coater

This processing unit is quite similar to the bottom-spray coater (Figure 3.5f). The main difference is that the particle motion is additionally facilitated by a motor driven rotor disc. The product is set into spiral motion by means of a rotating base plate that has air fed into the powder bed at its edge. The coating material is sprayed concurrently. The rolling motion of the particles provides high separation force that prevents agglomeration. This coater configuration is intended for coating high density grains or pellets with a very thick film layer. The high kinetic energy of accelerated particles makes it somewhat difficult to coat very small particles and is generally destructive for larger and non-spherical products, and so limits its application to coating materials that are not too crumbly. The capacities of batch coater are in a range from 500 g up to 250 kg/batch.

3.4.5 Fast Circulating Spout-Fluid Bed Coater

The new construction of the fast circulating spout-fluid bed apparatus (FCSFB), which is a modification of the Wurster coater intended for coating and encapsulation of fine particles, was developed by Szafran *et al.* [15, 36] (Figure 3.5g). It enables the application of multilayer coatings on fine particles by making use of the unique hydrodynamic parameters of the apparatus, formation of the so-called diluted fast-circulating bed, and feed of a negatively charged micropowder. The unique construction of the column ensures steady circulation of the bed, uniform distribution of mass and temperature in the work zones of the apparatus, and thus, constant in-time conditions for the conducting of the process. The spatial separation of the draft tube entrainment zone from the coating zone leads to the reduction of the effects of the particle-to-apparatus wall adhesion and pneumatic nozzle clogging. The high velocity of the particles in the coating zone allows for obtaining homogeneous coatings, and prevents material from granulation and from adhering to the walls of the apparatus and pneumatic nozzles.

The construction of the equipment allows for coating of fine particles of Geldart Groups A, B and C, with micro- and nanopowders. It is a Wurster-type apparatus composed of seven cylindrical sections and one conical section (Figure 3.7). The first section, the so-called gas distribution section, is fitted with an ejector that ensures a uniform bed feeding from the annular zone to the draft tube. Section S1 is provided with a cone-shaped bottom with the openings directing fluidizing air in a way that enables the formation of the axial swirling stream that supports the bed transfer to the ejector [37, 38]. The third conical section—where the coating of particle cores takes place—has a powder nozzle and a plasticizer atomizer. The

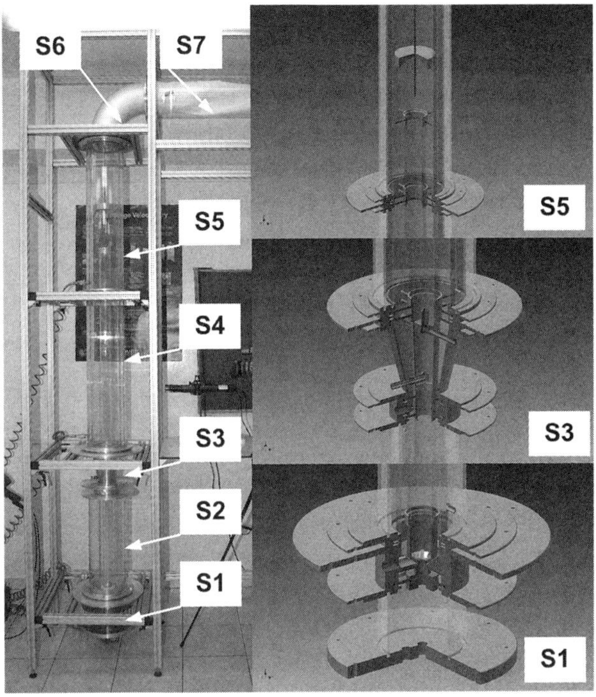

Figure 3.7 Column of (FCSFB) apparatus, S1- S8 – sections of column. Adapted from [15].

fifth section was equipped with a deflector enhancing the process of bed circulation in the apparatus. In the seventh section, there is a bag filter for separation of contaminants from the stream of exhaust gases. External walls of the cylindrical sections are made of glass with modified surface properties in order to limit electrostatic interactions with substrates. Additionally, they have an external jacket made of polycarbonate, thermostated with air. Inside the apparatus column, a draft tube was placed axially. The tube assures a smooth circulation of the diluted bed in the whole volume of the apparatus.

The apparatus may find application in pharmaceuticals, in particular at the final stage of manufacturing medicines containing substances sensitive to water and/or high temperature. The coater can be used for the preparation of drugs that are characterized by delayed or prolonged release, microcapsules, and drugs in the form of microparticles surrounded by the coating having controlled properties. The configuration of apparatus can also find application in CVD, MLD, ALD processes, where high mixing and homogeneity of fluidized bed is desired.

3.5 Fluid-Bed Coating and Encapsulation Processes

The term fluid-bed coating can refer to one of two different types of processes [39]. Objects to be coated can either be bed material or solid objects which are immersed into a bed of coating material. The most common application of the second type of the coating process is the treatment of metal objects that are immersed in fluidizing fine powder. When the temperature of the metal is above the melting point of a polymer powder, then a smooth, coherent film layer develops on the metal surface. This method is used for the painting of objects.

The basic principle of fluidized bed particle coating and encapsulation operations is to spray a liquid (solution, suspension, melt) or dry powder into a bed of fluidized particles. The spray consists of a substance which acts as a coating medium and usually a solvent in which the solute is dissolved or suspended; or it consists only of a plasticizer (in dry coating process). During the film coating, the atomized droplets impinge on the fluidized particles and spread on its surface. As the solvent evaporates, the solute remains on the surface of the particle. Several cycles of the layer-by-layer deposition of coating material and drying (or curing) result in the formation of a smooth and coherent layer (coat).

Depending on process duration and its parameters, the resultant coat morphology may vary significantly. It can yield [1]:

a. a monolayer coat of varying thickness with an onion like structure (Figure 3.8a);
b. a multilayer coat with varying coatings (Figure 3.8b);
c. a raspberry structure coat (Figure 3.8c);
d. a grape structure (granule) (Figure 3.8d).

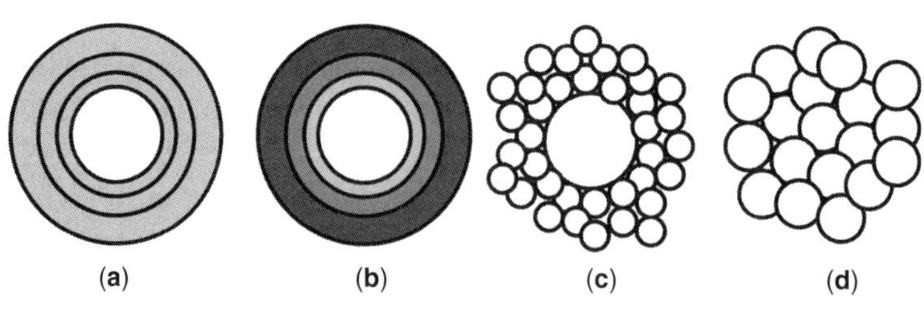

Figure 3.8 Morphology of coats; a) a monolayer coat of varying thickness with an onion-like structure, b) a multilayer coat with varying coatings, c) a raspberry structure coat, d) a grape structure (granule).

All previously mentioned types of fluidized and spouted-bed coaters can be used to perform film or dry coating on the surface of particles in a wide range of diameters. One can distinguish the following types of fluid-bed coating:

a. *Film coating*. The coating agent is dissolved or suspended in a solvent – usually water, organic solvent or supercritical CO_2. The coating medium is sprayed into the bed and forms a film on the particles surface. The solvent evaporates and is removed with a fluidizing air stream.
b. *Hot melt coating*. The coating agent is applied in its molten state. The coating medium is sprayed onto the bed and solidifies on the surface of the particles. The process is similar to that of the film coating, except that there is no solvent added to the coating medium. The cooling and solidification of the coating material on the particle surface occurs instead of a drying stage.
c. *Photocurable coatings*. The coating medium consists of functionalized liquid monomer/prepolymer and photoinitiator or photosensitizer. The coating medium is sprayed into the bed and polymerized under UV light irradiation. This is a kind of solventless technique used mainly in the pharmaceutical industry.
d. *Dry powder and electrostatic coating*. The film-coating polymer powder and liquid plasticizer are sprayed separately and directly into the bed in a coater chamber. The powder forms successive layers of coating. A curing stage completes film formation.
e. *Fluidized bed chemical vapor deposition (CVD), atomic layer deposition (ALD) and molecular layer deposition (MLD)*. The coating medium (precursor) is introduced to the apparatus in its gaseous form with an inert gas. As the precursor decomposes in an elevated temperature in the reaction chamber, the coating substance deposits on the particle surface and forms a coat.

3.5.1 Fluidized Bed CVD, ALD, MLD

Chemical vapor deposition is an important technique for surface modification of powders through grafting or deposition of films and coatings. In a typical CVD process, the substrate is exposed to

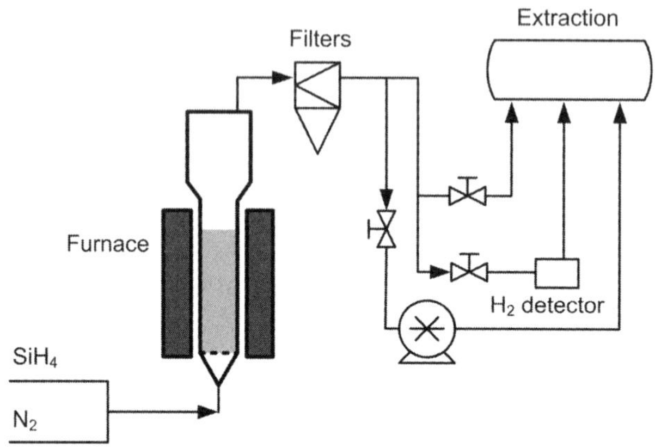

Figure 3.9 Typical setup of FBCVD used for deposition of silicon from SiH_4. Adapted from [67].

one or more gaseous precursors that react on a surface to produce the desired film. When a CVD process is combined with fluidization, it allows for deposition of thin layers on porous micro- and nanopowders. The comprehensive review on principles and applications of CVD powder technology can be found in the work of Vahlas *et al.* [25]. Beyond pioneering applications in the nuclear power industry, application domains, such as heterogeneous catalysis, microelectronics, photovoltaics and protection against wear, oxidation and heat are are of interest to the CVD processes [25].

A typical configuration of the FBCVD reactor is schematically presented in Figure 3.9. The principle of this method is that a bed of solid particles placed over a gas distribution plate (grid) is fluidized or spouted by a gas that passes through it, at a flow rate above the minimum fluidizing or spouting velocity. The precursor is added to the carrying gas during fluidization and then fed to the reactor (furnace). In contrast to CVD on flat surfaces, which often operates in the limited regime of surface kinetics, FBCVD is generally transport limited. This is due to the extremely high available ratios of the growth surface to the heated volume. Consequently, gaseous precursors are very often totally consumed a few centimeters after their entrance into the fluidized bed reactor, but the high degree of gas solid mixing that occurs in the FB or SB reactors compensates for this drawback, and ensures isothermal conditions and a uniform deposition.

Another technique closely related to CVD is the atomic layer deposition and molecular layer deposition. The CVD method has been developed for fabricating polymeric thin films. However, this method cannot control the order and location of molecular compounds on substrate surfaces that may inhibit the desired functionality of the coatings [27]. The ALD method has been employed to grow films with precise atomic layer control, and many inorganic materials have been grown via ALD, including binary compounds. The MLD method, which is similar to ALD and is also based on sequential, self-limiting surface reactions, can be utilized to deposit polymer films. In this process, molecules are stacked on substrates one by one in order of preference [27]. The MLD technique offers the same advantages for polymer film deposition as ALD does for ceramic films. In addition, MLD can deposit hybrid polymer films using suitable precursors, such as trimethylaluminum (TMA) and ethylene glycol (EG) for aluminum alkoxide (alucone) hybrid polymer [27].

In general, such new trends in micro- and nanopowders processing cover deposition of nanometric films on powders consisting of particles of meso- or microporosity and submicron size. Examples of FBCVD processes involving different types of powders can be found in literature [25]. Group A powders cover the preparation of supported catalysts on porous particles [40]. One of the best studied FBCVD processes in group B particles is the ultrapure silicon synthesis on 100 mm silicon particles, as a new way to produce electronic grade silicon for the microelectronic industry. A typical FBCVD process on group D particles covers the coating of radioactive particles by pyrolytic carbon and silicon carbide in order to obtain spherical fuel elements with a high qualification yield, i.e., uniform, defect-free coating on each particle [25]. The continuous growth of interest on nanoscience has led to an increasing demand for processes involving CVD on group C powders [41]. Those powders can be treated in dilute phase contactors, such as fast circulating fluidized beds.

The main limitations of the CVD process arise from [25]: a) the imposed CVD operating conditions and especially pressure and temperature, b) side deposition on the reactor walls and on or in the gas distributor, c) clogging of the bed due to high deposition rates and/or to low-quality fluidization, d) homogeneous nucleation, and e) handling of the CVD precursors.

Most of the technologies mentioned above use thermal activation of chemical deposition reactions. Alternatively, for coating when deposition on temperature-sensitive substrates is required, plasma-enhanced (PE) decomposition of the precursors is often used. Such cold plasma processes mainly find applications in biotechnology.

3.5.2 Dry Coating of Fine Particles

The basic principle of electrostatic coating, applied for years in powder painting technologies, makes use of electrostatic charge generation (positive or negative) onto the surface of the microparticles of coating powder. The process principles were discussed in detail by Bose and Bogner [42]. Coated cores should be electrically neutral (grounded). Powders for electrostatic coating may consist of a mixture of various substances. The resistivity of the powder should be higher than $10^{11}\Omega m$ in order to ensure charge stability on the surface of powder molecules until the layer formation on the coated core's surface is finished [42]. The obtained thickness of the dry-coating layer, at a level of 50μm, is usually larger than in the case of the layers formed by the solvent coating method (25μm). Its thickness may be controlled by the electric conductivity of powders. Powders with low resistivity ($10^{8}\Omega m$) lose the charge on the core surface, and—as a result—form thinner layers [42]. Powders with higher resistivity ($10^{12}\Omega m$) may cause the phenomenon of backward ionization and—as a result—prevent the deposition of subsequent layers on the surface, thus limiting the thickness of the layer. This phenomenon may also affect the creation of defects of the coating layer structure. Meanwhile, the electric resistivity of cores ought to be less than $10^{9}\Omega m$ in order to make it easier for the release of electric charges from their surface.

The elimination of the solvent and use of the so-called dry powder coating leads to the elimination of the basic factor that causes particle adhesion. In this process, apart from dry powder, a small amount of liquid plasticizer is added to the chamber of the apparatus. Obara *et al.* [43] used the process of dry powder coating for enteric tablets production in a fluidized bed and drum granulator. The authors obtained homogeneous, high-quality continuous coatings, and the solubility tests confirmed high usefulness of this method for the production of tablets that have prolonged or delayed release of the active component. Pearnchob and Bodmeier used a modified Wurster-type fluidized apparatus in the process of dry coating of pellets with diameters a little bit less than 1 mm [44] and tablets [45]. Plasticizer—a mixture of triethyl citrate (or acetylated monoglicerides, acetyl tributyl citrate) with 10% aqueous solution of hydroxypropylmethylcellulose (HPMC)—was added to the apparatus together with powder (dosed as a separate stream). The researchers obtained a high-quality product and gained a

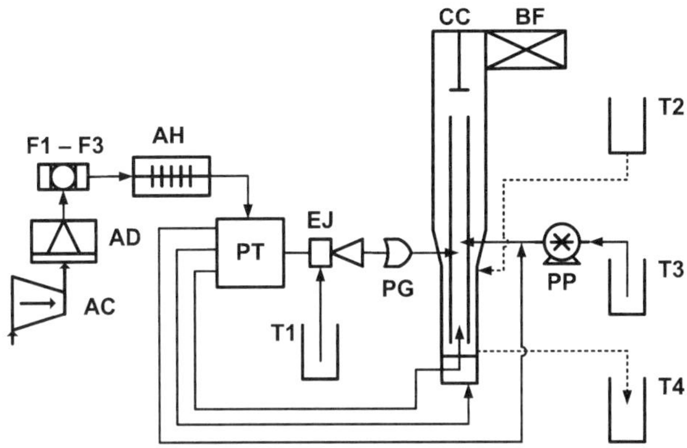

Figure 3.10 Process flow diagram of dry coating system, AC – air compressor; AD – air refrigerant dryer; F1 – F3 air filters (coarse, accurate, carbon); AH – air heater; PT – pneumatic table; EJ – ejector; PG – powder gun; CC – coating column; BF – bag filter; PP – plasticizer pump; T1 – powder container; T2 – particle container; T3 – plasticizer container; T4 – product storage tank. Adapted from [15].

significant coating time reduction as compared to the conventional solvent method.

The scheme of the installation for dry coating and encapsulation is presented in Figure 3.10. It is also described in detail in the patent applications [46, 47].

The installation is composed of the apparatus column CC, which, by means of pressure hoses, is connected to the distribution system of pneumatics PT, to which screw compressor AC is linked through air refrigerant dryer AD, coarse air filter F1, fine air filter F2 and carbon air filter F3. The distribution system of the pneumatics PT transfers the compressed air to: a) the spouting air connector at the bottom of the column, b) the fluidizing air connector – side connector at the bottom of the column, c) the atomizer, d) the powder nozzle, e) space of the thermostated jacket. The cores are periodically fed by means of the pneumatic transport from tank T2 to the interior part of the column in the upper part of section 2. Raw material is fluidized by dry air. Simultaneously, the bed is spouted, with the circulation facilitated by the deflector installed over the draft tube. In the ejector placed at the bottom of the column, the air sucks and lifts fluidized particles from the annular zone to the conical section of the column, where the powder nozzle is placed, by means of which dry and electrically charged powder is distributed to the column. Liquid plasticizer atomized by dry compressed air is fed to the formulated three-phase mixture with an atomizer in the conical section. The batch process is usually conducted for only 10 minutes.

The construction of the apparatus is especially intended for better operations with micropowders of Group C.

3.6 The Design, Optimization and Scale-Up of the Coating Process and the Apparatus

There are three phases present in the fluid bed: solid (coated particles), liquid (liquid coating material or plasticizer) or dry powder and gas (the fluidizing air). During the coating process many operations at the micro- and macro-level occur simultaneously resulting in the momentum, heat and mass transfer. This operations are as follows: bed fluidization or spouting, elutriation, liquid or powder spraying, drying, surface wetting and droplet coalescence, adhesion of particles. The resultant product quality depends on many factors and process parameters: physical and chemical properties of the material, the geometry of the apparatus, temperature, humidity and the flow rates of process streams, and the duration of the process. The complexity of the coating process makes it necessary to conduct a series of experimental trials as the theory of its modeling and scale-up is not sufficiently developed yet. The first requirement for a proper coating process is the ability of the coating liquid to wet a particles surface and to spread a droplet on the surface after droplet-particle collision. The wetting energy can be expressed as a wetting coefficient W_m:

$$W_m = \gamma_{SV} - \gamma_{SL} - \gamma_{LV} \tag{3.10}$$

The γ_{SV} is the interfacial tension between solid and vapor, γ_{SL} is the interfacial tension between solid and liquid, and γ_{LV} is the interfacial tension between liquid and vapor. A liquid can wet the particles surface when the wetting modulus is larger than zero $W_m > 0$.

It should be emphasized that the process is highly dependent upon micro-level processes: drying, droplet impact and adherence, droplet spreading and particle agglomeration. In addition to interfacial properties, the spreading of the liquid on the solid surface is also facilitated by low liquid viscosity and by droplets of a small diameter. The mean diameter of droplets d_d can be calculated from equation [48]:

$$d_d = \frac{585 \times 10^3 \sqrt[3]{\sigma}}{U_V \sqrt{\rho_l}} + 597 \left(\frac{\mu_l}{\sqrt{\sigma \rho_l}} \right)^{0.45} \left(\frac{1000\, Q_l}{Q_a} \right)^{1.5} \tag{3.11}$$

To calculate drying time t_{total} of droplets that is necessary to estimate spraying conditions one can use the equation:

$$t_{total} = \frac{\lambda\, \rho_l \left(d_0^2 - d_c^2\right)}{8K_d \left(T_a - T_s\right)} + \frac{\lambda\, d_c^2 \rho_p \left(X_c - X_f\right)}{12K_d \Delta T_{av}} \tag{3.12}$$

The calculated droplet evaporation time should be longer than the time needed to impact the particles surface by a droplet. Once droplets of the coating substance are spread on particles, they must dry quickly or else they will reach the annular zone of the apparatus, where they can undergo agglomeration.

The coating efficiency can be expressed in different ways, as material efficiency E_c, energy efficiency E_e, quality efficiency E_q or productivity efficiency E_p (kg product/hour). The most commonly used by authors, material efficiency (efficiency of adhesion), is defined as the ratio of the deposited mass of the coating to the total mass of the coating agent sprayed in the bed:

$$E_c = \frac{W_C}{W_{CS}\, C} \tag{3.13}$$

For empirical correlations for E_c see the relevant literature. Kucharski and Kmiec [49] analyzed the coating of tablets with sucrose solution and obtained:

$$\frac{E_c}{E_{c,in}} = 0.3253\, \mathrm{Re}_p^{1.089} \left(\frac{H_0}{d_p} \right)^{-0.0646} \left(\frac{W_{sp}}{W_{air}} \right)^{0.0393} (1 - C)^{1.0074}\, \phi^{-5.53} \tag{3.14}$$

Where $E_{c,in}$ is the efficiency of inertial fixation of the atomized droplets, given by:

$$E_{c,in} = \frac{Stk^2}{(Stk + 0.25)^{1.012}} \tag{3.15}$$

Here the Stokes number is defined as:

$$Stk = \frac{d_{saut}^2 \rho_{sp} u_H}{36\mu\, d_p} \tag{3.16}$$

Oliveira *et al.* [50] developed a correlation for the efficiency of coating alumina with aqueous solutions of sucrose and talc in a spouted bed:

$$\begin{aligned} E_c = 6.05\frac{Q_{air}}{Q_{ms}} - 1.944\left(\frac{Q_{air}}{Q_{ms}}\right)^2 + 174.156\left(\frac{W_{sp}}{W_{air}}\right) \\ -17977\left(\frac{W_{sp}}{W_{air}}\right)^2 - 4.204 \end{aligned} \tag{3.17}$$

The Eq. (3.17) is valid in the range $1.5 < Q_{air}/Q_{ms} < 1.7$; $0.00263 < W_{sp}/W_{air} < 0.00471$.

The most important hydrodynamic parameters of spouted-bed coaters that have to be estimated are the minimum spouting gas velocity U_{ms} and the maximum height of spoutable bed H_m. The former parameter can be calculated from the empirical equation proposed by Mathur and Gishler [2, 51]:

$$U_{ms} = \left(\frac{d_p}{D}\right)\left(\frac{D_i}{D}\right)^{1/3}\sqrt{\frac{2gH_0\left(\rho_p - \rho_f\right)}{\rho_f}} \tag{3.18}$$

The maximum height of spoutable bed H_m can be calculated from equation [2, 52]:

$$H_m = \frac{D^2}{d_p}\left(\frac{D}{D_i}\right)^{2/3}\frac{568\, b^2}{Ar}\left(\sqrt{1 + 35.9\times10^{-6}\, Ar} - 1\right)^2 \tag{3.19}$$

Where $b = 1.11$ is an adjustable parameter.

A successful design and optimization of the coating process and the apparatus calls for much attention from the engineer. In the first step a precise description of the objective of the coating operation is essential. This step leads to choosing a coating material and a method and a final form of the product—coat morphology. In the second step it is important to define methods of usage of capsules because this determines the size, shape and strength of the capsules.

Next, the formulation of the coating solution (coating material, solvent, plasticizer, additives, etc.), and some laboratory tests on particles wettability and adhesion should be performed. After we have obtained an "*in-vitro*" product with satisfactory properties, we can choose the proper equipment, operating mode (continuous, batch) and optimize its geometry and operating parameters regarding the required process yield and product quality. We have to determine the minimum and maximum spouting velocities, droplets diameters and their drying time that is necessary to determine the size and length of the apparatus zones. Finally, we can calculate process efficiency, costs and estimate profits.

3.7 Numerical Modeling of Fluid-Bed Coating

There are many publications on the Computational Fluid Dynamics (CFD) modeling of fluidized bed equipment and Discrete Element Method (DEM) for discrete phase flow simulation. However, CFD approaches to modeling of all aspects of coating process are noticeably missing from the literature probably because of the high complexity of the process. The approach needed for such simulations is to model the coating agent atomization simultaneously with the equations describing the movement of fluidizing gas and bed solids, interactions between coated (wet) particles and heat and mass transfer during solvent evaporation (drying). The interaction of the solids with the droplets from the nozzle could then be used to calculate the mass deposition of coating material.

The hydrodynamics of fluidizing gas and particle flow are usually described by the Eulerian-Eulerian two-fluid model [53]. In the Eulerian-Eulerian approach, both phases are treated as interpenetrating continua that is only a rough approximation to the granular phase. For each phase the continuity and momentum conservation equation (Navier-Stokes equation) is solved, and coupling is achieved through the applied pressure and interphase exchange terms. The model requires additional closure laws to describe the rheology of the granular phase and turbulence equations that describe effects of turbulent fluctuations of velocities on scalar quantities. Duarte *et al.* [54] used an Eulerian multiphase model to simulate the flow of particles in two-dimensional and cylindrical spouted beds. Magnusson *et al.* [55] developed a 3D Eulerian CFD model to simulate the movement of solids in a Wurster-type fluidized bed. Szafran and Kmiec [56] used the Eulerian-Eulerian approach to simulate the bed flow in a conical spouted-bed apparatus with a draft tube.

The flow hydrodynamics of the dispersed phase (particles or droplets) can be solved in the Lagrangian frame of reference (DEM) by tracking a large number of objects through the calculated flow field. Lagrangian models are solved by the Newtonian equations of motion for each individual object, taking into account effects of its collisions, breakage and coalescence (droplets). The discrete phase can exchange momentum with the fluid phase. The Lagrangian approach gives a direct physical interpretation of particle-particle and wall-particle interactions. However, this method is limited because it does not account for hydrodynamic forces (drag, lift, torque). Hence the simulation of the multiphase flow in coaters requires a coupling of the DEM method with that of CFD. In such models, a computational demand rises strongly with a number of traced objects. In addition to the two approaches for dispersed phase flow problems mentioned above, the population balance model was introduced to the CFD models as an alternative approach because of its reduced level of computational complexity. In the work of Link *et al.* [57] a discrete element model is presented for description of the gas–liquid–solid flow in a spout-fluidized bed including all relevant hydrodynamic phenomena, for the study of granulation. Buijtenen *et al.* [58] studied the effect of collisions of wet particles during granulation in a spout-fluid bed. The simulations are conducted with the CFD model that describes the dynamics of the continuous gas-phase coupled with the discrete particles and droplets (DEM models). Similarly, Fries *et al.* [59] proposed the DEM-CFD model to study the fluid and particle dynamics in a fluidized bed spray granulator. The atomization process was investigated and then improved using a combination between a population balance model and the CFD Eulerian multi-fluid model by Aly *et al.* [60–62]. Duangkhamchan *et al.* [63] developed a Eulerian–Lagrangian computational fluid dynamics model that was built to describe a two-fluid atomization in a tapered fluidized bed coater, using the air-blast/air-assisted atomizer model. In addition, a multi-fluid flow model (Eulerian–Eulerian framework) combined with a population balance model was used as an alternative approach for modeling the spray produced by a two-fluid nozzle.

Coupling of heat and mass transfer relationships with CFD models is necessary for correct modeling of solvent evaporation in a film coating process. Szafran and Kmiec [64] for the first time coupled a model of drying kinetics of particles in a spouted-bed apparatus with an Eulerian-Eulerian two-fluid approach. For a description of the heat and mass transfer occurring during the drying of grain, a partial differential equation of energy conservation was solved in conjunction with classical and diffusional drying kinetic models for periods I and II of drying, respectively. This model allows for the prediction of the rate of solvent (moisture) evaporation in various zones of the apparatus, depending on process conditions. The most complex model of the coating process in the Wurster bed coater describing particle and gas movement, particle wetting and drying was presented by Karlsson *et al.* [65]. The particles are modeled as a Eulerian phase and their rheology is described with the kinetic theory of granular flow. The continuous injection of liquid through a spray nozzle was modeled by specifying the moisture content for the particle phase when passing a region close to the liquid inlet.

The coating quality and the deposition of droplets on the tablets, the production and evolution of the liquid film on the surface of tablets are numerically analyzed by Suzzi *et al.* [66], where detailed computational fluid dynamics multiphase spray simulations were used. Spray droplets are simulated with the Discrete Droplets Method (DDM) Euler–Lagrange approach, whereas multi-component evaporation and particle/wall interaction phenomena are also included in the model. The wall film is treated with a two-dimensional model incorporating submodels for interfacial shear force, film evaporation and heat transfer between the film, solid wall and gas phase. The model allows for performing a detailed variation study and analyzing the impact of the system properties on the quality attributes of the resulting coat, but only for a single tablet.

Many works were concentrated on selected aspects of the coating process in fluid-bed coaters, such as hydrodynamics of phases flow, atomization, droplets deposition and drying, but there is still lack of a full-range numerical model of the coating process. The solution of the set of partial differential equations is usually obtained through commercially available control-volume-based solvers, e.g., Ansys Fluent or MFIX on the meshed 2D or 3D space of the apparatus. The accuracy of the results of computer simulations depends on several factors such as: a) the accuracy of the mathematical model, b) the accuracy and dimension of the modeled geometry (2D, 3D), c) the quality of the mesh, d) the quality of the solver, e) the convergence of numerical solution. As the final result of simulations depends on numerous independent factors, their usefulness is still limited and depends not only on the development of better mathematical models for the coating process, but also better computational fluid dynamics tools.

Nomenclature

C	coating solution dry mater content (solids concentration)	kg/kg
C_D	drag coefficient,	-
D	diameter of column	m
d_0	capillary diameter	m
d_c	droplet diameter at critical point	m
$\mathrm{d_d}$	mean droplets diameter	m
D_i	diameter of fluid inlet (inlet of column)	m
d_p	diameter of particle,	m
d_{saut}	Sauter diameter of the atomized droplets	m
E_c	material efficiency, eq. (3.13)	-
$E_{c,in}$	efficiency of inertial fixation of the atomized droplets, eq. (3.15)	-
g	gravitational acceleration = 9.81,	m/s^2
H_0	static bed depth	m
H_m	maximum height of spoutable bed	m
K_d	thermal conductivity	W/(m*K)
Q_a	air volumetric flow rate	m^3/s
Q_l	liquid volumetric flow rate	m^3/s
T_a	air temperature	°C
T_{av}	average temperature	°C
T_s	droplet surface temperature	°C
t_{total}	drying time of droplets	s
u_H	gas velocity at the central (spout) zone (can be taken as the orifice velocity),	m/s
U_{mf}	minimum fluidization velocity,	m/s
U_{ms}	minimum spouting gas velocity	m/s
U_p	particle velocity	m/s
U_{ter}	terminal velocity for single particle motion,	m/s
U_{tr}	transport velocity	m/s
$\mathrm{U_V}$	nozzle outlet air velocity	m/s
W_{air}	spouting gas mass flow rate	kg/s
W_c	deposited mass of the coating	kg

W_{cs}	mass of the sprayed coating solution	kg
W_m	wetting coefficient	J
W_{sp}	mass flow rate of atomized suspension	kg/s
X_c	critical moisture content	%
X_f	final moisture content of the dried particle	%

Greek letters

γ_{LV}	interfacial tension between liquid and vapor	J
γ_{SL}	interfacial tension between solid and liquid	J
γ_{SV}	interfacial tension between solid and vapor	J
λ	latent heat of vaporization	J/kg
μ	dynamic viscosity of fluidizing medium,	kg/(m*s)
μ_l	liquid viscosity	kg/(m*s)
ρ_f	density of fluidizing medium,	kg/m^3
ρ_l	liquid density	kg/m^3
ρ_p	density of particle,	kg/m^3
ρ_{sp}	density of suspension	kg/m^3
σ	liquid surface tension	N/m
φ	sphericity	-

Dimensionless numbers

Ar	Archimedes number, eq. (3.9)
Re_p	Particle Reynolds number, eq. (3.5)
Stk	Stokes number, eq. (3.16)

References

1. E. Teunou, and D. Poncelet. Fluid-bed coating. In *Encapsulated and powdered foods*. C. Onwulata, ed. Taylor & Francis, 2005.
2. N. Epstein, J.R. Grace. *Spouted and Spout-Fluid Beds*. Cambridge University Press, 2011.
3. B. Guignon, A. Duquenoy, E.D. Dumoulin. Fluid bed encapsulation of particles: Principles and practice. *Drying Technology* 20 (2002) 419–447.
4. M. Capece, R. Dave. Application of fluidized bed film coating for membrane encapsulation of catalysts. *Powder Technology* 211 (2011) 199–206.
5. H. Otsuka, Y. Nagasaki, K. Kataoka. PEGylated nanoparticles for biological and pharmaceutical applications. *Advanced Drug Delivery Reviews* 55 (2003) 403–419.
6. A. Ramanavicius, A. Kausaite, A. Ramanaviciene. Polypyrrole-coated glucose oxidase nanoparticles for biosensor design. *Sensors and Actuators B* 111–112 (2005) 532–539.

7. R. Pissinati, W.P. Oliveira. Enteric coating of soft gelatin capsules by spouted bed: Effect of operating conditions on coating efficiency and on product quality. *European J. Pharmaceutics & Biopharmaceutics* 55 (2003) 313–321.
8. K.G.H. Desai, H.J. Park. Recent developments in microencapsulation of food ingredients. *Drying Technol.* 23 (2005) 1361–1394.
9. M.W. Donida, S.C.S. Rocha, B.D. Castro, A.M.M. Marques. Coating and drying in spouted bed: Influence of the liquid-particle work adhesion. *Drying Technol.* 25 (2007) 319–326.
10. K. Dewettinck, A. Huyghebaert. Fluidized bed coating in food technology. *Trends in Food Sci. & Technol.* 10 (1999) 163–168.
11. D.E. Wurster. Means for applying coatings to tablets or like. *J. Am. Pharm. Assoc.* 48 (1950) 451–460.
12. D.E. Wurster. Method of applying coatings to edible tablets or the like. US Patent 2648609 (1953).
13. D.E. Wurster. Means for applying coatings to tablets or the like. US Patent 2799241 (1957).
14. D.E. Wurster, J.A. Lindlof. Particle coating apparatus. US Patent 3241520 (1966).
15. R.G. Szafran, W. Ludwig, A. Kmiec. New spout-fluid bed apparatus for electrostatic coating of fine particles and encapsulation. *Powder Technology* 225 (2012) 52–57.
16. K. Jono, H. Ichikawa, M. Miyamoto, Y. Fukumori. A review of particulate design for pharmaceutical powders and their production by spouted bed coating. *Powder Technology* 113 (2000) 269–277.
17. X.X. Cheng, R. Turton. The prediction of variability occuring in fluidized bed coating equipment. I. The measurement of particle circulation rates in a bottom-spray fluidized bed coater. *Pharmac. Dev. & Technol.* 5 (2000) 311–322.
18. S. Shelukar, J. Ho, J. Zega, E. Roland, N. Yeh, D. Quiram, A. Nole, A. Katdare, S. Reynolds. Identification and characterization of factors controlling tablet coating uniformity in a Wurster coating process. *Powder Technology* 110 (2000), 29–36.
19. M.P. Bender, J.P. Szczap, D.P. Verbarg. Wurster fluid bed coater with fluidizing gas distribution plate bypass. US Patent 7563325 B2 (2009).
20. D.M. Jones. Fluidized bed with spray nozzle shielding. US Patent 5437889 (1995).
21. S.I. Miyatake, S. Kawabata, N. Nonoguchi, K. Yokoyama, T. Kuroiwa, H. Matsui, K. Ono. Pseudoprogression in boron neutron capture therapy for malignant gliomas and meningiomas. *Neuro-Oncology* 11 (2009) 430–436.
22. S.I. Miyatake, S. Kawabata, K. Yokoyama, T. Kuroiwa, H. Michiue, Y. Sakurai, H. Kumada, M. Suzuki, A. Maruhashi, M. Kirihata, K. Onoc. Survival benefit of boron neutron capture therapy for recurrent malignant gliomas. *Applied Radiation and Isotopes* 7–8 (2009) S22–S24.
23. S.K. Lai, Y.Y. Wang, J. Hanes. Mucus-penetrating nanoparticles for drug and gene delivery to mucosal tissues. *Adv. Drug Deliv. Rev.* 61 (2008) 158–171.
24. J.R. van Ommen, J.M. Valverde, R. Pfeffer. Fluidization of nanopowders: A review. *J. Nanopart. Res.* 14 (2012) 1–29.
25. C. Vahlas, B. Caussatb, P. Serpc, G. N. Angelopoulos. Principles and applications of CVD powder technology. *Materials Science and Engineering* 53 (2006) 1–72.

26. L. Sanchez, F.J. Bolívar, M. del Pilar Hierro, J.A. Trilleros, F.J. Pérez. CVD in a fluidized bed reactor: A method of developing coatings at temperatures below 600°C. *Chem. Vap. Deposition* 13 (2007) 465–473.
27. X. Liang, D.M. King, P. Li, S.M. George, A.W. Weimer. Nanocoating hybrid polymer films on large quantities of cohesive nanoparticles by molecular layer deposition. *AIChE J.* 55 (2009) 1030–1039.
28. W.-C. Yang. *Handbook of fluidization and fluid-particle systems.* Marcel Dekker Inc. 2003.
29. D. Geldart. Types of gas fluidization. *Powder Technol.* 7 (1973) 285–292.
30. R. Dixit, S. Puthli. Fluidization technologies: Aerodynamic principles and process engineering. *Journal of Pharmaceutical Sciences* 98 (2009) 3933–3960.
31. W.R.A. Goossens. Classification of fluidized particles by Archimedes number. *Powder Technol.* 98 (1998) 48–53.
32. Y. Wang, G. Gu, F. Wei, J. Wu. Fluidization and agglomerate structure of SiO2 nanoparticles. *Powder Technol.* 124 (2002) 152–159.
33. J.M. Valverde, A. Castellanos. Types of gas fluidization of cohesive granular materials. *Phys. Rev. E.* 75 (2007) 031306-1-6.
34. http://www.glatt.com/cm/
35. F.N. Christensen, P. Bertelsen. Qualitative description of the Wurster based fluid bed coating process. *Drug Develop. & Ind. Pharm.* 23 (1997) 451–463.
36. R.G. Szafran, W. Ludwig, A. Kmieć. Coating device of fine grained materials with micro and nano powders. PL Patent application number: P392710 (2010).
37. R.G. Szafran, A. Witek-Krowiak. Bottom of apparatus for solventless coating of fine particles by micro- and nanoparticles I. PL Patent application number: P394263 (2011).
38. R.G. Szafran, A. Witek-Krowiak. Bottom of apparatus for solvent free coating of fine particles by micro- and nanoparticles II. PL Patent application number: P394264 (2011).
39. R. Turton, G.I. Tardos, B.J. Ennis. *Fluidized bed coating and granulation in fluidization solids handling and processing.* Y. Wen-Ching, ed. Noyes Publications (1999).
40. P. Serp, P. Kalck, R. Feurer. Chemical vapor deposition methods for the controlled preparation of supported catalytic materials. *Chem. Rev.* 102 (2002) 3085–3128.
41. P. Moravec, J. Smolik, V.V. Levdansky. Preparation of Al_2O_3–SiO_2 fine particles by CVD method in tube flow reactor. *Powder Technol.* 153 (2005) 159–165.
42. S. Bose, R.H. Bogner. Solventless pharmaceutical coating processes: A review. *Pharmaceutical Development & Technology* 12 (2007) 115–131.
43. S. Obara, N. Maruyama, Y. Nishiyama, H. Kokubo. Dry coating: An innovative enteric coating method using a cellulose derivative. *Eur. J. Pharm. Biopharm.* 1 (1999) 51–59.
44. N. Pearnchob, R. Bodmeier. Coating of pellets with micronized ethylcellulose particles by a dry powder coating technique. *Int. J. Pharm.* 1–2 (2003) 1–11.
45. N. Pearnchob, R. Bodmeier. Dry polymer powder coating and comparison with conventional liquid-based coatings for Eudragit RS, ethyl cellulose and shellac. *Eur. J. Pharm. Biopharm.* 3 (2003) 363–369.
46. R.G. Szafran, W. Ludwig, A. Kmiec. Coating system of fine grained materials with micro and nano powders. PL Patent application number: P392712 (2010).

47. R.G. Szafran, W. Ludwig, A. Kmiec. The way of dry coating of fine grained materials with micro and nano powders. PL Patent application number: P392711 (2010).
48. K. Masters. Drying of droplets/sprays. In *Spray drying handbook.* New York: John Wiley & Sons, 1988, pp. 298–342.
49. J. Kucharski, A. Kmiec. Kinetics of granulation process during coating of tablets in a spouted bed. *Chem. Eng. Sci.* 44 (1989) 1627–1636.
50. W.P. Oliveira, J.T. Freire, J.R. Coury. Analysis of particle coating by spouted bed process. *Intern. J. Pharmaceutics* 158 (1997) 1–9.
51. K.B. Mathur, P.E. Gishler. A technique for contacting gases with coarse solid particles. *AIChE J.* 1 (1955) 157–164.
52. G.S. McNab, J. Bridgwater. Spouted beds: Estimation of spouting pressure drop and the particle size for deepest bed. In *Proceedings of the European Congress on particle technology*, Nuremberg Germany (1977) 17 pages.
53. R.G. Szafran, A. Kmiec, W. Ludwig. CFD modeling of a spouted-bed dryer hydrodynamics. *Drying Technology* 23 (2005) 1723–1736.
54. C.R. Duarte, V.V. Murata, M.A.S. Barrozo. Study of the spouted bed fluid dynamics using CFD. *Proc. 14th Int. Drying Symp.* Sao Paulo, 22–25 Aug, Vol. A, 2004, pp. 581–588.
55. A.M. Magnusson, B.G.M. Van Wachem, A.E. Almstedt. CFD model development and experimental validation of the three-dimensional hydrodynamics of a Wurster-type fluidized bed. Paper 275a, Presented at the Annual AIChE Meeting, Indianapolis, Nov 3–8, 2002.
56. R.G. Szafran, A. Kmiec. Periodic fluctuations of flow and porosity in spouted beds. *Transport in Porous Media* 66 (2007) 187–200.
57. J.M. Link, W. Godlieb, N.G. Deen, J.A.M. Kuipers. Discrete element study of granulation in a spout-fluidized bed. *Chem. Eng. Sci.* 62 (2007) 195–207.
58. M.S. van Buijtenen, N.G. Deen, S. Heinrich, S. Antonyuk, J.A.M. Kuipers. A discrete element study of wet particle–particle interaction during granulation in a spout fluidized bed. *The Canadian Journal of Chemical Engineering* 87 (2009) 308–317.
59. L. Fries, S. Antonyuk, S. Heinrich, S. Palzer. DEM–CFD modeling of a fluidized bed spray granulator. *Chem. Eng. Sci.* 66 (2011) 2340–2355.
60. H.S. Aly, T.M. Lazin, Y.A. Eldrainy, M.N.M. Jaafar. (2009) Mathematical modelling of droplet atomisation using the population balance equation. In *Proceedings of International Conference on Signal Processing Systems, ICSPS 2009.* Institute of Electrical and Electronics Engineers, New York. pp. 955–959.
61. H.S. Aly, Y.A. Eldrainy, T.M. Lazim, M.N.M. Jaafar. On the contribution of drag and turbulent stresses in the fragmentation of liquid droplets: A computational study. *CFD Lett.* 2 (2010) 97–105.
62. H.S. Aly, Y.A. Eldrainy, K.M. Saqr, T.M. Lazim, M.N.M. Jaafar. A mathematical model for predicting spray atomisation characteristics in an Eulerian–Eulerian framework. *Int. Comm. Heat Mass Transfer* 37 (2010) 618–623.
63. W. Duangkhamchan, F. Ronsse, F. Depypere, K. Dewettinck, J.G. Pieters. CFD study of droplet atomisation using a binary nozzle in fluidised bed coating. *Chem. Eng. Sci.* 68 (2012) 555–566.
64. R.G. Szafran, A. Kmiec. CFD modeling of heat and mass transfer in a spouted bed dryer. *Ind. Eng. Chem. Res.* 43 (2004) 1113–1124.

65. S. Karlsson, A. Rasmuson, B. van Wachem, I. Niklasson Bjorn. CFD modeling of the wurster bed coater. *AIChE Journal* 55 (2009) 2578–2590.
66. D. Suzzi, S. Radl, J.G. Khinast. Local analysis of the tablet coating process: Impact of operation conditions on film quality. *Chem. Eng. Sci.* 65 (2010) 5699–5715.
67. B. Caussat, M. Hemati, J.P. Couderc. Silicon deposition from silane or disilane in a fluidized bed – Part I: Experimental study. *Chem. Eng. Sci.* 50 (1995) 3615–3624.

4

Use of Electrospinning for Encapsulation

Rocío Pérez-Masiá, Maria José Fabra, Jose Maria Lagarón and Amparo López-Rubio

Novel Materials and Nanotechnology Group, IATA-CSIC, Valencia, Spain

Abstract
The electrospinning technique, consisting of the application of an electrical voltage to a polymeric solution to generate fiber or capsule-like morphologies, has a tremendous potential for the development of encapsulation structures of interest in a number of areas such as biomedicine, food technology, bioremediation, energy storage, etc. Some interesting characteristics of the technique are that no temperature is required, which makes it suitable for the encapsulation of heat-sensitive substances, and that the size of the encapsulation structures span from the nano- to the microlevel. Both the size and morphology of the electrospun structures can be adjusted by changing the process parameters. The versatility of the technique together with the number of advantages over other well-established encapsulation methods, and the availability of industrial-scale equipment, presage its expansion as the preferred encapsulation technique for a number of applications.

Keywords: Electrospinning, electrospraying, controlled release, electrospun fibers

4.1 Introduction

4.1.1 Generalities About the Electrospinning Technique

The electrospinning process consists of the use of high electrostatic potentials for the fabrication of ultrathin polymer fiber mats. This process was first described in 1902 [1], however there was not

Vikas Mittal (ed.) Encapsulation Nanotechnologies, (107–136) © 2013 Scrivener Publishing LLC

widespread interest in the use of this technology until the 1990s. In recent years, much attention has been paid to the use of electrospinning in the field of nanoscience and nanotechnology, and thus many investigations in the production of nanofiber morphologies have been carried out.

Specifically, the electrospinning process uses high-voltage electric fields to produce electrically charged "jets" from viscoelastic polymer solutions which, on drying by means of evaporation of the solvent, produce diverse ultrathin structures. Generally, the basic setup for electrospinning consists of three components: a high-voltage power supply, a spinneret (a metallic needle) and a collector surface (a single piece of conductive substrate) [2]. An example of the typical setup of a lab-scale electrospinning apparatus is depicted in Figure 4.1.

For a more thorough description about the electrospinning theory and process, the interested reader is directed to some of the multiple reviews in the area, such as the one published by Subbiah and coworkers [3].

The electrospun nanostructures morphology and diameter are affected by different processing conditions. The most relevant factors can be divided in two categories: (i) those dependent on the intrinsic properties of the solution, such as the kind of polymer, the viscosity, the electrical conductivity, the polarity and the surface tension; and (ii) those related to the operational conditions of the electrospinning, such as the applied electric field, the distance between the spinneret and the collector and the feeding rate of the

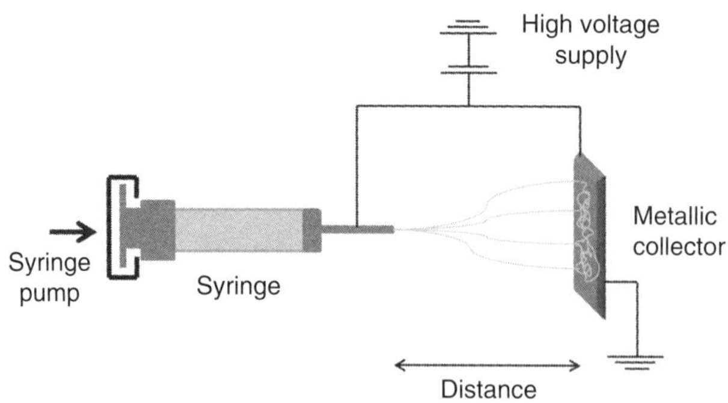

Figure 4.1 Schematic representation of the electrospinning process.

polymer solution [4]. Therefore, by changing these parameters, multiple morphologies can be attained and continuous polymeric fibers and capsules (beads) with diameters ranging from a few nanometers to a few microns can be obtained.

The important advantages of the electrospinning technique, which are further outlined in the next section, are the production of very thin fibers to the order of few nanometers with large surface areas, ease of functionalization for various purposes, superior mechanical properties and ease of processing as suggested by many experts in this field. The possibility of large-scale productions combined with the simplicity of the process makes this technique very attractive for many different applications.

Because of their small surface areas and small pore size in comparison with commercial textiles, the electrospun materials are excellent candidates for many applications. For instance, they can be used in filtration or separation membranes, since the submicrometer-size fibers produce a layer that has high porosity but very small pore size [5]. Due to the ultrathin size of these materials, they can also be used as reinforcement in composite materials, since they can provide superior structural properties which generally cannot be achieved by microfibers of the same material [6]. Besides, the biomedical field is one of the important application areas among others utilizing the technique of electrospinning. Electrospun fibers have been successfully developed for the encapsulation and the delivery of bioactive compounds within the body for therapeutic treatments. Moreover, the topographical similarity of electrospun matrices with the extracellular matrix was realized as favorable for tissue engineering purposes and medical implants [7]. Finally, the electrospinning technology can be used as an encapsulation technique creating small droplets of solid or liquid particles (core material) which are packed into a matrix (wall material) designed to protect the core or release it under desired conditions.

4.1.2 Advantages of Electrospinning for Encapsulation

Although electrospinning is not yet used commercially for encapsulation purposes, at least in the food area, it has a number of advantages over other well-established encapsulation technologies. For instance, it does not require the use of high temperatures for solution electrospinning, and thus, temperature-sensitive ingredients may be encapsulated using this processing technique without suffering from any activity loss due to the temperature effect. Moreover, although many polymers are required to be dissolved in organic solvents for a stable electrospinning process, one can also produce electrospun structures from some biopolymers using aqueous solutions, mainly by adjusting the process parameters and/or changing the solution properties through the addition of proper additives. This is of special interest in food-related applications, where the use of organic solvents for the development of edible food ingredients can pose reasonable concerns regarding the toxic effects due to the presence of remaining solvents in the structures.

Another advantage of the electrospinning technique is that the morphology of the encapsulation structures obtained can be varied by adjusting the process parameters, and for a certain material, apart from fiber-like morphologies, reduced size capsules can be obtained when lowering the polymer concentration and/or increasing the tip-to-collector distance (process known as electrospraying due to the noncontinuous nature of the polymer jet). In Figure 4.2, for example, several encapsulation morphologies obtained through electrospinning and electrospraying are shown.

Moreover, there is no limitation in terms of the substance to encapsulate independent of the chemical nature of the encapsulating matrix, as coaxial electrospinning might be employed. The configuration in coaxial electrospinning, which consists of two concentrically arranged dies connected to two reservoirs containing different spinning solutions, presents a number of advantages, such as the possibility of including as core material a favorable

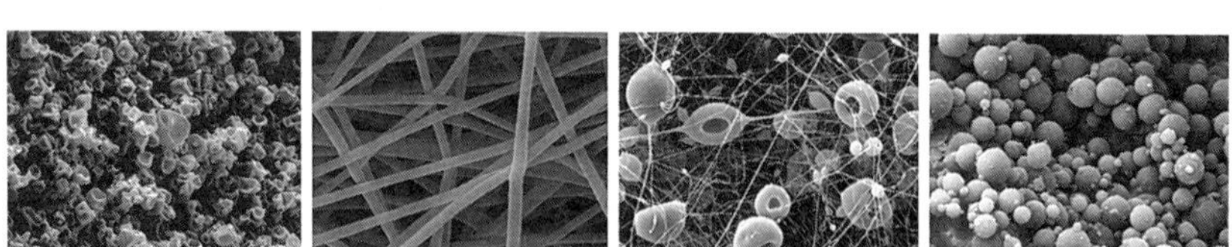

Figure 4.2 Examples of different encapsulation morphologies attained through electrospinning and electrospraying.

fluid medium for the functional component to encapsulate, which does not have to be spinnable as it becomes entrained by the outer polymeric shell [8].

Furthermore, most encapsulation technologies commercially available give rise to capsules of a considerable size (the smallest sizes obtained being over a micron), while electrospinning can generate structures with diameters between 10 and 1000 nm depending on the solution and the process conditions. The key advantage of producing fibers with very small diameters is their large surface-to-mass ratio, high porosity and superior mechanical performance [9, 10] It is recognized that for specific applications, such as targeted controlled release, nanoencapsulation technologies can offer a number of advantages. In general, encapsulation offers improved stability and targeting, and thus, the amount of material required to exert a specific effect when encapsulated is much less than the amount required when non-encapsulated. This is particularly useful when dealing with expensive bioactive agents. But, apart from that, a timely and targeted release, which can be accomplished by a rational design of the encapsulation system, improves the effectiveness of the bioactives, broadens the application range of the ingredients and ensures optimal dosage, thereby improving cost-effectiveness of the product. Moreover, the properties of the electrospun polymeric structures can be modified, either by tailoring the fiber or capsule surface composition and morphology, or by using polymer blends to create composite materials for encapsulation that may be able to better fulfill specific industrial requirements in terms of their material properties, thereby increasing the potential applications. Recently, investigations have focused on the inclusion of other nanoscale structures within the nanofibers in order to produce structures with added functionalities. For instance, silver nanoparticles have been included in synthetic polymer fibers to produce potent antimicrobially active materials [11]. Likewise, a combination of nanofibers and self-assembled structures such as micelles, liposomes and microemulsions, could also create novel delivery systems with superior properties for encapsulation properties [12].

Electrospinning as an encapsulation technique, as mentioned before, is still in an exploratory phase and most of the equipment used is lab-scale. However, there are a number of companies, such as Bioinicia S.L. (through its engineering brand Fluidnatek®) that are already commercializing pilot plant scale and even industrial scale equipment, which can be tailor-made to match the specific requirements for a certain application.

4.2 Electrospun Structures for the Encapsulation of Bioactive Substances in the Food Area

The development of functional foods containing bioactive ingredients is an area of increasing interest not only for the scientific community, but also for the food industry. These bioactive ingredients are expected to impart a health benefit to consumers in addition to the nutrition that the food itself offers. However, both the physiological benefits and the effectiveness in reducing the risk of diseases depend on preserving the bioavailability of the active ingredients. This represents a formidable challenge for scientists, as the functional substances are known to lose effectiveness either during processing, storage or in the gastrointestinal tract. The development of nano- and microstructures able to protect the active ingredients acting as carriers and delivery vehicles for controlled release is undoubtedly a plausible option. When the bioactive substances are surrounded by a suitable matrix, they can have improved stability to diverse factors such as pH and temperature changes. Microencapsulation of food ingredients is well established, but nanoencapsulation can offer a number of advantages such as increased bioavailability, controlled release properties and better dispersion in aqueous systems for water-insoluble food ingredients and additives [13, 14]. Electrospinning is one of the available techniques that can be used for the nanoencapsulation of food ingredients. Although it has not been used yet commercially, it has attracted enormous interest in recent years for this purpose, reflected in the increased number of scientific publications dealing with encapsulation of bioactives using this versatile technique.

Specifically, aiming at the development of electrospun structures for the encapsulation of food bioactives, biopolymers are the preferred choice because they may be nontoxic, edible and digestible. Biopolymers are also of great interest in other areas, such as the biomedical field, as they are considered to be biocompatible and biodegradable. However, the production of electrospun structures from biopolymers has been rather limited due to several technical challenges. However, it is not the aim of this section to review the electrospinning of biopolymers, and the interested reader is directed to the work of Kriegel and coworkers [12] for more information in this area.

4.2.1 Enzyme Encapsulation

Enzymes have multiple applications in the food area, not only for food processing, but also for use as antioxidant or antimicrobial additives and for food quality control. It is widely recognized that enzyme immobilization on solid substrates offers advantages over the use of free enzymes, enhancing the stability, and hence applicability, of these biomolecules as reusable and robust biocatalysts. Immobilization can stabilize enzymes, enable better control of the enzymatic reaction and allow their repeated use. Encapsulation for the immobilization of enzymes might, thus, improve their properties because substrate specificity might be enhanced and the effect of inhibitors might be reduced. However, many methods of encapsulation cause significant structural deformation of the enzyme, leading to reduction in activity. Significant optimization of the immobilization method is therefore often required [15].

The use of electrospinning for the incorporation of diverse enzymes has gained increasing attention. Electrospun nanofibers are excellent candidates for hosting enzymes for several reasons: (i) their small size confers a large surface area and makes possible the creation of materials with high concentrations of an enzyme; (ii) the porosity of the fibers can be tailored, and thus, the movement of molecules into and out of the fibers can be controlled according to specific requirements; (iii) the use of non-soluble fibrous mats in aqueous medium provides the ability to recover the mat for reuse; and (iv) multiple enzymes from diverse sources can be encapsulated together [16].

For instance, laccase was successfully encapsulated into electrospun microfibers made of poly(D,L-lactide) (PDLLA) and a triblock copolymer by emulsion electrospinning [17]. Laccase is an unspecific copper-containing oxidase with potential applications, not only in the food industry [18], but also in the textile, pulp and paper industries, for biodegradation and biotransformation of pollutant, etc. The obtained core–shell structure and porosity of the electrospun fiber were beneficial for preserving the activity and stability of immobilized laccase. The immobilized laccase maintained

50% of its initial activity after 10 successive runs and a broadening in the pH range of catalysis activity compared to the free laccase was observed [17]. Liu and coworkers [19] also developed laccase-containing electrospun structures as biosensors for phenolic compounds. Polyvinyl alcohol (PVA) was used as the encapsulation matrix. The results showed that the enzyme retained its high catalytic activity and good sensing performance for several polyphenolic compounds. In addition, the biosensor exhibited good repeatability and reproducibility, implying that the electrospun nanofibers were appropriate for the immobilization of the enzymes. Porous silica electrospun fibers containing horseradish peroxidase were also developed for use as biosensors, demonstrating a good catalytic activity [20].

Other enzymes encapsulated using coaxial electrospinning have been alkaline phosphatase (AP) and β-galactosidase (β-gal) [16]. In this case the shell consisted of a blend of polycaprolactone (PCL) with poly(ethylene glycol) (PEG), which gave rise to a pore-containing fiber structure, thus allowing the movement of molecules into or out of the fibers. Enzyme assays showed that especially with the encapsulated β-gal, the fibers acted as an efficient enzymatic microreactor with a relative enzymatic activity reaching a level of about 50% [16].

4.2.2 Encapsulation of Probiotic Bacteria

Probiotics are defined as living microorganisms which, when administered in adequate amounts, confer health benefits to the host, including the prevention and treatment of some pathologies. These include reduction of gastrointestinal infections, improvement of lactose metabolism, reduction of serum cholesterol, and improvement of immune system defenses [21]. Amongst probiotics, the genus *Bifidobacterium* have been the subject of intense research due to its predominance in breastfed infants and the beneficial effects attributed to some strains, leading to their incorporation into diverse food products and pharmaceutical formulations for commercialization. Microencapsulation has been suggested to ensure their survival during product storage and marketing, as probiotics must be alive, metabolically active and abundant in the product to guarantee their efficacy. However, encapsulation technologies that do not involve severe conditions, both in terms of temperature and solvents used, and that give rise to small capsule sizes are highly

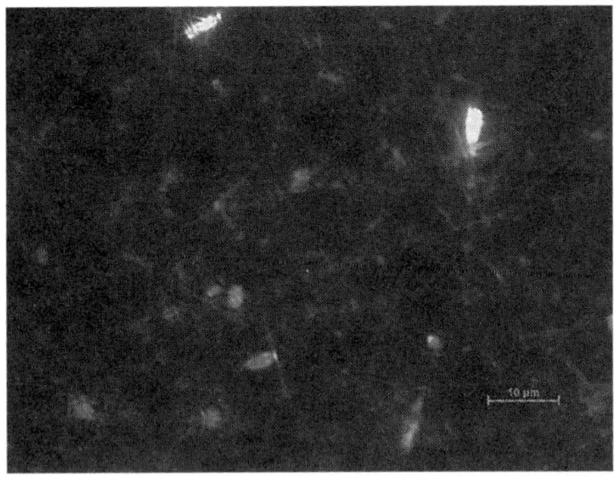

Figure 4.3 Optical micrograph using a fluorescence source of hybrid PVOH/bifidobacteria electrospun fibers. The bifidobacteria were previously stained with fluorescein.

desired. Thus, the electrospinning technique is an ideal tool for this purpose. The suitability of electrospinning for generating probiotic-containing encapsulation structures was initially proven using polyvinyl alcohol (PVA) and a coaxial configuration of the equipment [22]. Fiber-like morphologies with the bacteria distributed along the fibers (as observed in Figure 4.3) were obtained which considerably extended the viability of the cells at various storage temperatures.

Later on, protein-based (whey protein concentrate) and carbohydrate-based (pullulan) electrosprayed capsules were developed for the encapsulation of a bifidobacterial strain. These electrosprayed hydrocolloid-based encapsulation structures demonstrated the ability to prolong bifidobacterial survival during storage at 4 and 20°C and at various relative humidity conditions (0, 11, 53 and 75% RH) [23].

4.2.3 Antioxidant Encapsulation

In foods, antioxidants are added to minimize changes in flavor, aroma, color or nutritional value. But, moreover, antioxidants can protect the body against damages caused by free radicals and degenerative diseases, and thus, are increasingly studied for their inclusion in functional foods. However, due to their intrinsic sensitivity to several factors, such as light, oxygen or temperature, natural antioxidants should be protected from the surrounding medium or the processing conditions during food production. Recently, the electrospinning technique has been evaluated for the encapsulation of antioxidants, as no temperature is required in the process, and thus, the antioxidant activity of the molecules is thought to remain unchanged during encapsulation. An interesting natural antioxidant is β-carotene, a terpene with pro-vitamin A activity, and has been encapsulated through electrospinning using either zein (a prolamine) [24] or a whey protein concentrate (WPC) [25], giving rise to fiber or capsule morphologies, respectively. Both works demonstrated an increased stability of the antioxidant within the encapsulation matrices (in comparison with the non-encapsulated compound), and very high encapsulation efficiency was obtained when using glycerol as a vehicle for the β-carotene incorporation in WPC [25]. Zein fibers were also developed to encapsulate and protect a polyphenolic compound, specifically epigallocatechin-gallate (EGCG), which is a catechin from green tea with diverse health benefits (oxidative stress protection and reduced risk of CVD and certain types of cancer) [26]. Both relative humidity and aging time after electrospinning were important in determining the stability of EGCG upon subsequent contact with water. A very good immobilization and stability of the antioxidant compound was observed after aging the fibers for at least 1 day under dry conditions at ambient temperature [26].

4.2.4 Encapsulation of Other Food Compounds

4.2.4.1 *Antimicrobials*

Active polymer fibers can also be developed through electrospinning to improve food safety by means of the encapsulation of antimicrobial compounds. For instance, a naturally occurring antimicrobial compound, allyl isothiocyanate (AITC), with known bactericidal activity, was encapsulated into electrospun fibers from soy protein isolate/poly(ethylene oxide) blend and poly(lactic acid). A controlled release of the antimicrobial from the fibers as a function of relative humidity was achieved, rendering promising structures for use in active packaging applications for foods [27].

4.2.4.2 *Omega-3 Fatty Acids*

Polyunsaturated fatty acids (PUFAs), and more specifically, omega-3 fatty acids (ω -3), have become popular as food supplements due to the beneficial health effects supported by a variety of epidemiological and interventional studies of fish consumption, including a reduction in blood pressure, modulation of the response to endogenous and exogenous thrombolytic agents, antiarrhythmic actions, inhibition of platelet activation, modulation of inflammation, triglycerides reduction, and decrease of cardiovascular diseases [28]. Docosahexaenoic acid (DHA), a long chain polyunsaturated fatty acid of the ω -3 group, was encapsulated in zein ultrathin capsules produced by electrospraying [29]. Zein ultrathin DHA encapsulation was observed by ATR-FTIR spectroscopy to be more efficient against degradation under both ambient conditions and in a confined space (so-called headspace experiment). In the latter case, which more closely simulates a sealed food packaging situation, the bioactive DHA was considerably more stable. Moreover, the ultrathin zein-DHA capsules resulted to be more stable across relative humidity and temperature and released much less off-flavors [29].

4.2.4.3 *Flavors*

Flavors are very valuable ingredients in any food formula. Even small amounts of some aroma substances can be expensive, and because they are usually delicate and volatile, preserving them is often a top concern of food manufacturers. Encapsulation of flavors has been carried out using many different methods such as spray drying, spray chilling, extrusion, coacervation and molecular inclusion [30]. Cyclodextrin inclusion complexes (CD-IC) have also been used to improve flavor stability [31]. The encapsulation of these CD-IC within PVA electrospun fibers has been proven to enhance the durability and provide high temperature stability of flavors, and specifically, of vanillin [32].

4.3 Electrospun Encapsulation Structures for Biomedical Applications

Although electrospinning has been traditionally focused on textile applications, the use of electrospun nanofibrous scaffolds for biomedical applications has attracted great attention in recent years [33]. For instance, nanofibrous scaffolds have been demonstrated as suitable substrates for tissue engineering [34, 35], immobilized enzymes and catalyst [36, 37] and artificial blood vessels [38]. They have also been used as barriers for the prevention of post-operative induced adhesion and vehicles for controlled drug delivery [39, 7]. Polymeric drug delivery systems are able to improve therapeutic efficacy, reduce toxicity and enhance compliance of the patients by delivering drugs at a controlled rate over a period of time to the site of action. In particular, biodegradable polyesters and their copolymers have demonstrated their potential as effective carriers for drug delivery applications [40, 41]. Among the different methods used for preparing bioactive loaded polymer structures for drug delivery, the electrospinning technique presents a number of advantages such as the possibility to produce high specific surface area structures in a facile approach requiring mild preparation [42].

For electrospun nanofibrous scaffolds in biomedical applications, its physical and biological properties, such as hydrophilicity, mechanical modulus and strength, biodegradability, biocompatibility, and specific cell interactions, are largely determined by the materials' chemical compositions. Besides taking advantage of the materials compositions, the fabrication process, through which the fiber diameter, morphology and scaffold porosity can be manipulated, also plays an important role in the scaffold properties and functionality.

The encapsulation and controllable release of bioactive agents such as drugs are crucial for maximizing the safety, effectiveness, and reliability of these agents [43]. The incorporation of bioactive agents into electrospun fibers could lead to a biofunctional tissue engineering scaffold, and biofunctionalization of electrospun fibers will determine the efficiency of these fibers for regenerating biological functional tissues. Tissue engineering scaffolds with the incorporation of drugs or bioactive proteins have been investigated using, among other techniques, post-spinning modifications, electrospinning drug/polymer or nanoparticles blends, emulsion electrospinning and core-shell electrospinning [7]. Table 4.1 includes a summary of the characteristics of these fabrication techniques, together with the advantages, drawbacks and some of the published works using them.

4.3.1 Post-Spinning Modification

Loading drugs into the electrospun matrices as post-spinning modification allows easy variation of drugs, mixtures and concentrations starting from a common matrix. The simplest setup of drug loading is adsorption to the large surface of the scaffolds. This is a versatile drug delivery platform to release different drugs from

Table 4.1 Drug loading techniques for generating electrospun bioactive mats for biomedical applications, including their advantages, drawbacks and some of the scientific publications dealing with them.

	Drug loading techniques	Benefits	Drawbacks	References
Post-spinning modification	-Electrospinning of polymer in the first step followed by drug adsorption to the electrospun matrix - Specific immobilization of drug molecules on the scaffold surface: covalent modification of electrospun matrix followed by drug adsorption	- Versatile drug delivery platform to deliver different drugs from the same matrix. - Drug molecules are not exposed to the electrospinning process. - Variable release profile depending on the matrix-drug interaction	- When it comes to sustaining high concentrations of drugs locally and controlling drug release over extended time periods, adsorptive drug loading is usually insufficient. Instead, specific immobilization of drug molecules on the scaffold surface is needed.	Bolgen et al., 2007; Fu et al., 2008 Lu et al., 2009

(Continued)

Table 4.1 *(cont.)*

	Drug loading techniques	Benefits	Drawbacks	References
Electrospinning of drug/ polymer blend	- Electrospinning of drug/polymer blends from drug solution, emulsion or suspension in the polymer solution.	- Modified drug release. - Encapsulation of low molecular weight substances. - Possibility to electrospun directly on the site of action.	-Drug functionality may be affected by exposure to organic solvents, as well as by electric charge and mechanical stress during the electrospinning process. - Encapsulation of high molecular weight substances is more difficult - The influence of the electrospinning process and release on the structure and bioactivity of the incorporated proteins	Kenawy et al., 2002 Jiang et al., 2004 Qi et al., 2006 Xu et al., 2005 Xu et al., 2006
Coaxial or "core-shell" electrospinning	-Two different polymer solutions may be electrospun by utilizing a coaxial setup of an inner and an outer capillary tube in order to better control the release kinetics of the drugs contained in either the core or the shell of electrospun fibers	- Core-shell fibers have great potential to preserve proteins during the electrospinning process. - It has been successfully demonstrated with various drugs ranging from small molecules to macromolecules. - Programmable release. - Encapsulation of virus, bacteria, cell, etc.	- The operational conditions have to be judiciously adjusted and it is often difficult to ensure the desired results.	Jaysinghe et al., 2007 Saraf et al., 2009 Micknova et al., 2012 Kowalczyk et al., 2008

the same matrix, and the drug is not exposed to the electrospinning process [44]. Loading of growth factors or other proteins into electrospun scaffolds can also be achieved by a covalent modification of the electrospun matrix followed by drug adsorption. However, this technique could induce a variable release profile depending on the matrix-drug interaction [45]. The concept of post-spinning modification of electrospun scaffolds offers numerous opportunities for localized and controlled delivery of drugs, and in the case of sensitive biomolecules such as growth factors (GFs), the major advantage of this technique is the avoidance of destabilizing conditions during the electrospinning process. However, to date, only a limited number of reports in this direction are available.

4.3.2 Blending and Emulsion Electrospinning

Most publications studying drug-loaded fibrous matrices prefer direct electrospinning of drug/polymer blend from drug solution, emulsion or suspension in a suitable polymer solution.

For the application of blending electrospinning, the incorporated drugs or proteins in nanofibers have a burst phenomenon in the initial stage because drug particles tend to locate on the surface of nanofibers under the impelling electric force during the process of electrospinning. Furthermore, the incorporated drugs or proteins tend to change their complex physical and chemical properties under the impacts of electrospinning, storage and release processes, and the inherent structure of proteins could be modified, thus affecting their bioactivity. Blend electrospinning involves mixing of proteinaceous biomolecules with the polymer solution. Some researchers have also termed this method "emulsion electrospinning" because the aqueous protein solution was first emulsified by ultrasonication, and then the protein emulsion was mixed with the polymer solution for electrospinning.

Electrospinning of emulsions has attracted growing interest [46, 47]. The emulsions (particularly water-in-oil type of emulsions) usually contain a continuous phase that is constituted by the polymer (generally a biocompatible/biodegradable polymer) dissolved in organic solvent(s), and a separated/isolated phase (emulsion particles/droplets with sizes ranging from sub-microns to microns) that is the bioactive agent (e.g., a drug) dissolved in water. Electrospinning of emulsions can produce composite nanofibers with nanoscaled drug particles surrounded/coated by emulsifiers/surfactants and impregnated in biocompatible and/or biodegradable polymers. This type of composite nanofiber mats possesses the combined characteristics of a tissue engineering scaffold and a controllable drug encapsulation/release vehicle. In this sense, encapsulation of low molecular weight substances like tetracycline hydrochloride [48] or ibuprofen [49] into electrospun nanofibers has already been demonstrated to be successful. In most cases, the drug was dissolved or dispersed in the polymer solution and was encapsulated using the electrospinning. However, when electrospinning drug/polymer blends, drug functionality may be affected by exposure to organic solvents, which are required for dissolution of many polymers, as well as by the electric charge and mechanical stress during the electrospinning process. It is obvious that blending polymer solutions with drugs must be considered to affect the properties of electrospun fibers. Furthermore, drug solubility in the polymer solution is also likely to have an effect on the drug distribution within the electrospun fibers and also on the extent of burst release.

In contrast, encapsulation of higher molecular weight substances is more difficult because the electrospinning of macromolecular dispersions is more challenging than electrospinning of homogeneous polymer solutions. In this case, the concept of coaxial electrospinning led to core-shell structured fibers which proved their suitability as drug delivery devices for larger molecules.

4.3.3 "Core-Shell Electrospinning" or "Coaxial Electrospinning"

The major challenge of protein encapsulation by electrospinning is that the exposure of hydrophilic proteins to organic solvents and hydrophobic polymers could lead to protein destabilization and inactivation. Blend electrospinning could simply entrap the bioactive agents within ultrafine fibers by dispersing the protein into the polymer solution. However, the major disadvantages are the severe burst release phenomenon, the reduction in effective lifetime and the influence of the electrospinning process and release on the structure and bioactivity of the incorporated proteins. So, apart from the use of blends, core-shell electrospinning is an attractive strategy for the delivery of susceptible biomolecules because the produced core-shell fibers have great potential to preserve protein structure, and thus, bioactivity during the electrospinning process. As a result, the coaxial electrospinning method has proven to be successful with various drugs ranging from small molecules to macromolecules showing retained biological activity, and even for the encapsulation of whole cells, revealing maintained viability upon electrospinning [50–54]. As previously outlined before in the chapter, for core-shell or coaxial electrospinning, two different solutions may be electrospun by utilizing a coaxial setup of an inner and an outer capillary tube in order to better control the release kinetics of the drugs contained in either the core or the shell of electrospun fibers. Usually, the drug is embedded in the core part and released through the shell material or it can be released through aqueous pores, both against a concentration gradient. In addition, programmable release can be achieved by using an impermeable but degradable shell, providing temporal protection of drugs in the core and deferring drug action until shell degradation starts [7]. So, the hydrophilic core solution facilitates the loading and preservation of protein bioactivity, whereas the hydrophobic polymer shell allows fiber formation [56, 55]. Kowalczyk and coworkers (2008) [57] showed that, in general, aqueous biological solutions are very difficult to electrospin due to their low viscosity. So, in both blend and coaxial electrospinning, different compounds, such as poly(ethylene glycol), poly(ethylene oxide), poly(ethylene imine) or dextrans, are usually added to the aqueous biological solution to improve its fiber-forming properties [54, 58, 59]. Sun and coworkers [60] reported, for the first time, the formation of core-shell nanofibers by coaxial electrospinning and this technique proved to be very versatile for encapsulation of relevant biomolecules and nanocomposites. Zhang and coworkers [51] also demonstrated the successful encapsulation of a model protein, fluorescein isothiocyanate-conjugated bovine serum albumin, along with poly(ethylene glycol) within biodegradable polycaprolactone (PCL) nanofibers using a coaxial electrospinning technique. Ji and coworkers [54] produced PCL-based nanofibrous scaffolds with incorporated protein (bovine serum albumin) via either the blend or coaxial electrospinning technique, and they compared both techniques with respect to processing set-up and scaffold characteristics as well as the release kinetics and biological activity of the loaded protein. These authors concluded that coaxial electrospinning was superior to blend electrospinning for the preparation of nanofibrous scaffolds with a uniform fibrous structure and protein distribution, and sustained protein release kinetics as well as higher preservation of the protein activity. It was also demonstrated that the core-shell structured ultrafine fibers could protect the structural integrity and bioactivity of encapsulated lysozyme, and an increase in the protective effect was demonstrated for fibers prepared from poly(ethylene glycol)-PLA matrices [59]. More recently, Micknova and coworkers [55] also studied two different nanofibers-liposome systems: blending and core/shell electrospinning. Concretely, they produced liposomes dispersed within blended nanofibers and core/shell nanofibers with embedded liposomes, and they found that the greatest potential was also shown by intact liposomes incorporated into fibers by coaxial electrospinning, in contrast with blend electrospinning.

Although the coaxial electrospinning technique can result in the formation of nanofibers having core-shell structures with sheaths being biocompatible/biodegradable polymers and cores being encapsulated bioactive agents [51], the operational conditions have to be judiciously adjusted and it is often difficult to ensure the desired results.Coaxial electrospinning has also been used to encapsulate biological moieties like bacteria, virus, cells, etc., generating living membranes. In this sense, [61] the potential of using coaxial electrospinning technology for the generation of scaffolds comprised of living organism in the form of threads and scaffolds has been demonstrated. Bacteria (Escherichia coli, Staphylococcus) and viruses (T7, T4, λ) [62] have also been encapsulated in electrospun polymer nanofibers and have been shown to survive the electrospinning process and remain viable for three months at low temperatures like -20 and -55°C. Furthermore, dispersions of M13 viruses in water-soluble poly(vinyl pyrrolidone) (PVP) have also been processed into nanofibers by electrospinning [63], and the resulting virus-PVP electrospun fibers maintained their ability to infect bacterial hosts after re-suspending in a buffer solution.

Therefore, polymer nanofibers containing biological agents can be directly prepared without a detrimental effect in their biological functionality by electrospinning.

4.4 Other Uses of Electrospinning for Encapsulation

4.4.1 Energy Storage Devices

The development of energy conversion and energy storage systems has been intensified over the last years because of the economic and environmental problems associated with the increasing world population and the energy sources used nowadays. In this area, nanoscale dimensions achieved through electrospinning technology provide specific properties such as high surface area and aspect ratios, low density and high pore volume, which allow performance improvements in these systems. Therefore, the use of electrospinning in energy devices has increased in recent years [64]. Moreover, electrospinning has been used specifically for encapsulation applications in energy storage systems, such as thermal energy or electrochemical energy storage systems.

4.4.1.1 Thermal Energy Storage Systems

Recently, the use of phase change materials (PCMs) for thermal energy storage has gained extensive attention due to increasing energy consumption and environment pollution problems [65]. PCMs are able to absorb and release a large amount of latent heat during their phase transition process over a narrow temperature range, and thus, they can be used to enhance the energy storage capability of different materials. PCMs are generally classified into two categories: inorganic materials, such as salt hydrates, and organic materials, such as paraffins or fatty acids. A large number of compounds can be identified as PCMs from their melting temperature; however, they should also present suitable physical, chemical and kinetic properties. Nevertheless, the use of these materials in thermal energy storage applications presents some drawbacks, such as weak thermal stability, low thermal conductivity and the fact that some of them are liquid at ambient temperature, and thus, they are not easy to handle [66]. The encapsulation of the PCM is a plausible solution to avoid these problems. Some of the advantages of introducing these materials inside a shell material are: (i) the PCM is protected against the influences of the outside environment; (ii) the heat transfer area is increased; (iii) the changes in volume of the PCM, as the phase transition occurs, are withstood; (iv) a solid matrix which allows an easier handling of the materials is provided, and; (v) small and portable energy storage systems can be designed. In conclusion, the encapsulation of the PCMs makes them more suitable to be applied in many fields, such as building materials, packaging of temperature-sensitive products, air conditioning applications, solar energy storage systems, greenhouses, temperature regulating textiles, electronics devices and biomedical systems [67].

There are many methods developed for the encapsulation of PCMs. The most common techniques are interfacial polymerization [68], emulsion polymerization [69], *in-situ* polymerization [70], layer-by-layer deposition of polyelectrolytes [71], spray drying and coacervation [72]. However, very little PCM can be encapsulated by some of these techniques, and for some applications a large particle size is also obtained, which could reduce the efficiency of the heat transfer [73]. Therefore, the electrospinning technique is an innovative approach to encapsulate PCMs [74] and to design novel thermal energy storage devices. Electrospinning can encapsulate materials from the melt as well as from polymer solutions, enhancing even further the number of encapsulation matrices that can be used. A significant advantage of the technique is the suitable use of biomass-derived materials and of biodegradable polymers as encapsulating elements, with the corresponding environmental benefits associated with their use. Biomass-derived materials not only present encapsulation flexibility and efficiency but can also help reduce the environmentally meaningful parameter, the so-called carbon footprint. Recently, heat management materials with potential applications in food biopackaging (for keeping the cold chain) were developed by means of electrospinning. These structures consisted on a zein matrix containing encapsulated dodecane (a PCM paraffin which has a transition temperature at −10°C). The thermal characteristics and encapsulation efficiency varied with the morphology of the encapsulation structures [75]. As an example of this type of heat management structure, Figure 4.4 presents some polymeric encapsulates with different morphologies obtained

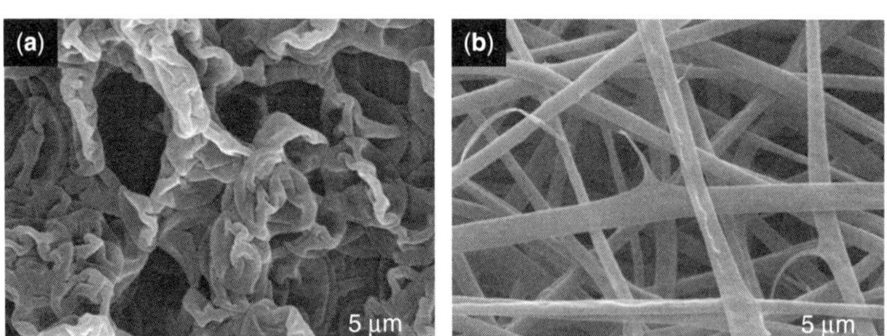

Figure 4.4 SEM images of: a) PLA/PCM beads, and b) zein/PCM fibers. Scale markers correspond to 5 μm.

through electrospinning. Figure 4.4a shows PLA/PCM capsules (beads) and Figure 4.4b shows zein/PCM fibrilar encapsulates.

4.4.1.2 Electrochemical Energy Storage Systems

In the past decades considerable attention has been paid to electrochemical energy storage systems because of their application in small and portable electronic devices. In this area there are future challenges regarding these systems for use in more demanding applications such as electric or hybrid vehicles. Therefore, significant advances and improvements are needed in various aspects of these materials. Until now, rechargeable Lithium-ion batteries (LiB) have been the most employed systems in this field. However, some features of LiB, such as energy density, cycling life, charge/discharge rate, safety and cost, must be improved in order to achieve a satisfactory performance and a widespread commercialization in various fields of these energy storage systems [64, 76].

One strategy to improve the efficiency and the durability of LiB is to maintain a low weight, volume and cost by designing nanostructured materials to be used as electrodes in the batteries. The use of electrospinning to encapsulate cathode and anode compounds has been reported to be a versatile alternative approach for making these instruments, since this technology allows nanometric geometries which significantly increase the rate capability and power density of the batteries, favors a high electrode/electrolyte contact area, and, moreover, reduces manufacturing costs [64]. Specifically, MgO have been used as shell material to encapsulate $LiCoO_2$, which is the cathode compound commonly used in most commercial batteries. The encapsulation increased the stability and cycling performance of $LiCoO_2$ [77]. Additionally, a carbon coating ensures a higher conductivity which makes a faster ionic transport possible. Thus, carbon electrospun nanofibers have been loaded with metal or oxide particles in order to be used as anode materials. In this area, the most studied materials are Si, Sn and Ni [76, 78–80].

4.4.2 Optical and Electronic Devices

Recently, wires consisting of metal particles have been the focus of much scientific research due to their potential use as active components for interconnects which could be employed in the production of optical and electronic devices [81]. However, it has been reported that these metallic wires are very sensitive to ambient conditions, such as air and moisture, and therefore the degradation of the devices where they are incorporated could occur [82]. Until now, synthetic approaches for the construction of metal–insulator nanostructures have focused on methods such as pulsed laser deposition [83, 84], ion-beam sputtering deposition [85] and chemical vapor deposition [86]. However, most of these methods are usually troublesome and high-cost. Thus, new approaches should be developed to meet the application demands. Among other encapsulation technologies, electrospinning is a simple and low-cost method for the preparation of large-scale ultrafine nanofibers which could act as coatings for the metallic components. The shell could protect the metal wires from oxidation and corrosion caused by the environmental conditions, and therefore could improve the performance of the devices over a longer period of time. Some examples of the use of electrospinning in this ambit are the encapsulation of silver particles inside a polymeric shell made of polyethylene oxide (PEO) and polyethylene glycol (PEG), and the encapsulation of gold nanoparticles into polyvinylpyrrolidone (PVP) nanofibers [87].

More recently, photosynthetic biological materials have been receiving much attention for potential use, not only in optoelectronic devices, but also for organic photovoltaic (OPV) and sensor applications given their superior photo responsive properties and inherent biodegradability and renewability [88]. The pigment-containing proteins in photosynthetic biological materials are part of a double membrane envelope called the thylakoid, which houses the light reactions of photosynthesis that are responsible for the synthesis of ATP. The inclusion of thylakoids in a material matrix for photoelectronic and sensor applications is of particular interest because the encapsulation of intact and functioning thylakoids would be a step toward a photosynthetic "living material." In this sense, a recent work has demonstrated that electrospinning can be a useful technique for this purpose, and nanofibers from a solution of thylakoids, poly(3,4-ethylenedioxythiophene) / poly(styrene sulfonate (PEDOT) and poly(ethylene oxide) (PEO) were developed, generating electrically conductive nanofibers with changes in electronic properties as a response to light [89].

Electrospinning has also proven very useful in generating optical sensors, which are interesting alternatives to electrochemical sensors for monitoring biological parameters such as oxygen and pH, as they are easy to miniaturize, cost-effective and can be read without physical contact [90]. A multifunctional material was developed by co-electrospinning, in which hydrophobic suspensions formed by PMMA melt, magnetic nanoparticles and a hydrophobic luminescent oxygen indicator were encapsulated in a pH-fluorescent sensing copolymer. These core-shell fiber mats were magnetic and had a well-organized structure which allowed, simultaneously, the optical monitoring of pH and O_2 *in situ* and in real time [91].

4.4.3 Biotechnical Plant Protection Systems

The release of female pheromones in order to cause the confusion of male insects, and thus avoid destructive plagues in crops, has been successfully achieved and is currently used in the plant protection area. However, this technique presents some drawbacks such as the heterogeneous distribution of the pheromone along the field and the low maintenance of the required concentration of the pheromone over a long period of time.

The microencapsulation of the pheromones inside a shell material could make the pheromone less prone to being swept away by storms and heavy rains, could control the rate at which they are released, and could cause a homogeneous distribution of the pheromone over the field, cutting down the large amount of the pheromone otherwise needed in case of dispensers [92]. Therefore, electrospinning could also be used in this area to produce biotechnical plant protection systems based on the encapsulation of pheromones. A significant advantage of the technique is the suitable use of biomass-derived materials and of biodegradable polymers as encapsulating elements. These materials not only present encapsulation flexibility and efficiency but can also help to preserve the agricultural environment and reduce the meaningful parameter, the so-called carbon footprint. An example of the use of electrospinning in this field is the production of oligolactide (OLA)-pheromones microcapsules immobilized inside biodegradable polyester nanofibers [92].

4.5 Outlook and Conclusions

Electrospinning, which consists of the formation of solid structures (fibers or capsules) using electrostatic forces, is a versatile technique with great potential in the encapsulation of compounds for a number of applications, such as biomedical scaffolds for controlled drug release, functional foods, bioremediation, energy storage systems, etc. The number of research papers dealing with the electrospinning technique has exponentially increased since the mid 90s, also broadening the research areas where the technology has been applied. This is a reflection that the materials generated using this type of technology, due to their unique characteristics and the ease of the process, are attracting increased interest in many areas of knowledge. Moreover, significant advances in the technique and design of equipment, and the strategies that can be used to generate different encapsulation morphologies and even simultaneously encapsulate diverse substances, augur well for the expansion of electrospinning for encapsulation purposes. Furthermore, the extrapolation from the electrospun structures developed at the research stage for a commercial scale can be carried out rather easily and there are already industrial electrospinning apparatus available.

References

1. W.J. Morton. (1902). Method of dispersing fluids. US Patent 705, 691.
2. D. Li, and Y. Xia. (2004). Electrospinning of nanofibers: Reinventing the wheel? *Advanced Materials* 16:1151–1170.
3. T. Subbiah, G.S. Bhat, R.W. Tock, S. Parameswaran, S.S. Ramkumar. (2005). Electrospinning of nanofibers. *Journal of Applied Polymer Science* 96:557–569.
4. D.H. Reneker, and I. Chun. (1996). Nanometre diameter fibers of polymer, produced by electrospinning. *Nanotechnology* 7:216–223.
5. P.W. Gibson, H.L. Schreuder-Gibson, and D. Rivin. (1999). Electrospun fiber mats: Transport properties. *AIChE Journal* 45:190–195.
6. J.M. Lagaron, L. Cabedo, D. Cava, J.L. Feijoo, R. Gavara, and E. Gimenez. (2005). Improving packaged food quality and safety. Part 2: Nanocomposites. *Food Additives and Contaminants* 22:994–998.
7. A.J. Meinel, O. Germershaus, T. Luhmann, H.P. Merkle, and L. Meinel. (2012). Electrospun matrices for localized drug delivery: Current technologies and selected biomedical applications. *European Journal of Pharmaceutics and Biopharmaceutics* 81, 1–13.
8. A. Greiner, J.H. Wendorff, A.L. Yarin, E. Zussman. (2006). Biohybrid nanosystems with polymer nanofibers and nanotubes. *Applied Microbiology and Biotechnology* 71:387–393.
9. A. Frenot, and I.S. Chronakis. (2003). Polymer nanofibers assembled by electrospinning. *Current Opinion in Colloid & Interface Science* 8:64–75.
10. J.S. Kim, and D.H. Reneker. (1999). Mechanical properties of composites using ultrafine electrospun fibers. *Polymer Composites* 20:124–131.
11. W.K. Son, J.H. Youk, and W.H. Park. (2006). Antimicrobial cellulose acetate nanofibers containing silver nanoparticles. *Carbohydrate Polymers* 65:430–434.

12. C. Kriegel, A. Arrechi, K. Kit, D.J. McClements, and J. Weiss. (2008). Fabrication, functionalization, and application of electrospun biopolymer nanofibers. *Critical Reviews in Food Science and Nutrition* 48:775–797.
13. Q. Chaudhry, M. Scotter, J. Blackburn, B. Ross, A. Boxall, L. Castle, R. Aitken, and R. Watkins. (2008). Applications and implications of nanotechnologies for the food sector. *Food Additives & Contaminants* 25:241–258.
14. M.R. Mozafari, J. Flanagan, L. Matia-Merino, A. Awati, A. Omri, Z.E. Suntres, and H. Singh. (2006). Recent trends in the lipid-based nanoencapsulation of antioxidants and their role in foods. *Journal of the Science of Food and Agriculture* 86:2038–2045.
15. L. Betancor, and H.R. Luckarift. (2008). Bioinspired enzyme encapsulation for biocatalysis. *Trends in Biotechnology* 26 (10): 566–572.
16. Y. Dror, J. Kuhn, R. Avrahami, and E. Zussman. (2008). Encapsulation of enzymes in biodegradable tubular structures. *Macromolecules* 41:4187–4192.
17. Y. Dai, J. Niu, J. Liu, L. Yin, and J. Xu. (2010). In situ encapsulation of laccase in microfibers by emulsion electrospinning: Preparation, characterization and application. *Bioresource Technology* 101:8942–8947.
18. R. Minussi, G.M. Pastore, and N. Duran. (2002). Potential applications of laccase in the food industry. *Trends in Food Science and Technology* 13:205–216.
19. J. Liu, J. Niu, L. Yin, and F. Jiang. (2011). In situ encapsulation of laccase in nanofibers by electrospinning for development of enzyme biosensors for chlorophenol monitoring. *Analyst* 136:4802–4808.
20. A.C. Patel, S. Li, J.-M. Yuan, and Y. Wei. (2006). In-situ encapsulation of horseradish peroxidase in electrospun porous silica fibers for potential biosensor applications. *Nano Letters* 6:1042–1046.
21. R. Havenaar, and J.H.J. Huis in't Veld. (1992). The lactic acid bacteria in health and disease. In *The lactic acid bacteria*, Vol. 1, ed. B.J.B. Wood, (1992), (pp. 209–224). London: Chapman & Hall.
22. A. Lopez-Rubio, E. Sanchez, Y. Sanz, and J.M. Lagaron. (2009). Encapsulation of living bifidobacteria in ultrathin PVOH electrospun fibers. *Biomacromolecules* 10:2823–2829.
23. A. Lopez-Rubio, E. Sanchez, S. Wilkanowicz, Y. Sanz, and J.M. Lagaron. (2012). Electrospinning as a useful technique for the encapsulation of living bifidobacteria in food hydrocolloids. *Food Hydrocolloids* 28:159–167.
24. A. Fernandez, S. Torres-Giner, and J.M. Lagaron. (2009). Novel route to stabilization of bioactive antioxidants by encapsulation in electrospun fibers of zein prolamine. *Food Hydrocolloids* 23:1427–1432.
25. A. Lopez-Rubio, and J.M. Lagaron. (2012). Whey protein capsules obtained through electropraying for the encapsulation of bioactives. *Innovative Food Science and Emerging Technologies* 13:200–206.
26. B.N. Singh, S. Shankar, and R.K. Srivastava. (2011). Green tea catechin, epigallocatechin-3-gallate (EGCG): Mechanisms, perspectives and clinical applications. *Biochemical Pharmacology* 82:1807–1821.
27. C. Vega-Lugo, and L.-T. Lim. (2009). Controlled release of allyl isothiocyanate using soy protein and poly(lactic acid) electrospun fibers. *Food Research International* 42:933–940.
28. L.A. Horrocks, and Y.K. Yeo. (1999). Health benefits of docosahexaenoic acid (DHA). *Pharmacological Research* 40:211–225.

29. S. Torres-Giner, A. Martinez-Abad, M.J. Ocio, J.M. Lagaron. (2010). Stabilization of a nutraceutical omega-3 fatty acid by encapsulation in ultrathin electrosprayed zein prolamine. *Journal of Food Science* 75:N69–N79.
30. A. Madene, M. Jacquot, J. Scher, and S. Desobry. (2006). Flavour encapsulation and controlled release: A review. *International Journal of Food Science & Technology* 41:1–21.
31. H.M.C. Marques. (2010). A review on cyclodextrin encapsulation of essential oils and volatiles. *Flavour and Fragrance Journal* 25:313–326.
32. F. Kayaci, and T. Uyar. (2012). Encapsulation of vanillin/cyclodextrin inclusión complex in electrospun polyvinyl alcohol (PVA) nanowebs: Prolonged shelf-life and high temperatura stability of vanillin. *Food Chemistry* 133:641–649.
33. S. Agarwal, J.H. Wendorff, and A. Greiner. (2008). Use of electrospinning technique for biomedical applications. *Polymer* 5603–5621.
34. S.A. Riboldi, M. Sampaolesi, P. Neuenschwander, G. Cossu, and S. Mantero. (2005). Electrospun degradable polyesterurethane membranes: Potential scaffolds for skeletal muscle tissue engineering. *Biomaterials* 26:4606–4615.
35. F. Yang, R. Murugan, S. Wang, and S. Ramakrishna. (2005). Electrospinning of nano/micro scale poly(L-lactic acid) aligned fibers and their potential in neural tissue engineering. *Biomaterials* 26:2603–2610.
36. Y. Wang, and Y.-L. Hsieh. (2004). Enzyme immobilization to ultra-fine cellulose fibers via amphiphilic polyethylene glycol spacers. *Journal of Polymer Science. Part A, Polymer Chemistry* 42:4289–4299.
37. L. Wu, X. Yuan, and J. Sheng. (2005). Immobilization of cellulose in nanofibrous PVA membranes by electrospinning. *Journal of Membrane Science* 250:167–173.
38. Z. Ma, M. Kotaki, T. Yong, W. He, and S. Ramakrishna. (2005). Surface engineering of electrospun polyethylene terephthalate (PET) nanofibers towards development of a new material for blood vessel engineering. *Biomaterials* 26:2527–2536.
39. T.J. Sill, and H.A. Von Recum. (2008). Electrospinning: Applications in drug delivery and tissue engineering. *Biomaterials* 29:1989–2006.
40. R. Langer. (1990). New methods of drug delivery. *Science* 249 (4976): 1527–1533.
41. L. Youxin, C. Volland, and T. Kissel. (1994). In vitro degradation and bovine serum albumin release of the ABA triblock copolymers consisting of poly(L(+) lactic acid) or poly(L(+) lactic acid-co-glycolic acid) A-blocks attached to central polyoxyethylene B-blocks. *Journal of Controlled Release* 32:121–128.
42. N. Bhardwaj, and S.C. Kundu. (2010). Electrospinning: A fascinating fiber fabrication technique. *Biotechnology Advances* 28 (3): 325–347.
43. R. Langer. 2003. Where a pill won't reach. *Scientific American* 288 (4): 50–57.
44. N. Bolgen, I. Vargel, P. Korkusuz, Y.Z. Menceloglu, and E. Piskin. (2007). In vivo performance of antibiotic embedded electrospun PCL membranes for prevention of abdominal adhesions. *Journal of Biomedical Materials Research Part B: Applied Biomaterials* 81:530–543.
45. Y. Lu, H. Jiang, K. Tu, and L. Wang. (2009). Mild immobilization of diverse macromolecular bioactive agents onto multifunctional fibrous membranes prepared by coaxial electrospinning. *Acta Biomaterials* 5:1562–1574.
46. X.L. Xu, L.X. Yang, X.Y. Xua, X. Wanga, X. Chena, Q. Lianga, J. Zengc, X. Jinga. (2005). Ultrafine medicated fibers electrospun from W/O emulsions. *Journal of Controlled Release* 108:33–42.

47. X.L. Xu, X.L. Zhuang, X.S. Chen, X.R. Wang, L.X. Yang, and X.B. Jing. (2006). Preparation of core-sheath composite nanofibers by emulsion electrospinning. *Macromolecular Rapid Communications* 27 (19): 1637–1642.
48. el-R. Kenawy, G.L. Bowlin, K. Mansfield,J. Layman, D.G. Simpson, E.H. Sanders, and G.E. Wnek. (2002). Release of tetracycline hydrochloride from electrospun poly(ethylene-co-vinylacetate), poly(lactic acid), and a blend. *Journal of Controlled Release* 81 (1–2): 57–64.
49. H. Jiang, D. Fang, B. Hsiao, B. Chu, and W. Chen. (2004). Preparation and characterization of ibuprofen-loaded poly(lactide-co-glycolide)/poly(ethylene glycol)-g-chitosan electrospun membranes. *Journal of Biomaterials Science Polymer Edition* 15 (3): 279–296.
50. Y. Zhang, X. Huang, B. Duan, L. Wu, S. Li, and X. Yuan. (2007). Preparation of electrospun chitosan/poly(vinyl alcohol) membranes. *Colloid and Polymer Science* 285:855–863.
51. Y.Z. Zhang, X. Wang, Y. Feng, J. Li, C.T. Lim, and S. Ramakrishna. (2006). Coaxial electrospinning of (fluorescein isothiocyanate-conjugated bovine serum (albumin)-encapsulated poly(epsilon-caprolactone) nanofibers for sustained release. *Biomacromolecules* 7:1049–1057.
52. I.C. Liao, S.Y. Chew, and K.W. Leong. (2006). Aligned core-shell nanofibers delivering bioactive proteins. *Nanomed* 1:465–471.
53. Z.M. Huang, C.L. He, A. Yang, Y. Zhang, X.J. Han, J. Yin, and Q. Wu. (2006). Encapsulating drugs in biodegradable ultrafine fibers through co-axial electrospinning. *Journal of Biomedical Materials Research, Part A.* 77:169–179.
54. W. Ji, F. Yang, J.J.J.P. Van Den Beucken, Z. Bian, M. Fan, Z. Chen, and J.A. Jansen. (2010). Fibrous scaffolds loaded with protein prepared by blend or coaxial electrospinning. *Acta Biomaterialia* 6 (11): 4199–4207.
55. A. Mickova, M. Buzgo, O. Benada, M. Rampichova, Z. Fisar, E. Filova, M. Tesarova, D. Lukas, and E. Amler. (2012). Core/shell nanofibers with embedded liposomes as a drug delivery system. *Biomacromolecules* 13 (4): 952–962.
56. A. Saraf, G. Lozier, A. Haesslein, F.K. Kasper, R.M. Raphael, L.S. Baggett, and A.G. Mikos. (2009). Fabrication of nonwoven coaxial fiber meshes by electrospinning. *Tissue Engineering, Part C: Methods* 15 (3): 333–344.
57. T. Kowalczyk, A. Nowicka, D. Elbaum, and T.A. Kowalewski. (2008). Electrospinning of bovine serum albumin: Optimization and the use for production of biosensors. *Biomacromolecules* 9:2087–2090.
58. S. Maretschek, A. Greiner, and T. Kissel. (2008). Electrospun biodegradable nanofiber nonwovens for controlled release of proteins. *Journal of Controlled Release* 127 (2): 180–187.
59. Y. Yang, X. Li, S. He, L. Cheng, F. Chen, S. Zhou, and J. Weng. (2011). Biodegradable ultrafine fibers with core-sheath structures for protein delivery and its optimization. *Polymers for Advanced Technologies* 22 (12): 1842–1850.
60. Z. Sun, E. Zussman, A.L. Yarin, J.H. Wendorff, and A. Greiner. (2003). Compound Core–Shell Polymer Nanofibers by Co-Electrospinning. *Advanced Materials* 15:1929–1932.
61. S.N. Jayasinghe, S. Irvine, and J.R. McEwan. (2007). Cell electrospinning highly concentrated cellular suspensions containing primary living organisms into cell-bearing threads and scaffolds. *Nanomedicine* 2:555–567.

62. W. Salalha, J. Kuhn, Y. Dror, and E. Zussman. (2006). Encapsulation of bacteria and viruses in electrospun nanofibres. *Nanotechnology* 17 (18): 4675–4681.
63. S.W. Lee, and A.M. Belcher. (2004). Virus-based fabrication of micro- and nanofibers using electrospinning. *Nano Letters* 4:387–390.
64. S. Cavaliere, S. Subianto, I. Savych, D.J. Jones, and J. Rozière. (2011). Electrospinning: Designed architectures for energy conversion and storage devices. *Energy and Environmental Science* 4:4761–4785.
65. A. Sari, C. Alkan, and A. Karaipekli. (2010). Preparation, characterization and thermal properties of PMMA/n-heptadecane microcapsules as novel solid-liquid microPCM for thermal energy storage. *Applied Energy* 87:1529–1534.
66. G. Fang, H. Li, F. Yang, X. Liu, and S. Wu. (2009). Preparation and characterization of nano-encapsulated n-tetradecane as phase change material for thermal energy storage. *Chemical Engineering Journal* 153:217–221.
67. N. Sarier, E. Onder, S. Ozay, and Y. Ozkilic. (2011). Preparation of phase change material-montmorillonite composites suitable for thermal energy storage. *Thermochimica Acta* 524:39–46.
68. L.Y. Chu, R. Xie, J.H. Zhu, W.M. Chen, T. Yamaguchi, and S.I. Nakao. (2003). Study of SPG membrane emulsification processes for the preparation of monodisperse core-shell microcapsules. *Journal of Colloid and Interface Science* 265:187–196.
69. C.J. McDonald, and M.J. Devon. (2002). Hollow latex particles: Synthesis and applications. *Advances in Colloid and Interface Science* 99:181–213.
70. R. Yang, H. Xu, and Y. Zhang. (2003). Preparation, physical property and thermal physical property of phase change microcapsule slurry and phase change emulsion. *Solar Energy Materials and Solar Cells* 80:405–416.
71. G.B. Sukhorukov, D.G. Shchukin, W.F. Dong, H. Möhwald, V.V. Lulevich, and O.I. Vinogradova. (2004). Comparative analysis of hollow and filled polyelectrolyte microcapsules templated on melamine formaldehyde and carbonate cores. *Macromolecular Chemistry and Physics* 205:530–535.
72. M.N.A. Hawlader, M.S. Uddin, and M.M. Khin. (2003). Microencapsulated PCM thermal-energy storage system. *Applied Energy* 74:195–202.
73. L. Sánchez-Silva, J.F. Rodríguez, A. Romero, A.M. Borreguero, M. Carmona, and P. Sánchez. (2010). Microencapsulation of PCMs with a styrene-methyl methacrylate copolymer shell by suspension-like polymerisation. *Chemical Engineering Journal* 157:216–222.
74. J.M. Lagaron, R. Perez-Masia, and A. Lopez-Rubio. (2011). P201131063 Patent application (2011). Procedimiento de encapsulación de PCMs. Inventors: J.M. Lagaron, R. Perez-Masia, and A. Lopez-Rubio. Holder entity: CSIC.
75. R. Perez-Masia, A. Lopez-Rubio, and J.M. Lagaron. (2013). Development of zein-based heat-management structures for smart food packaging. *Food Hydrocolloids* 30:182–191.
76. L. Ji, Z. Lin, A.J. Medford, and X. Zhang. (2009). In-situ encapsulation of nickel particles in electrospun carbon nanofibers and the resultant electrochemical performance. *Chemistry - A European Journal* 15:10718–10722.
77. Y. Gu, D. Chen, X. Jiao, and F. Liu. (2007). LiCoO2-MgO coaxial fibers: Co-electrospun fabrication, characterization and electrochemical properties. *Journal of Materials Chemistry* 17:1769–1776.

78. H.S. Choi, J.G. Lee, H.Y. Lee, S.W. Kim, and C.R. Park. (2010). Effects of surrounding confinements of Si nanoparticles on Si-based anode performance for lithium ion batteries. *Electrochimica Acta* 56:790–796.
79. Y. Yu, L. Gu, C. Wang, A. Dhanabalan, P.A. Van Aken, and J. Maier. (2009). Encapsulation of Sn@carbon nanoparticles in bamboo-like hollow carbon nanofibers as an anode material in lithium-based batteries. *Angewandte Chemie - International Edition* 48:6485–6489.
80. L. Zou, L. Gan, F. Kang, M. Wang, W. Shen, and Z. Huang. (2010). Sn/C nonwoven film prepared by electrospinning as anode materials for lithium ion batteries. *Journal of Power Sources* 195:1216–1220.
81. S.R. Samarasinghe, K. Balasubramanian, and M.J. Edirisinghe. (2008). Encapsulation of silver particles using co-axial jetting. *Journal of Materials Science: Materials in Electronics* 19:33–38.
82. H. Cao, Z. Xu, H. Sang, D. Sheng, and C. Tie. (2001). Template synthesis and magnetic behavior of an array of cobalt nanowires encapsulated in polyaniline nanotubules. *Advanced Materials* 13:121–123.
83. B. Burteaux, A. Claye, B.W. Smith, M. Monthioux, D.E. Luzzi, and J.E. Fischer. (1999). Abundance of encapsulated C60 in single-wall carbon nanotubes. *Chemical Physics Letters* 310:21–24.
84. B.W. Smith, M. Monthioux, and D.E. Luzzi. (1999). Carbon nanotube encapsulated fullerenes: A unique class of hybrid materials. *Chemical Physics Letters* 315:31–36.
85. J.S. Wu, S. Dhara, C.T. Wu, K.H. Chen, Y.F. Chen, and L.C. Chen. (2002). Growth and optical properties of self-organized Au2Si nanospheres pea-podded in a silicon oxide nanowire. *Advanced Materials* 14:1847–1850.
86. H.Y. Chun, J.S. Goh, and Y.H. Kim. (2007). Characteristics of inertio-gravity waves revealed in rawinsonde data observed in Korea during 20 August to 5 September 2002. *Journal of Geophysical Research D: Atmospheres* 112:D16108–D16123.
87. W. Shi, W. Lu, and L. Jiang. (2009). The fabrication of photosensitive self-assembly Au nanoparticles embedded in silica nanofibers by electrospinning. *Journal of Colloid and Interface Science* 340:291–297.
88. I. Wilner, E. Katz. (2005). *Bioelectronics*. Wiley-VCH: Weinheim, Germany, 2005.
89. N.M. Bedford, G.D. Winget, S. Punnamaraju, and J. Steckl. (2011). Immobilization of stable thylakoid vesicles in conductive nanofibers by electrospinning. *Biomacromolecules* 12:778–784.
90. C. McDonagh, C.S. Burke, and B.D. MacCraith. (2008). Optical Chemical Sensors. *Chemical Reviews* 108:400–422.
91. A.L. Medina-Castillo, J.F. Fernandez-Sanchez, and A. Fernandez-Gutierrez. (2011). One-step fabrication of multifunctional core-shell fibers by co-electrospinning. *Advanced Functional Materials* 21:3488–3495.
92. P. Bansal, K. Bubel, S. Agarwal, and A. Greiner. (2012). Water-stable all-biodegradable microparticles in nanofibers by electrospinning of aqueous dispersions for biotechnical plant protection. *Biomacromolecules* 13:439–444.

5

Microencapsulation by Interfacial Polymerization

Fabien Salaün[1,2]

[1]*University of Lille Nord de France, Lille, France*
[2]*ENSAIT, GEMTEX, Roubaix, France*

Abstract

Microencapsulation is recognized as an effective method to protect various types of active agents in a variety of application fields such as medicine, agrochemicals, industrial chemicals, etc., and more recently textiles. Interfacial polymerization, including polycondensation, polyaddition, *in situ* polymerization as well as other heterophase polymerization processes, is defined by the formation of the capsules shell at or on a droplet or particles by polymerization of reactive monomers. This technology allows encapsulating a wide range of core materials, such as aqueous solutions, water-immiscible liquids and solid particles. In all cases, the phase containing the core substance is dispersed until it reaches the desired droplet size in a continuous phase. A key feature of the encapsulation is the diffusion of the reagents to the interface to react; and during the wall formation, the polymeric species create a barrier to diffusion and begin to limit the rate of the interfacial polymerization reaction.

Keywords: Microencapsulation, interfacial polymerization, particle formation, polycondensation, polyaddition, *in situ* polymerization

5.1 Introduction

Microencapsulation refers to the formation of polymeric particles with a range of diameters from nanometers to millimeters enclosing an active substance whatever its physical state, i.e., solid, liquid or gaseous form; and that exhibits several kinds of morphologies.

Vikas Mittal (ed.) Encapsulation Nanotechnologies, (137–174) © 2013 Scrivener Publishing LLC

Microparticles range in size between 1 and 1000 μm, and while they are greater than 1 mm they can be termed macroparticles, and those smaller than 1 μm are qualified as nanoparticles. Furthermore, particles having a mean diameter from 100 μm to 1000 μm are sometimes defined as milliparticles. Their morphologies depend mainly on the physico-chemical characteristics of the core material and the deposition process or formation of the membrane around it. Thus, microparticles may have regular or irregular shapes, and on the basis of their morphology, several classifications may be done as mononuclear or core/shell structure, multinuclear or polynuclear particles, and matrix particle or microsphere (Figure 5.1). Microspheres consist of polymeric network structure in which an active substance is distributed homogeneously, whereas microcapsules or core/shell structures exhibit a reservoir structure, i.e., the core substance is surrounded by a distinct polymeric layer [1, 2]. Furthermore, the layer and the core numbers are not limited to a single one, and double layered microcapsules shell, multilayer microcapsules or dual core particle are found in the literature; and the microparticles can also be obtained from clusters of microcapsules [3, 4].

More than 200 microencapsulation methods have been described in scientific literature and patents, most of them include three basic steps, i.e., enclosure of core component, formation of the microparticles, and hardening of it. Several routes have been developed for the synthesis of microcapsules, and these can be classified into two main categories, i.e., chemical processes and physical or mechanical processes [2]. This classification can be somewhat misleading since some methods classified as mechanical might involve a chemical reaction, and some chemical processes

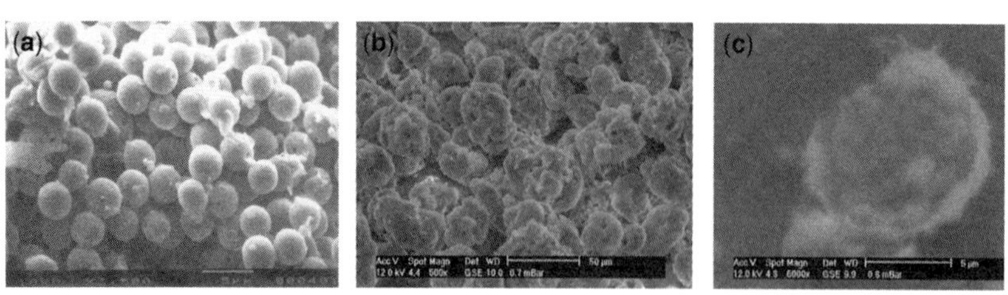

Figure 5.1 SEM micrographs of three representative types of microcapsules, (A) Core/shell microcapsules, (B) porous microspheres , and (C) crushed multinuclear microcapsules.

are only based on physical events. Whereas, in most of the microencapsulation techniques used as coating materials lipids, wax or polymers, chemical processes are based on the *in situ* formation of the polymeric shell where the starting materials are either monomers or pre-polymers. Whatever the chemical techniques used, such as suspension, dispersion, precipitation and emulsion polymerization or interfacial and *in situ* polycondensations, a chemical reaction is induced between one or several complementary monomers leading to the formation of the shell or a matrix to entrap the active substance. Then, even if the most popular process is interfacial polycondensation, when water is used as the continuous and storage phase, this method is operationally and economically attractive; anionic or radicalar polymerization can also be used to improve the electro-static stability and the macromolecular chain crosslinking or to work at room temperature according to the polymeric shell choice.

The choice of one method over another is not only based on the cost of processing, and the use of organic solvents for health and environment considerations; but also because of the nature of the active substance and the required properties of the obtained microparticles. Depending on the use of the microparticles, microencapsulation technology may be used for controlled release, protection, immobilization, structuration or functionalization [5]. Microencapsulation is an effective tool to obtain a desired delay or a burst effect of the active substance when the desired stimulus is encountered [6]. One of the main objectives of the microencapsulation is to limit the contact, to prevent undesired interactions between parts of a system, to separate the active substance from potential reaction partners, or to protect volatile or unstable substance from the surrounding medium until its release. Thus, microencapsulation is used for isolating substances until their activity is needed. This technology allows protection core compounds against oxidation, heat, moisture or humidity, alkali and acidity conditions, etc., to increase and to improve its shelf life. Artificial cells and enzyme immobilization have been earlier reported by Chang in 1964 [7]. The particle structuration allows turning liquid into a pseudo-solid state to improve flowdability, dispersibility and solubility. According to the final use, it is desirable to enhance the microparticle performance with their surface functionalization. Thus, the click chemistry concept was one of the recent concepts adapted by researchers to succeed in [8].

The functional performance of the microcapsules depends on the morphology, the chemical nature and the surface characteristics of the polymeric shell influenced by the process parameters [9]. The choice of a particular process is determined by the solubility characteristics of the active compound and the shell material. Thus, many factors such as polymer nature and concentration [10], emulsifiers concentration [11], stirring speed [12], temperature [13], and ratio of the volumes of the dispersed to the continuous phase [14] are selected as parameters controlling the encapsulation efficiency and the size distribution. Concerning the choice of the shell material, the diversity of natural, artificial and synthetic polymers provides a wide scope to design the membrane, It may be permeable for release application, semi-permeable for controlled release or for use as a micro-reactor, or impermeable to protect the core material from the external environment before it can be ruptured, melted, dried out, degraded or dissolved in a determined solvent.

Interfacial polymerization designates the cases where the polymerization reaction is located at the interface of two phases. According to Thies [15], interfacial polymerizations are polymerization reactions which are made to occur at interfaces, or to produce polymers that concentrate at interface to produce microcapsules. Thus, from this definition, he proposes five types of encapsulation processes, i.e., (i) the reagents for the shell formation are present in two mutually immiscible liquids; (ii) the reactant dissolved in the dispersed phase reacts with the continuous phase to produce a co-reactant which can react with the unreacted reactant at the dispersed side of the interface to form the shell; (iii) a reactant only present in the continuous phase is transported to the interface where polymerization occurs; (iv) the *in situ* polymerization, where the monomer or pre-polymer is dispersed in the continuous phase, the modification of the physico-chemical parameters of the system promotes the formation of the shell at the interface; and (v) a solution of water immiscible vinyl monomer, initiator, and core material is dispersed in an aqueous phase containing a dispersing agent, and the polymerization is initiated.

The objective of this chapter is to illustrate the use of interfacial polymerization to encapsulate liquid or solid core compounds. In the first section, general considerations associated with the formation of the microcapsules are drawn. The second part of this chapter considers the formation of polymeric particles through heterophase polymerization including emulsion polymerization, suspension polymerization, dispersion polymerization and miniemulsion polymerization, which are briefly described. In the last two parts, the microencapsulation methods carried out by interfacial polycondensation and *in situ* polycondensation are detailed. The shell formation mechanisms and the process parameters influencing it are discussed through the examples of polyamide, polyurethane and aminoplast resin microcapsules.

5.2 Generalities

The polymerization method, in which monomers polymerize around a droplet of an emulsion to form a solid polymeric shell, is one of the most often used methods to synthesize microparticles. This family has two subcategories, namely the polymerization *in situ*, where monomers or precondensate are usually added only to the aqueous phase of the emulsion either before, to perform it, or after according to the formulation parameters used; and the interfacial polymerization in which one of the monomers is solubilized in the continuous phase and the other in the dispersed phase. In most cases, in the first stages of the reaction, polymerization leads to the formation of prepolymer, with a relatively low molecular weight, and during its growth in size, it tends to be deposited onto the droplet surface of the core compound to form a continuous core/shell structure, also called microcapsule.

The microencapsulation process includes two main steps, e.g., the emulsification step which determines the size and the size distribution of the microcapsules; and the formation of the capsules. The emulsification step may be influenced at once by physical parameters such as apparatus configuration, stirring rate and volume ratio of the two phases, and by physicochemical properties such as interfacial tension, viscosities, densities and the chemical compositions of the two phases. The formation of microcapsules is greatly affected by the surfactant, which influences not only the mean diameter but also the stability of the dispersion. The surfactants used in the system have two roles, one to reduce the interfacial tension between oil and aqueous phases allowing formation of smaller microcapsules, and the other to prevent coalescence by its adsorption on the oil-water interface and therefore by forming a layer around the oil droplets [16–20]. The formation of a stable dispersion should be obtained either from a direct dispersion, an oil in water emulsion for an organosoluble active substance, or from an inverse dispersion, a water in oil emulsion for a hydrosoluble active substance. Thus, the choice of the surfactant formulation is mainly influenced by the kind of dispersion. A hydrophilic active agent having a HLB between 8 and 15 is used for a direct dispersion, while a HLB ranging from 3 to 6 is required for an inverse dispersion. Furthermore, the mean size and the size distribution are also affected by the process parameters such as the stirring rate and emulsification time, the nature and the concentration of the surfactant, the vessel configuration and the homogenization apparatus, the physico-chemical properties of the phases (nature, viscosity, density, etc.), the emulsification temperature, etc. [21, 22]. It has been reported in the literature that the decrease of the mean diameter may be obtained with the increase of the stirring rate [12], the decrease of the interfacial tension which can be realized with a increase of the surfactant concentration [23] as well as by the adding of a co-surfactant [11], a decrease of the dispersed phase volume ratio [24], and an increase of the temperature that leads to a decrease of the phase viscosities. The second step, or the synthesis of a core/shell particle or other possible morphologies, is mainly governed by the kinetic factors, i.e., the ability of the monomers, pre-polymer or polymer to react or to crosslink, and thermodynamic factors, indicating the minimum total free energy exchange in the system. However, Wakamatsu *et al.* also observed that the size of the microcapsules was dependent on the conditions of the polycondensation [25].

The interfacial polymerization method is one of the widely used microencapsulation methods, which is characterized by the fact that the obtained microparticles show high strength and stability, and the membrane permeability can be adjusted or modified by selecting appropriate combinations of monomers or crosslinking agents. The use of this method is usually done so as to obtain particle having a mean diameter between 1 to 30 μm, to enhance the structural anti-permeability to bring up a solid protection and to improve the thermal stability of these particles. The selection of the microencapsulation process is mainly governed by the choice of the chemical nature of shell materials and by the desired mean diameter. Furthermore, the polymeric shell represents only 5 to 15% in weight of the capsule, and it is possible to adjust the porosity and then the functionality of the shell to control the permeation properties. The main drawbacks of this technique are its complexity, the slowness of the reaction, the existence of parasite or secondary reactions which may disturb the system and create some unwanted reactive sides, the use of organic solvent and in some cases the nonbiocompatible carrier materials. The emulsification step of this process usually yields a broad size distribution influenced by the type of impeller used, the agitation rate as well as the concentration of emulsifier, temperature, etc. [26]. Furthermore, the chemical nature of the active substance is an important factor in designing the microencapsulation process, even though most of the syntheses concern non-water soluble active substance, the latter does not have some labile hydrogen to avoid reaction with isocyanate or acid chloride. Microcapsules with higher concentration cannot be easily produced by this process. It seems that the surfactant selection is one of the key parameters to limit the formation of aggregated or agglomerated structure. One of the strategies described in the patent literature is the use of the salt of partial ester of styrene-maleic anhydride copolymer as surfactant to encapsulate liquid or solid with a low melting point active substance [27].

The morphology of the microparticles is mainly determined by the solubility of the polycondensate molecules or oligomers formed in the dispersed phase. Indeed, highly insoluble oligomers lead to the formation of microcapsules since they deposit themselves around the droplets to form a primary shell; while they are entrapped they can grow inside the particles to form microcapsules or microspheres if they are soluble in the dispersed droplets [28].

From 1944, interfacial polymerization was extensively studied. Prior to its use to synthesize microcapsules, it was used to find new soft routes to synthesize polymer. One of the first descriptions was done by Smith in 1946 [29]. This method was widely described and reviewed by Morgan and Wittbecker who studied the formation of polyurethanes and polyamides at Dupont [30–33]. They were the first to describe the principles of interfacial polycondensation for the formation of a polymeric film. In 1965, Morgan proposed a list of the polymers carried out by this method with the process conditions [34]. This method was thereafter adapted to produce nylon microcapsules by Chang [7]. Interfacial polymerization was also patented in 1961, in which MacKinney described the formation of the shell around microcapsules [35]. The use of emulsifying agents to form dispersion of internal phase into the continuous phase in the microencapsulation process was assigned to Ruus in 1969 [36]. *In situ* polymerization was patented in 1961 [37, 38]. In this invention, monomers were dispersed only in the dispersed oil phase and polymerized, *in situ*, without co-reactive monomers in the water phase. A second shell wall was then formed by coacervation of the polymers used to disperse the oil phase. A review of the *in situ* encapsulation methods was provided by Baxter [39], Thies [2, 40], and Arshady and George [41].

5.3 Encapsulation by Heterophase Polymerization

5.3.1 Emulsion Polymerization

Emulsion polymerization is a method used for the preparation of nanoparticles, and generally involves emulsification of a hydrophobic monomer in an aqueous phase with the monomer polymerized using either a free radical initiator or high energy irradiation. This polymerization method was first reported in 1932 by Luther and Heuck [42], and later became a successful industrial process. The emulsion polymerization involves the formation of large monomer droplets emulsified with a surfactant above its critical micelle concentration (CMC) in aqueous phase. Polymerization begins with the introduction of a water soluble initiator by the formation of free radical and the addition of the first monomer units. These species diffuse through the monomer-swollen micelles. The propagation polymerization step is supported by the absorption of monomer molecules in the aqueous phase to maintain equilibrium. From the formation of stabilized nuclei to form primary particles, the polymerization is insured until all the monomers are consumed and the polymeric chains grow in the micelles. This process leads to the formation of nanoparticles having a mean diameter between 50 nm to 1 μm.

Emulsion polymerization was used in the 80s by Couvreur *et al.* to develop biodegradable polyalkylcyanoacrylate nanospheres [43–46]. Cyanoacrylic monomers are emulsified in the aqueous phase, and the anionic polymerization of these monomers occurs spontaneously at room temperature in the micelles to lead to the formation of colloidal nanospheres in acidic conditions. From the same kind of monomer, nanocapsules have been developed by Al Khoury *et al.* [47] and by Damgé *et al.* for insulin delivery [48] via an interfacial polymerization process in emulsion. Furthermore, emulsion polymerization is widely used for the encapsulation of inorganic particles in the presence or absence of surfactant. These methods are useful for modifying the surface of the inorganic particles and improving the physical properties of the polymers. These polymerization reactions are performed using either cationic active monomers [49], or non-ionic monomers such as vinyl acetate, methyl methacrylate [50] and styrene [51].

Emulsion polymerization techniques have also been used for the encapsulation of an antibiotic in polyacrylate nanoparticles [52, 53]. Yan *et al.* have reported the synthesis of porous microspheres of poly(styrene-*co*-acrylic acid) (PS-*co*-PAA) carried out by one-step soap-free emulsion polymerization [54]. They also demonstrated that the synthesis of their particles is ascribed to the phase separation between the encapsulated hydrophilic PAA segment and the hydrophobic PS domain within the PS-*co*-PAA microspheres. Microcapsules with a narrow size distribution containing liquid oily core can also be obtained by a two-step process as described by Ma *et al.* [55]. They observed that for a complete encapsulation, high oily core fraction, high monomer conversion and the addition of hydrophilic monomer are required. This process mainly allows the encapsulation of relatively hydrophobic solvent or active liquid substances [56]. Thus, in recent years polymethyl methacrylate, polyvinyl acetate, polystyrene and polyethyl methacrylate were mainly used as shell materials for phase change materials encapsulation by emulsion polymerization [57, 58].

5.3.2 Suspension Polymerization

The suspension polymerization technique leads to the formation of particle with an average diameter between 10 μm to 2 mm, close to the initial droplet. Most of the time, this process is referred to as bead polymerization or pearl polymerization. The reaction mixture containing initiator, water insoluble monomer and active agent is suspended as droplets in the aqueous phase. The stabilization of these droplets in the continuous medium is ensured by the use of vigorous agitation and hydrophilic polymeric stabilizers such as poly(vinyl alcohol), cellulosic derivative or polyvinylpyrrolidone. The aqueous phase may also contain fillers, buffers or electrolytes. A washing step is needed after completion of the process to recover the particles. The advantages of this method, mainly used for styrene, methyl methacrylate and vinyl chloride monomers, are the heat of polymerization absorption by the continuous phase, the formation of uniform spherical beads in size and their release characteristics [59–62]. Nevertheless, the coalescence of the particle during the polymerization process is one the main drawbacks.

Sanchez *et al.* reported the development of a microencapsulation process based on the suspension polymerization technique to entrap organic phase change material by a polystyrene shell [59]. They observed that the loading content and the particle size distribution vary with the kind and the nature of the core materials used. Furthermore, the method was more suitable for active substance with a hydrophobic nature than with a hydrophilic one. They also denote that the reaction temperature affects the particle morphology, and it should be contained between 98 to 113°C to obtain spherical morphology. The particle size is closely related to the stirring rate. And from the investigation of the paraffin/polymer mass ratio, they observed that the encapsulation was difficult for a ratio higher than 2 [60]. Furthermore, this encapsulation process was mainly governed by multiple simultaneous mechanisms, i.e., coalescence, break-up, nucleation and diffusion of monomer to the interface, which confers the size, the structure, as well as the surface properties of the particles. To improve these properties, they also copolymerized methyl methacrylate with styrene, which led to a decrease in reaction time and particle size. They also observed that the use of methyl methacrylate improved the loading content due to it higher reactivity and solubility in water. Amidst the strategies to decrease the mean diameter and to improve the uniformity of the particles, Li *et al.* proposed the use of ultrasonic dispersion to assist the suspension polymerization [63]. They obtained styrene-divinylbenzene porous microsphere in the range of 5–50 μm for cosmetic or pharmaceutical uses.

Suspension polymerization is also used for the encapsulation of inorganic particles. Thus, in 1985 the encapsulation of carbon black by butyl methacrylate copolymer was reported by Bakhshaee *et al.* [64]. Kim *et al.* employed this method to encapsulated calcium carbonate particles with PMMA and PS in 1995 [65]. Silica particles were also encapsulated in PMMA by Cooper & Vincent [66]. Duguet *et al.* studied the encapsulation by aqueous suspension polymerization in which they modified the surface of alumina through the condensation of 3-(trimethoxysilyl) propylmethacrylate [67]. The treated particles were dispersed in the initiator/methyl methacrylate solution, and then re-dispersed in aqueous solution containing poly(vinyl alcohol) as stabilizer.

5.3.3 Dispersion Polymerization

In a dispersion polymerization, all the reactants are dissolved in the continuous phase to form a homogeneous solution, and the polymerization is carried out in a single step. The process is based on precipitation polymerization, since at the end an insoluble polymer in spherical form is obtained. Dispersion polymerization is also recognized as an attractive alternative compared to other polymerization methods since monodisperse particles in a single batch can be obtained. The polymerization medium is a poor solvent for the resulting polymer, and then the macromolecules swell rather than precipitate which leads to locating the polymerization reactions within these particles. The microparticles formation occurs in two steps, i.e., the macromolecular chains collapse and coagulate to form particle nuclei stage, and particle growth stage. To maintain a good dispersion, suitable water soluble polymeric stabilizer is required. The particle size is much larger than obtained in emulsion polymerization (0.1–15 μm). The starting monomers mainly used in this process include styrene, methacrylate, divinylbenzene, ethylcyanoacrylate, hydroxyethylmethacryate and chlorostyrene. Nevertheless, the presence of the stabilizer considered as undesirable contaminants for certain applications is one of the limitations of this process [68].

Dispersion polymerization has been recognized as an alternative method for obtaining a micrometer-sized particle distribution and is used to obtain magnetic polymer composite from the polymerization of styrene [69], styrene and glycidyl methacrylate [70], or glycidyl methacrylate [71]. Goldshtein and Margel also proposed this method to formulate new flame retardant particles by polymerization of the pentabromobenzyl acrylate monomer [72]. One of the most frequently used methods to encapsulate inorganic particle involves the adsorption of monomer, prepolymer or coupling agent to initiate the polymerization. Thus, this method was used to encapsulate silica beads by polystyrene in a polar medium of ethanol and water by Bourgeat-Lami and Lang, where they demonstrated that polymerization occured only when the silica particles were modified with a coupling agent [73, 74]. PMMA was also used to encapsulate silica in supercritical carbon dioxide by Park *et al.* [75]. A two step dispersion polymerization was also employed for the encapsulation of titania particles either with poly[(St-*co*-DVB)-MAA], poly[(MAA-*co*-EGDMA)-MAA] or poly(St-*co*-MAA) [76–79].

5.3.4 Miniemulsion Polymerization

Miniemulsions are aqueous stable dispersions of oil droplet in the size range of 50 to 500 nm formed by shearing a system containing the dispersed phase (e.g., a water insoluble monomer), water, a surfactant and highly hydrophobic compound preventing or suppressing Ostwald ripening of the droplets [80]. This process allows all type of monomers to be used to form the particles, even if they are miscible with the continuous phase. Each droplet acts as a nanoreactor, and the polymerization occurs without changing their identity. The formation of the polymeric particles may be obtained by radical polymerization for styrene or acrylate derivatives, for example, by polyaddition for epoxy or polyurethane latex, by polycondensation which allows the formation of polyester, by anionic polymerization for polyamide or polybutylcyanoacrylate, etc. [81]. Furthermore, this technique is particularly attractive since it has an adjustable size under 500 nm, low surfactant concentration. It offers various possibilities for the encapsulation of different kind of materials, ranging from solid or liquid, organic or inorganic, or a hydrophobic or hydrophilic material, into a polymer shell [82–84]. Thus, crosslinked polystyrene, polymethacrylate, crosslinked poly(butyl acrylate), poly(styrene-*co*-γ-methacryloxypropyletrimet hoxysilane) hybrid shells were synthesized to encapsulate paraffin [84], nematic liquid crystals [85], *n*-hexadecane [86] and octane [87], respectively. Furthermore, polymeric nanocapsules can also be used as controlled delivery agents for dyes, fragrances, enzymes and protection of light sensitive components, etc.

5.4 Microencapsulation by Polyaddition & Polycondensation Interfacial

The microencapsulation of active substance by interfacial polycondensation or polyaddition involves the dispersion of the liposoluble phase in an aqueous continuous phase, or an aqueous phase in an organic phase, depending on the solubility medium of the core compound, and also induces the precipitation of the polymeric materials at the droplet interface. Each phase contains a dissolved specific monomer suitable to react with the other present in the other phase. The dispersed phase acts as a good solvent for the monomers but also serves as a non-solvent for the produced polymer. Therefore during polymerization, the system is composed of three mutually immiscible phases. Once the various monomers are added to the system, the reactions occur at the interface resulting in the formation of insoluble oligomers in the droplet with the tendency to precipitate at the interface to form primary shell around the droplets. The polymer formed is soluble neither in the dispersed phase nor in the continuous phase and precipitates at the interface, where it can grow. Further crosslinking reactions lead to the formation of growing shell by diffusion of monomers. When multifunctional monomers are used, a three-dimensional crosslinked system is obtained. Nevertheless, the thickness of the shell increases slowly due to the restricted diffusion of the starting monomers inducing the changes in layer morphology. The porosity of the capsules increases with the precipitation of the polymer at the interface and the solvent molecule diffusion through the wall. However, the main drawback of this method is the use of organic solvent, e.g., toluene or ethyl acetate, to solubilize both core material and reactive liposoluble monomer. The formation of the membrane around the droplets is governed by the swelling power of both phases, a porous structure may be obtained when the solvency of the medium for the polymer is low [28]. Furthermore, the morphology of the particles is influenced by the rate of precipitation of the polymer, and a higher rate promotes the formation of less uniform and more porous membrane. Therefore, the knowledge of the mechanism of the shell formation and polymerization reactions which occur during the synthesis is necessary to control the shape and the morphology of the particles [88, 89]. Various studies have shown that the polycondensation reactions mainly occur in the organic phase [90]. Nevertheless, it is also noticed that the location of the growth of the shell depends on the chemical compositions of the polymer, and for polyester the growth occurs in the aqueous side of the membrane [30]. Using the interfacial polycondensation method, active core compounds are encapsulated with different wall polymers such as polyamide, polyester and polyethyleneimine, while polyurea and polyurethane are synthesized from polyaddition reactions (Table 5.1). Even if most of the reported methods employ

Table 5.1 Main polymers and monomers used during the synthesis of microparticles through interfacial polycondensation (and polyaddition) – Principal application fields of microcapsules.

Polymeric wall	First shell wall component	Second shell wall component	Microcapsules applications - examples
Polyamide	**Amine (di-, poly-)** 1,6-hexamethylene diamine, Diethylenetriamine, Ethylenediamine L-lysine, —	**Acid chloride (di-, poly-)** Sebacoyle chloride, Terephtaloyl chloride, 1,3,5-benzene tricarbonyl trichloride, Phosgene, —	**Purpose (& mechanism)** **Core material released** • Permeable wall (diffusion • Semipermeable wall (retention of larger and release of smaller molecules) • Impermeable wall (external pressure, explosion, burning, mechanical abrasion, swelling…) **Core material permanently protected** • Impermeable wall **Fields** • Phytosanitary • Chemical industry • Biomedical • Biotechnology • Pharmaceutical industry • Buildings • Textile industry • Electronics • Graphics and printing • Agriculture
Polyurea	**Amine (di-, poly-)**	**Isocyanate (di-, poly-)** Toluene 2,4-diisocyanate, Methylene diisoyanate, Diphenyl methylene diisocyanate, Hexamethylene 1,6-diisocyanate, Isophorone diisocyanate, —	
Polyurethane	**Amine (di-, poly-)**	**Chloroformate (di-, poly-)** 1,3,5-benzene trichloroformate, Hexamethylene chloroformate, Phenylene – bis-chloroformate, —	
Polyurethane	**Diol, polyol** Polycaprolactone , Xylitol, di-, tri-methyl propanediol, Poly(ethylene glycol),	**Isocyanate (di-, poly-)**	

(Continued)

Polymeric wall	First shell wall component	Second shell wall component	Microcapsules applications - examples
	Poly(propylene glycol), Castor oil 1,4-butane diol, 1,6-hexane diol, Ethylene glycol, 2,2-bis (4-hydroxyphenyl propane), Bisphenols A, —		**Applications** • Proteins, enzymes, • Cosmetics (UV absorbers, sunscreens,…) • Pesticides, agrochemicals, … • Dyes (pressure sensitive copying papers), toners, thermochromic ink • Adhesives, catalysts, self healing • Fragrances, essential oils • Phase change materials, cooling agent, • Electronick ink displays, liquid crystals displays, • Chelating agent, hydrogels, • Flame retardant, …
Polysulphonamide	Amine (di-, poly-)	Sulphonyl chloride (di-, poly-)	
Polyester	Diol, polyol	Acid chloride (di-, poly-)	
Polycarbonate	Diol, polyol	Chloroformate (di-, poly-)	
Polyethyleneimine			
Other polymeric walls	Gelatin Chitosan Gelatin Albumine Polymine Acid carboxilic (di-, poly-)	Diisocyanate Diisocyanate Terephtaloyl chloride Sebacoyl chloride Epoxy resin Epoxy resin	

oil-in-water or water-in-oil systems, oil-in-oil systems may also be used to prepare microcapsules especially for polyurethane and polyurea microcapsules; in this case, the continuous medium is often a paraffin oil [91]. Kobašlija and McQuade studied the preparation of polyurea microcapsules carried out by an interfacial polycondensation in methanol-in-cyclohexane system [92].

5.4.1 Location of the Film Formation

Microencapsulation by interfacial polycondensation can be carried out in two systems, i.e., in direct emulsion (oil in water-O/W) with the organic phase dispersed in water, and; in inverted emulsion (water in oil-W/O) with the aqueous phase dispersed in the organic phase. The polymerization reactions occur at, or in a thin region adjacent to, the interface of the two immiscible phases, and since the polymer formed is insoluble in both the phases, it accumulates as a film at the surface of contact between the phases. The location of the polymerization is determined by the partition coefficient of each monomer in both solvents used. This coefficient depends on the chemical nature of the monomers and the solvents, the monomer concentrations, and the pH of the solution which controls the availability of the aqueous monomer. Thus, the reaction begins where the product of the monomer concentrations is highest. The reaction occurs in a thin layer in the organic phase close to the interface, since the solubility in water of the monomer dispersed in the organic phase is negligible.

5.4.2 Reaction Rate

The reaction rate depends on the chemical nature of monomers and organic solvent as well as the diffusion factors of the reactive compounds. Nevertheless, during the microencapsulation, the factors limiting the polycondensation rate are not the same, since the monomers diffusion is hampered and slowed by the film formation. Then, the rate of monomer transfer decreases, and it accumulates at the interface region. Therefore, the encapsulation yield and the molecular polymer weight are a function of reaction time. For homogenous polycondensation, Morgan [30] estimated a rate value in the range of 10^2 to 10^6 $m^3/kmol\ s$; for capsules from condensation of terephtaloyl dichloride (TDC) and diethylenetriamine (DETA) in the Janssen and Nijenhuis study [93], the polycondensation rate constant was in between 10^4 and 10^6 m^3/kmol s, meaning in the same range of those used by Dhumal *et al.* [94] and Yadav *et al.* [95] for polyurethane microcapsules.

5.4.3 Shell Formation

As described previously, the formation mechanism of the microcapsules is complex due to the simultaneous occurrence of polymer phase separation and film formation, and occurs in two consecutive steps, i.e., formation of the primary shell by precipitation of the initially-formed oligomer molecules and membrane growth by diffusion of one of the monomers through the membrane. Thus, the type of organic phase, and especially the organic solvent, play an important role in the microencapsulation process. Indeed, the two steps are governed by the solvency of the medium [28], and the solvent should favor the precipitation of the polymer while allowing the aqueous monomer diffusion through the membrane to provide its growth. Therefore, the choice of the solvent is important since it should sufficiently swell the polymer to allow the diffusion [96], and the polymer-solvent interactions also influence the morphology of the resulted membrane as well as the wall thickness. Thus, for the production of polyamide microcapsules, a binary mixture of cyclohexane-chloroform in the ratios 4:1 or 3:1, deduced from sedimentation tests, has been widely used. Indeed, the polymer was swollen by chloroform and precipitate in cyclohexane [97]. For polyurethane microcapsules, toluene [98, 99] or a mixture of xylene and Miglyol 812 [90] is selected as lipophilic phase.

Polyamides, and more specially Polyamide 6–10, are widely studied in the microcapsules formation by interfacial polycondensation. The reaction is based on the Schotten-Bauman reaction which takes place at interface of the aqueous/organic phases, between 1,6-hexamethylène diamine and sebacoyl chloride. In the first step, the acid chloride reacts with an amine to form an amide. Addition of a base and pH control is required to neutralize the acid formed. For the production of polyamide microcapsules, the pH control plays an important role since it is not limited to the elimination of hydrochloric acid, but also influences the polycondensation rate since an increase leads to an increase of activity of the diamine and then favors its partition to the organic phase [97]. Crosslinking agents are also used in addition to the raw monomers to improve the thermomechanical properties of the capsules [100, 101]. Furthermore, the choice of the starting monomers, such as linear or aromatic chloride, influences the membrane permeability and therefore the release properties [101–103]. The mechanism of polyamide microcapsule formation from reaction between terephtaloyldichloride and diethylenetriamine was studied by Janssen and Nijenhuis [93, 104, 105]. They showed that the rate of polyamide production in the organic phase was limited by the DETA diffusion through this membrane after the formation of the first layer. Furthermore, the transfer rate of the DETA, inversely proportional to membrane thickness, was found to be linked to the reaction time. They also observed that the rate of wall formation decreased as the reaction time proceeded. The permeability of the membrane increased as the monomer concentration ratio increased, and the adding of a diamine reduced it. Danicher *et al.* showed that the membrane thickness was not only a function of time but also of the crosslinker concentration [106].

Polyurea and polyurethane microcapsules were widely studied in the 90s [9, 14, 16, 88, 89, 95, 107–111]. For the formation of the polyurethane, the mechanism of the polyaddition of the diisocyanate at the droplet interface can be illustrated through the following reaction schemes (Figure 5.2). Once polyisocyanate is added to the system, reactions occur at the interface resulting in the formation of insoluble oligomers in the droplet, with the tendency to precipitate at the organic side of the interface to form primary shell around

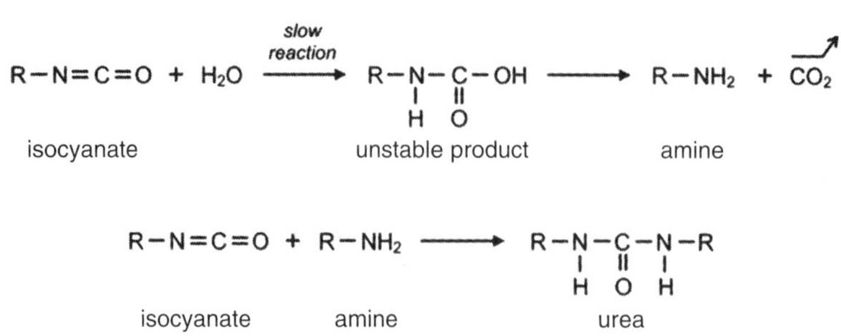

Figure 5.2 Reactions of isocyanate functions.

the droplets. Further crosslinking reactions lead to the formation of growing shell by diffusion of monomers. Nevertheless, the thickness of the shell increases slowly due to the restricted diffusion of the starting monomers inducing layer morphology changes. The porosity of the capsules increases with the precipitation of the polymer at the interface and the solvent molecule diffusion through the wall. In the first reaction, diisocyanate or isocyanate end groups react with hydroxyl groups of polyol to form a urethane linkage, and therefore the polyurethane chains. In the second reaction, isocyanate monomers can be slowly hydrolyzed at the interface to form an unstable amino acid group which dissociates in amine end group and carbon dioxide. This reaction occurring in the oil side of the interface depends mainly on the water molecules diffusion in the medium or through the polymer shell network. The formation and release of CO_2 during the membrane formation contribute to increase the porosity of the particles. The amine end group reacts with the isocyanate end group to form a urea linkage in the third reaction. Other reactions can occur during the shell growth, as the reaction between an isocyanate end group and urethane or urea unit results in the formation of an allophanate or a biuret, respectively, creating interconnections between the polymer chains.

In the same way, the polyurethane shell can also be formed by reaction of the hydroxyl groups of cellulose acetate butyrate (CAB) with isocyanate groups at the interface [112]. Furthermore, Cho *et al.* [113] observed that the formation of a polyurethane shell should also be provided from the reaction of the isocyanate with the hydroxyl groupments of the surfactant. This particularity was also used by Saihi *et al.* to formulate polyurethane microcapsules from Span 85 and diphenyl methylene diisocyanate (MDI) [114]. To enhance the reactivity of the synthesis, isocyanate monomers can be replaced by polyurethane prepolymer, which can reduce the porosity of the thicker shell since the isocyanate hydrolysis is limited, and allows obtaining a thermoplastic rather than a thermosetting with no covalent bond between the shell and the active substance. The chemical nature of the monomers has a significant effect on pore morphology and therefore on release behavior of these particles. Thus, Jabbari *et al.* showed that the porosity and the pore size of the shell significantly decreased when the amount of chain-extending agent increased [115]. Hong and Park also observed that a decrease of the molecular weight of the polyol led to the formation of more porous and permeable membrane due to an increase of the hydrophobic hard segment [89]. The temperature of the reaction is one of the most important parameters to consider during the process since it controls the reaction kinetics and allows the formation of an external porous layer as described by Frère *et al.* [111]. Polyurethane, as well polyamide microcapsules, can also be formulated in direct or inverse emulsion. One of the last trends for an inverse emulsion is to replace toluene, xylene, cyclohexane or hexadecane by a nontoxic solvent such as Miglyol 812. Even if the isocyanate is easily solubilized in Miglyol, the chemical shell composition differs. Indeed, it was reported that during the synthesis urea and urethane bonds are created, and the diol used has as much affinity with Miglyol than with other organic solvent, inducing a better diffusion that leads to a higher molar amount of urethane functions [116].

5.4.4 Influence of the Synthesis Parameters on the Formation of the Shell

The influence of the monomer concentration on the shell formation was reported by Yadav *et al.* [95], Dhumal *et al.* [94] and Wagh *et al.* [117] for a polyurea system based on the reaction of hexamethylene diamine (HMDA) and methylenebis(cyclohexyl isocyanate) (HMDI). They showed that the rate of the polycondensation was controlled by the kinetics until the limiting monomer conversion of about 80%; and during this stage, the rate was proportional to the product of the initial monomers concentrations. This fact was also observed by Bouchemal *et al.* [118] for the synthesis of polyamide nanocapsules from TDC and DETA.

Wagh *et al.* [117] also discussed the effect of the organic solvent nature constituting the dispersed phase. They compared the reaction rates obtained with cyclohexane, p-xylene, CCl_4 and toluene, and they showed that the reaction rate was not related to the partition coefficient of the monomer in the aqueous phase, but it increased with the decrease of solvent polarity. Moreover, the fact that the kinetic depends on the organic solvent nature also justifies that the reaction occurs in the organic side of the interface.

In most cases the interfacial polycondensation is carried out at room temperature. While some authors mention the influence of the temperature of the reaction kinetics, few of them take it into account in the models. Nevertheless, it seems that a increase leads to an increase of the secondary reactions and decrease in the molecular weight of the resulted polymer with a lower encapsulation yield, even if Frère *et al.* denote a faster reaction rate [111].

The stirring rate applied during the formation of the polymeric shell can sometimes lead to the formation of aggregated structure as described by Choi *et al.* [119]. This phenomenon can also occur in the formation of polyamide microcapsules when the stirring rate is too high. In their study, Siddhan *et al.* propose a reduction after the formation of the primary shell from toluene diisocyanate and diethylene triamine monomers [120].

5.4.5 Influence of the Synthesis Parameters on the Particles Properties

The properties of microcapsules obtained by interfacial polymerization may be controlled by a number of factors: the chemical nature of monomer(s) and the conditions under which the polycondensation reaction is performed determine the chemical composition and the porosity of the microcapsule membrane and the degree of polymer crosslinking. The microcapsule size distribution can also be controlled by appropriate modifications of the process conditions (surfactant type and concentration, stirring rate, etc.). These characteristics affect the release of the core substance through the shell [14, 105, 109, 115, 121] or by rupture related to its mechanical properties. The mechanical resistance of the polymeric shell depends on the capsules' size and can be adjusted with crosslinkers or by an increase of the shell thickness.

For a release system by diffusion, the shell permeability, which depends on the shell thickness, surface morphology, crosslinking density, crystallinity index, as well as the chemical nature of the polymer, is a key parameter, since its structure governs the release kinetics of the encapsulated substance. Most previous cited parameters are related to the nature of the monomers used. Thus, the shell thickness depends on the amount of monomers as well as their chemical structure. According to Persico *et al.* [122], the use of trifunctional monomers leads to the crosslinked shell and is therefore thicker, while the use of bifunctional monomers increase the polymer crystallinity. The crosslinking density can be adjusted by the adding of crosslinkers, which enlarge the size pores and then affect the kinetics of the release. The crystallinity index depends on the reaction rate, and an increase of it decreases the release of the core compound.

5.4.6 Nanoencapsulation by Interfacial Polycondensation

Since the last decade, methods derived from interfacial polymerization are also used to produce nanocapsules. Then, to encapsulate an active ingredient sensitive to light, heat and oxygen, Bouchemal *et al.* [123] used an interfacial polycondensation coupled to a spontaneous emulsification of oil in water emulsion to obtain polyurethane or poly(ether urethane) shell. Furthermore, Montasser *et al.* [124–126] showed that the stability of nanocapsules was enhanced by the use of shell based on crosslinked polymer. The permeability of this later is related to its crystallinity and contributes to the growth of nanocapsule membrane by the diffusion of the hydrophilic monomers to get stable colloidal suspensions. Polyurea nanoparticles containing curcumin from various diamine chain length were synthesized by using MDI as an oil-soluble monomer and various diamines (i.e., EDA, BDA, and HMDA) as the water-soluble monomers through spontaneous emulsion, emulsion diffusion and interfacial polymerization [127]. It was also observed that the thermal properties and thermal stability were influenced by the processes choice and the diamine chain length. Thus, it was found that the suitable curcumin loaded nanoparticles were synthesized with polyurea shell based on EDA or HMDA by spontaneous emulsion.

5.5 Microencapsulation by *In Situ* Polymerization

Encapsulation carried out by an *in situ* polymerization, e.g., polycondensation or polyaddition, is based on the presence of monomer or pre-polymer only in a single phase. According to the monomer, pre-polymer and resulting polymer solubilities in the continuous medium, Arshady and George denoted three distinct types of polymerization: (i) suspension polycondensation when the starting monomer was insoluble in the polymerization medium; (ii) precipitation polycondensation if the continuous phase was a solvent and a precipitant for the monomer and polymer, respectively; (iii) dispersion polycondensation for a system when the polymerization medium is a good and poor solvent for the monomer and polymer, respectively [41]. Furthermore, in the *in situ* microencapsulation class, the microcapsules' walls can be formed from starting monomers or pre-condensates present only in the discontinuous phase or in the continuous phase. During the polymerization, they migrate to the interface between the continuous and the discontinuous, resulting in the formation of the microcapsule shell. This technique also includes free radical polymerization and the incorporation of polyisocyanate and polyol compounds within the discontinuous phase [128].

Among various shell materials presumably impermeable, amino resins, more especially melamine–formaldehyde and urea-formaldehyde resins, play a main role in the patent literature [129]. Searches in "freepatentsonline," a patent database, revealed that in September 2012, there were more than 2500 patents on microencapsulation carried out by *in situ* polymerization (keywords used "microcapsules" & "*in situ* polymerization"). In 1989 and 1990, Dietrich *et al.* published a series of reports on amino resin microcapsules including literature and patent reviews [129], preparation and morphology [130], release properties [131] and surface tension of the resins and mechanism of capsules formation [132]. This process was used to produce microcapsules for various applications, such as fragrances or essential oils [133–135], pesticides [136], animal repellents [137], fire retardants [138], pressure-sensitive copying papers, photosensitive color-producing microcapsules, electronic ink [139, 140], phase change materials [20], adhesives, curing agent, and self-healing materials [141], enzyme electrodes, and extraction and separation of precious metals. The polymerization *in situ* allows the formation of microcapsules containing water-immiscible dispersed phase, with improved mechanical properties [142] and thermal stability [143, 144]. The use of melamine-formaldehyde resin has attracted many researchers to try to improve the thermal stability of microencapsulated core compound. Furthermore, melamine-formaldehyde prepolymers offer some advantages to the synthesis of microcapsules due to their high reactivity, and therefore a short reaction time and a controlled amount of polymer are required to form the shell with a high-loading content. The properties of the membrane depend not only on its chemical structure but also on all the synthesis conditions. The polycondensation of the amino resin occurs in the continuous phase, and the phase separation is linked to the pH and the formaldehyde/melamine molar ratio [20, 130, 132, 134].

The first step of *in situ* polymerization is to disperse a water immiscible liquid or solide core materials in an aqueous phase containing monomers (i.e., melamine and formaldehyde; urea and formaldehyde; urea, melamine and formaldehyde), or commercial prepolymers (i.e., partially methylated trimethylolmelamine, dimethylolomelamine, hexamethoxy-methylolmelamine condensates), surfactant and water at a pH of 4 (Figure 5.3). This dispersion is the determining step for establishing the size distribution of the final particles having the desired physical properties. The pH value of 4 helps to reduce surface tension of the continuous phase since the intermolecular distance between surfactant molecules is

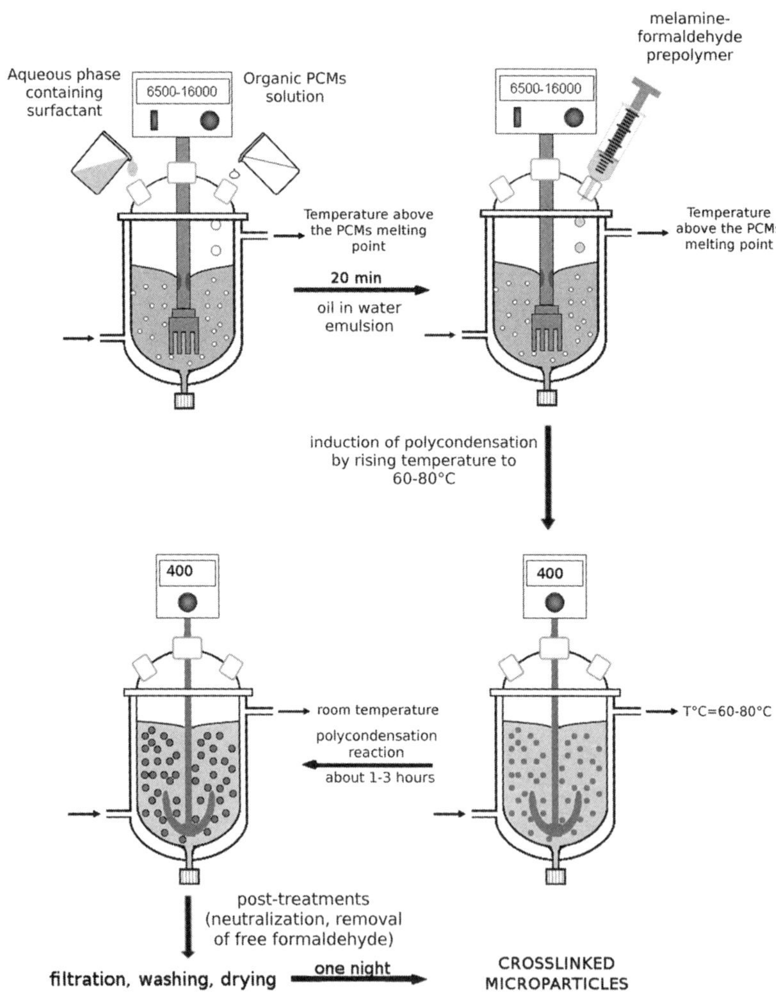

Figure 5.3 Example of the production of encapsulated phase change material.

decreased, leading to an enhanced emulsification [20]. Furthermore, the phase volume ratio was established in order to obtain a narrow size distribution and a mean diameter within the range of 1 to 10 μm in most studies. In the second step of the synthesis, the amino pre-polymers which are initially soluble in the continuous phase are activated under acidic catalyst action and undergo etherification reactions. This gives rise to amino pre-polymer of relatively low molecular weight in the continuous phase. In the third step, the reduction of hydroxyl content corresponding to a decrease of the water solubility of the amino resin can promote the phase separation from the continuous phase as a liquid solution relatively is rich in active pre-polymer. Thus, this phase can deposit itself as a continuous primary shell on the core material droplet by the formation of hydrogen bonds with the hydrophilic groups of the nonionic surfactant as the pre-polymer molecular weight increases. Finally, in the fourth step, due to enhanced resin concentration in the boundary layer, polycondensation reaction occurs to form a crosslinked shell either by ether or methylene linkages. Since the polycondensation occurs entirely on the aqueous phase side of the interface, the reactive agent does not have to be dissolved in the core material and thus capsular morphology is obtained.

5.5.1 Melamine-Formaldehyde Microcapsules

The formation of the microcapsule shell occurs in three consecutive stages. In the first step, the melamine-formaldehyde pre-polymers obtain H^+ by changing into active pre-polymers under acidic condition, which results in an increase of the etherification degree due to a reduction in hydroxyl group concentration. Then, the water solubility of the pre-polymer decreases and the material separates from the continuous phase as a liquid solution relatively concentrated in active pre-polymer. During the second step, the amino resins wet the dispersed core compound droplets to create primary shell around them. The concentration of resin in the boundary layer is enhanced by the hydrophilic/hydrophobic interactions of the partial methylolated melamine, and therefore it occurs by an enrichment of resin molecules within the interface. Thus, the resin condensation proceeds much faster in the boundary layer than in the volume phase, allowing the formation of tougher capsule walls. From this step, it is possible to recover particle under powder form. Nevertheless the capsule walls are not yet thermo-mechanically stable and not completely hardened, and the particles might have collapsed during drying. In the last step the reaction rate of the polycondensation at the interface is increased with the result of microcapsule shell formation. During the polycondensation process, the particle surface becomes more and more hydrophobic, and according to the pH level, the shell is crosslinked either by ether linkage or methylene bridges as shown in Figure 5.4. Furthermore, the surface morphology depends mainly on the pH value, thus, a low pH value promotes the formation of methylene bridges affecting the amino resin solubility and therefore obtains a rough surface. The formation of higher oligomers of melamine-formaldehyde polymer with the formation of methylene bridges can be described as the reaction of bound CH_2OH group with H (Figure 5.5).

(a) $\text{-NCH}_2\text{OCH}_3 + \text{ROH} \overset{H^+}{\rightleftharpoons} \text{-NCH}_2\text{OR} + \text{CH}_3\text{OH}$

(b) $\text{-NCH}_2\text{OR} + \text{HOCH}_2\text{N-} \overset{H^+}{\rightleftharpoons} \text{-NCH}_2\text{OCH}_2\text{N-} + \text{ROH}$

(c) $\text{-NCH}_2\text{OR} + \text{HN-} \xrightarrow{H^+} \text{-NCH}_2\text{N-} + \text{ROH}$

(d) $\text{-NCH}_2\text{OR} + \text{HOCH}_2\text{N-} \xrightarrow{H^+} \text{-NCH}_2\text{N-} + \text{ROH} + \text{CH}_2\text{O}$

(e) $\text{-NCH}_2\text{OR} + \text{ROCH}_2\text{N-} \xrightarrow{H^+} \text{-NCH}_2\text{N-} + \text{CH}_2(\text{OR})_2$

(f) $\text{-NCH}_2\text{OH} + \text{HN-} \xrightarrow{H^+} \text{-NCH}_2\text{N-} + \text{H}_2\text{O}$

Figure 5.4 Crosslinking reactions of melamine resin.

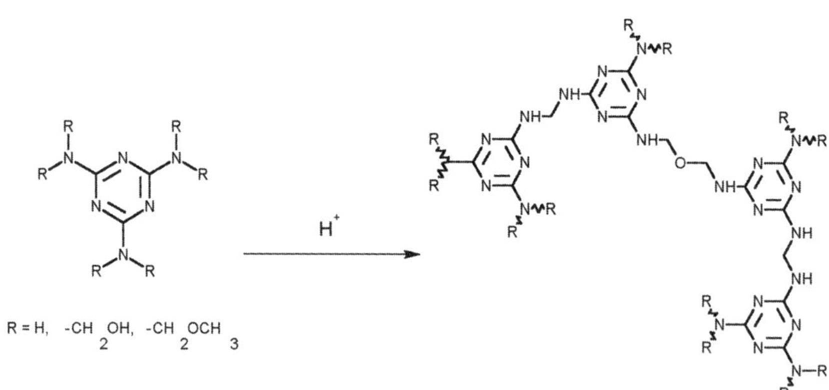

Figure 5.5 Formation of the amino-shell.

The use of an *in situ* method to prepare microcapsules results in a high loading content (from 60–80 wt.%) and a narrow size distribution; nevertheless the weight ratio of the core/shell materials also affected the particle size, its distribution and the surface morphology of the microcapsules [20]. These particles have better thermal and mechanical stability properties than those synthesized from other polymers [145]. To improve their toughness, resorcinol can be added to the system [146]. However, the presence of free-formaldehyde after forming the shell may cause environmental and health problems as it is relatively difficult to eliminate all formaldehyde which can be continuously released from the resultant microcapsules. To solve this problem, Li *et al.* [147] proposed the incorporation of formaldehyde once, and urea or melamine three times; on the other hand, Šumiga *et al.* [148] observed that the use of ammonia during the post-treatment process allowed the decrease of the formaldehyde content level in the suspension.

The morphology of melamine-formaldehyde microcapsules is deeply influenced by the pH, the temperature and the core content. The surface of the particles is sometimes found with increased roughness due to the presence of fragments, tiny particles or unreacted amino resin deposited during the recovery (Figure 5.6). Salaün & Vroman in their study observed that the introduction of a complementary bifunctional monomer to

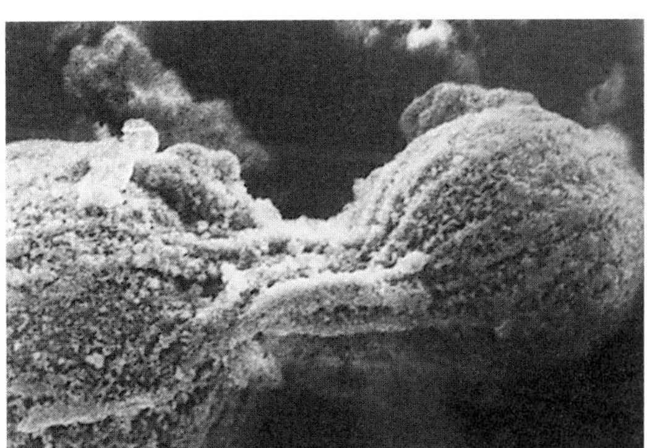

Figure 5.6 SEM micrograph of MF microcapsules with tiny particles on the surface.

increase the chain length during the synthesis limited the interpenetration between the core compound and the amino resin, and therefore the surface appeared smoother [144].

This process is not restricted to very hydrophobic core active substance, since it was widely studied for the encapsulation of intumescent flame retardant, especially in the case of ammonium polyphosphate (APP) by Wu *et al.* These authors proposed several amino polymers, i.e., melamine-formaldehyde [149] melamine-formaldehyde and dipentaerythritol [150, 151], urea-melamine-formaldehyde [152], PVA-melamine-formaldehyde [153], starch-melamine-formaldehyde [154], urea-formaldehyde and melamine formaldehyde to succeed in the formation of a double shell [155], and melamine-poly(ethylene glycol)-formaldehyde [156]. APP was firstly dispersed in ethanol under stirring, before adding a suitable amount of amino prepolymer. Then, the pH was adjusted to 4–5 with sulphuric acid, and the temperature was kept constant at 80°C for 2 h. The particles were recovered by filtration, washing and drying at 105°C. The shell polymer prevented the core from the attack of moisture, and moreover, the lowering of particles size resulted from the increase in the hydrophobic nature of shell polymer, and thus, the lowest size distribution was established for amino resin modified with PEG and starch which was in correlation with the water solubility. Furthermore, recovered particles have a rougher surface than raw APP due to the deposition of melamine-formaldehyde macromolecular chains onto the surface, and then the shell appears similar to a multilayer structure.

5.5.2 Urea-Formaldehyde Microcapsules

Urea is also used to form the capsule wall by condensation polymerization with formaldehyde. The process consists of the reaction of urea and formaldehyde to produce methylol urea, which further condenses under acidic conditions to form the shell material [141, 157–160]. The microencapsulation process is divided in two steps in which firstly, the active substance is emulsified in urea-formaldehyde resin solution, and then the pH of emulsion liquid is adjusted into acidic conditions to promote the reaction of urea with formaldehyde. Two reactions occur when urea reacts with formaldehyde. In the first addition reaction, formaldehyde reacts with H of amine to form methylol. In the second reaction, condensation takes place between hydroxyl groups of methylol and H of amine leading to the formation of methylene link between two amines of two urea molecules. Both reactions are catalyzed either by OH^- or H^+. It was also shown that the rate of the addition reaction in basic condition was as high as the rate in acidic condition, while the rate of condensation reaction was faster in acidic than in basic condition [161]. Some authors reported the presence of both porous and nonporous zone as a common feature of urea-formaldehyde microcapsules. The roughness is also attributed to the deposition of the nanoparticles on the surface during the process, thus to obtain smooth surface capsules a high final pH value, low wall material and high surfactant concentration are required to minimize the presence of nanoparticles [160]. Furthermore, it was noticed that polymeric surfactant, such as poly(ethylene-alt-maleic anhydride), plays a main role in the formation of capsules by phase separation, since it should have reactive functional groups to provide reaction footholds and can adsorb at the interface to give reaction sites [162].

5.5.3 Silica Microcapsules

The sol-gel process coming from the ceramic industry can also be regarded as an *in situ* polymerization encapsulation process. This field of encapsulation is relatively new. This kind of encapsulation involves the evolution of inorganic networks through the formation of a colloidal suspension also called sol, and gelation of the sol to form a network in a continuous liquid phase was labeled as gel. In each case, the precursor used to synthesize the particles consists of a metal or metalloid element surrounded by various active ligands. Alkoxysilane such as tetramethoxysilane, 3-aminopropyl triethoxysilane and tetraethoxysilane are the most appropriated metal alkoxides due to their low toxicity and to the formation of glass capsules. The silica precursor is often dissolved in ethanol or a similar alcohol, and is there hydrolyzed to silicic acid, which condenses to give a silica gel network [163]. The gelation of the sol is accomplished through low-temperature hydrolysis and condensation reactions. The most popular use of the sol-gel process is the production of immobilized biomaterials such as enzymes or microorganism, but it can also be used in the food industry for food ingredient such as flavors, preservative agents, vitamins and nutrients [164]. Other uses include the encapsulation of dye [165, 166], of phase change material [167], and of water soluble drug [168]. The versatility of this process allows encapsulation of hydrophilic as well as hydrophobic active substances. Furthermore, according to the hydrophobic or hydrophilic characteristics of the encapsulation precursors, this process can be classified into two different methods, i.e., in the case of the hydrophobic encapsulation precursors, the water mixture solutions containing the active compounds and the gelling agents (acid or base) are emulsified into oil phase, and then the emulsions are solidified by adding the precursors into systems [169]; and in the hydrophilic encapsulation precursor, the water mixture solutions of the hydrophilic precursors and the hydrophilic active compounds are emulsified into oil solutions, and then the emulsions in liquid states are solidified by adding gelling agents into the systems [170]. One of the main advantages of this method is the very mild processing conditions, e.g., room temperature, slightly acidic or basic pH, the small particle size (from submicron to a few tens of microns), and the affordable raw material [171]. Furthermore, the advantageous properties of inorganic shell materials are expected in terms of higher physical strength and higher thermal conductivity than those of the polymeric one [163].

5.6 Conclusion

In this chapter, it has emerged that a number of methods based on interfacial polymerization are available for the preparation either of microparticles or nanoparticles. These methods are based on the polymerization of a monomer, prepolymer or various complementary monomers into a homogenous or heterogeneous phase, or with the precipitation of the preformed polymer. Some of these processes present drawbacks from a technological and environmental standpoint, and should be studied by the book of specifications regarding the final product end-use. Furthermore, the performances of the capsules are affected by the choice of the polymeric shell, the degree of crosslinking, the wall thickness, the mean diameter and size distribution, as well as the physical form of the final product and the presence of additive. Thus, within each of the polymer categories, e.g., polyamide, polyurethane, polyurea, etc., a range of polymers can be formulated according to the desired properties. Interfacial polymerization methods are more attractive to prepare microcapsules with higher concentrations and higher core loading. In the future, research should include the elucidation of membrane formation mechanism to optimize the process parameters, and therefore, the microcapsules properties and the development of new microencapsulation processes to lead to the creation of new functionalized products. One of the latest trends is the modification of the particle surface to obtain functionalized microcapsules either to enhance their incorporation on a substrate or to obtain particles with a desired release rate. Thus, the application fields of these microcapsules may be extended in the near future with the use of new processes such as supercritical CO_2, or with the development of a new microcapsules classes such as complexing materials.

References

1. S.K. Ghosh. Functional coatings and microencapsulation: A general perspective. In *Functional coatings by polymer microencapsulation*, S.K. Ghosh, ed. WILEY-VCH Verlag GmbH & Co. KGaA, 2006.
2. C. Thies. A survey of microencapsulation processes. In *Microencapsulation methods and industrial applications*, S. Benita, ed. Marcel Dekker, Inc, pp. 1–19, 1996.
3. F. Salaün, I. Vroman, and C. Aubry. *Powder Technol.* Vol. 192, p. 375, 2009.
4. O.I. Vinogradova. *J. Phys. Condens. Matter* Vol. 16, p. R1105, 2004.
5. D. Poncelet, C. Dreffier, P. Subra-Paternault, and T.F. Vandamme. Introduction aux techniques de microencapsulation. In *Microencapsulation des sciences aux technologies*, T.F. Vandamme, D. Poncelet, and P. Subra-Paternault, eds. Éd. Tec & Doc, pp. 1–7, 2007.
6. R.C. Koestler. Microencapsulation by interfacial polymerization techniques - Agricultural applications. In *Controlled release technologies : Methods, theory, and applications*, A.F. Kydoniens, ed. CRC Press, pp. 117–132, 1980.
7. T.M.S. Chang. *Science* Vol. 146, p. 524, 1964.
8. A.S. Goldmann, L. Barner, M. Kaupp, A.P. Vogt, and C. Barner-Kowollik. *Prog. Polym. Sci.* Vol. 37, p. 975, 2012.
9. S.K. Yadav, A.K. Suresh, and K.C. Khilar. *AIChE J.* Vol. 36, p. 431, 1990.
10. Z. El Bahri, and J.L. Taverdet. *Powder Technol.* Vol. 172, p. 30, 2007.
11. S. Alexandridou, and C. Kiparissides. *J. Microencapsulation* Vol. 11, p. 603, 1994.
12. Y.F. Maa, and C. Hsu. *J. Controlled Release* Vol. 38, p. 219, 1996.
13. G. Fundueanu, M. Constantin, F. Bortolotti, R. Cortesi, P. Ascenzi, and E. Menegatti. *Eur. J. Pharm. Biopharm.* Vol. 66, p. 11, 2007.
14. S.K. Yadav, K.C. Khilar, and A.K. Suresh. *J. Membr. Sci.* Vol. 125, p. 213, 1997.
15. C. Thies. Microencapsulation. *Encyclopedia of polymer science and technology.* John Wiley & Sons, Inc., 2004.
16. P. Ni, M. Zhang, and N. Yan. *J. Membr. Sci.* Vol. 103, p. 51, 1995.
17. N. Yan, M. Zhang, and P. Ni. *J. Membr. Sci.* Vol. 72, p. 163, 1992.
18. N. Yan, M. Zhang, and P. Ni. *J. Microencapsulation* Vol. 11, p. 365, 1994.
19. M. Zhang, P. Ni, and N. Yan *J. Microencapsulation* Vol. 12, p. 425, 1995.

20. F. Salaün, E. Devaux, S. Bourbigot, and P. Rumeau. *Chem. Eng. J.* Vol. 155, p. 457, 2009.
21. Y.F. Maa, and C. Hsu. *J. Microencapsulation* Vol. 13, p. 53, 1996.
22. Y.F. Maa, and C. Hsu. *J. Microencapsulation* Vol. 13, p. 419, 1996.
23. B. Poncelet De Smet, D. Poncelet, and R.J. Neufeld. *Can. J. Chem. Eng.* Vol. 68, p. 443, 1990.
24. H.S. Tan, T.H. Ng, and H.K. Mahabadi. *J. Microencapsulation* Vol. 8, p. 525, 1991.
25. Y. Wakamatsu, M. Koishi, and T. Kondo. *Chem. Pharm. Bull.* Vol. 22, p. 1319, 1974.
26. B. Poncelet De Smet, D. Poncelet, and R.J. Neufeld. *Enzyme Microb. Technol.* Vol. 11, p. 29, 1989.
27. C.-C. Lo. Microcapsule suspension and a process for its preparation, EP0551796, assigned to Novartis AG, August 13, 1997.
28. R. Arshady. *J. Microencapsulation* Vol. 6, p. 13, 1989.
29. L.R.H. Smith. *Synthetic fiber developments in Germany.* New York, Textile Research Institute (Princeton, N.J.), 1946.
30. P.W. Morgan, and S.L. Kwolek. *Journal of Polymer Science* Vol. 40, p. 299, 1959.
31. E.L. Wittbecker, and M. Katz. *Journal of Polymer Science* Vol. 40, p. 367, 1959.
32. E.L. Wittecker, and P.W. Morgan. *Journal of Polymer Science* Vol. 40, p. 289, 1959.
33. P.W. Morgan. *Society of Plastics Engineers Journal* Vol. 15, p. 485, 1959.
34. P.W. Morgan. *Condensation polymers : by interfacial and solution methods.* New York, Interscience Publishers, 1965.
35. H.W. MacKinney. Procédé de microencapsulation. FR1278621, assigned to IBM, December 15, 1961.
36. H. Russ, Method of encapsulation. US Patent 3429827, assigned to Moore Business Forms Inc, February 25, 1969.
37. C. Brynko. Oil containing capsules and method of making them. US Patent 2969330, assigned to NCR CO, January 24, 1961.
38. C. Brynko, and J.A. Scarpelli. Process of making dual-walled oil containing capsules. US Patent 2969331, assigned to NCR CO, January 24, 1991.
39. G. Baxter. Microencapsulation processes in modern business forms. In *Microencapsulation : Processes and application,* J.E. Vandegaer, ed. Plenum Press, pp. 127–143, 1974.
40. C. Thies. Microencapsulation. In *Encyclopedia of polymer science and engineering,* H.F. Mark, N. Bikales, C.G. Overberger, G. Menges, and J.I. Kroschwitz, eds. Wiley, pp. 724–745, 1987.
41. R. Arshady, and M.H. George. *Polym. Eng. Sci.* Vol. 33, p. 865, 1993.
42. M. Luther, and C. Heuck. Products of latex character and a process for producing the same. US Patent 1864078, assigned to IG Farbenindustrie AG, June 21, 1932.
43. P. Couvreur, M. Roland, and P. Speiser. Biodegradable submicroscopic particles containing a biologically active susbtance and compositions containing them. Assigned May 11, 1982.
44. P. Couvreur, M. Roland, and P. Speiser. Process for preparing biodegradable submicrometric particles containing a biologically active substance and their use. US Patent 4489055, assigned to N.V. Sopar S.A., December 18, 1984.

45. P. Couvreur, M. Roland, and P. Speiser. Preparation of submicroscopic particles, particles thus obtained and pharmaceutical compositions containing them. US Patent 4913908, assigned to N.V. Sopar S.A., April 3, 1990.
46. C. Verdun, P. Couvreur, H. Vranckx, V. Lenaerts, and M. Roland. *J. Controlled Release* Vol. 3, p. 205, 1986.
47. N. Al Khouri Fallouh, L. Roblot-Treupel, H. Fessi, J.P. Devissaguet, and F. Puisieux. *Int. J. Pharm.* Vol. 28, p. 125, 1986.
48. C. Damgé, C. Michel, M. Aprahamian, and P. Couvreur. *Diabetes* Vol. 37, p. 246, 1988.
49. K. Nagai, Y. Ohishi, K. Ishiyama, and N. Kuramoto. *J. Appl. Polym. Sci.* Vol. 38, p. 2183, 1989.
50. A. Zhu, H. Cang, C. Yu, and J. Shen. *Eur. Polym. J*, Vol. 39, p. 851, 2003.
51. E.A.W.G. Janssen, A.M. van Herk, and A.L. German. *Polymer Preprint* Vol. 34, p. 532, 1993.
52. E. Turos, J.-Y. Shim, Y. Wang, K. Greenhalgh, G.S.K. Reddy, S. Dickey, and D.V. Lim. *Bioorg. Med. Chem. Lett.* Vol. 17, p. 53, 2007.
53. J.C. Garay-Jimenez, and E. Turos. *Bioorganic & amp; Medicinal Chemistry Letters* Vol. 21, p. 4589, 2011.
54. R. Yan, Y. Zhang, X. Wang, J. Xu, D. Wang, and W. Zhang. *J. Colloid Interface Sci.* Vol. 368, p. 220, 2012.
55. G.H. Ma, Z.G. Su, S. Omi, D. Sundberg, and J. Stubbs. *J. Colloid Interface Sci.* Vol. 266, p. 282, 2003.
56. J. Berg, D. Sundberg, and B. Kronberg. *J. Microencapsulation* Vol. 6, p. 327, 1989.
57. A. Sarı, C. Alkan, and A. Karaipekli. *Appl. Energy* Vol. 87, p. 1529, 2010.
58. R. Yang, H. Xu, and Y. Zhang. *Sol. Energy Mater. Sol. Cells* Vol. 80, p. 405, 2003.
59. L. Sánchez, P. Sánchez, A. de Lucas, M. Carmona, and J. Rodríguez. *Colloid & Polymer Science* Vol. 285, p. 1377, 2007.
60. L. Sánchez, P. Sánchez, M. Carmona, A. de Lucas, and J. Rodríguez. *Colloid & amp; Polymer Science* Vol. 286, p. 1019, 2008.
61. L. Sánchez-Silva, J.F. Rodríguez, A. Romero, A.M. Borreguero, M. Carmona, and P. Sánchez. *Chem. Eng. J.* Vol. 157, p. 216, 2010.
62. M. Laus, C. Dinnella, G. Lanzarini, and A. Casagrande. *Polymer* Vol. 37, p. 343, 1996.
63. L. Li, J. Cheng, X. Wen, P. Pi, and Z. Yang, *Chin. J. Chem. Eng.* Vol. 14, p. 471, 2006.
64. M. Bakhshaee, R.A. Pethrick, H. Rashid, and D.C. Sherrington. *Polymer Communications* Vol. 26, p. 185, 1985.
65. D.K. Kim, K.-T. Kim, and Y.-W. Chang. *Korea Polymer Journal* Vol. 3, p. 82, 1995.
66. E.C. Cooper, and B. Vincent. *J. Colloid Interface Sci.* Vol. 132, p. 592, 1989.
67. E. Duguet, F. Morvan, P. Maheu, M. Fontanille, and M. Aboud. *Macromolecular Symposia* Vol. 151, p. 353, 2000.
68. E.S. Dragan and C.D. Vlad. New developments in the synthesis of cross linked (Co) polymers as beads particles. In *New trends in noionic (Co) polymers and hybrids*, E.S. Dragan, ed. Nova Science Publishers Inc., pp. 121–166, 2006.
69. M.A. Ushakova, A.V. Chernyshev, M.B. Taraban, and A.K. Petrov. *Eur. Polym. J.* Vol. 39, p. 2301, 2003.

70. J. Zhang, D. Yu, W. Chen, Y. Xie, W. Wan, H. Liang, and C. Min. *J. Magn. Magn. Mater.* Vol. 321, p. 572, 2009.
71. D. Horák, M. Trchová, M.J. Beneš, M. Veverka, and E. Pollert. *Polymer* Vol. 51, p. 3116, 2010.
72. J. Goldshtein, and S. Margel. *Eur. Polym. J.* Vol. 45, p. 2987, 2009.
73. E. Bourgeat-Lami, and J. Lang. *J. Colloid Interface Sci.* Vol. 197, p. 293, 1998.
74. E. Bourgeat-Lami, and J. Lang. *J. Colloid Interface Sci.* Vol. 210, p. 281, 1999.
75. E.J. Park, W.S. Kim, H.S. Hwang, C. Park, and K.T. Lim. *Macromolecular Symposia* Vol. 249–250, p. 196, 2007.
76. J. Zhang, J. Gao, X. Sun, Z. Peng, and J. Diao. *Iran. Polym. J.* Vol. 16, p. 39, 2007.
77. D.-G. Yu, and J.H. An. *Colloids Surf., A* Vol. 237, p. 87, 2004.
78. D.-G. Yu, and J.H. An. *Polymer* Vol. 45, p. 4761, 2004.
79. D.-G. Yu, J.H. An, J.Y. Bae, S. Kim, Y.E. Lee, S.D. Ahn, S.-Y. Kang, and K.S. Suh. *Colloids Surf., A* Vol. 245, p. 29, 2004.
80. J.M. Asua. *Prog. Polym. Sci.* Vol. 27, p. 1283, 2002.
81. K. Landfester, A. Musyanovych, and V. Mailänder. *J. Polym. Sci., Part A: Polym. Chem.* Vol. 48, p. 493, 2010.
82. K. Landfester. *Angew. Chem. Int. Ed.* Vol. 48, p. 4488, 2009.
83. F. Tiarks, K. Landfester, and M. Antonietti. *Langmuir* Vol. 17, p. 908, 2001.
84. Y. Luo, and X. Zhou. *J. Polym. Sci., Part A: Polym. Chem.* Vol. 42, p. 2145, 2004.
85. H.-D. Koh, and J.-S. Lee. *Macromol. Rapid Commun.* Vol. 28, p. 315, 2007.
86. A.J.P. van Zyl, D. d. Wet-Roos, R.D. Sanderson, and B. Klumperman. *Eur. Polym. J.* Vol. 40, p. 2717, 2004.
87. K.-F. Ni, G.-R. Shan, and Z.-X. Weng. *Macromolecules* Vol. 39, p. 2529, 2006/04/01 2006.
88. J. Lukaszczyk, and P. Urbas. *React. Funct. Polym.* Vol. 33, p. 233, 1997.
89. K. Hong, and S. Park. *React. Funct. Polym.* Vol. 42, p. 193, 1999.
90. A.M. Pensé, C. Vauthier, and J.P. Benoit. *Colloid & Polymer Science* Vol. 272, p. 211, 1994.
91. P.G. Shukla, and S. Sivaram. *J. Microencapsulation* Vol. 16, p. 517, 1999.
92. M. Kobašlija, and D.T. McQuade. *Macromolecules* Vol. 39, p. 6371, 2006.
93. L.J.J.M. Janssen, and K. te Nijenhuis. *J. Membr. Sci.* Vol. 65, p. 59, 1992.
94. S.S. Dhumal, S.J. Wagh, and A. K. Suresh. *J. Membr. Sci.* Vol. 325, p. 758, 2008.
95. S.K. Yadav, K.C. Khilar, and A.K. Suresh. *AlChE J.* Vol. 42, p. 2616, 1996.
96. T.L. Whateley. Microcapsules by polymerization and complexation. In *Microencapsulation : Methods and industrial applications*, S. Benita, ed. Marcel Dekker, Inc, pp. 349–376, 1996.
97. N. Zydowicz, P. Chaumont, and M.L. Soto-Portas. *J. Membr. Sci.* Vol. 189, p. 41, 2001.
98. S. Giraud, S. Bourbigot, M. Rochery, I. Vroman, L. Tighzert, and R. Delobel. *Polym. Degrad. Stab.* Vol. 77, p. 285, 2002.
99. F. Salaün, G. Bedek, E. Devaux, D. Dupont, and L. Gengembre. *J. Membr. Sci.* Vol. 370, p. 23, 2011.
100. B. Tylkowski, M. Pregowska, E. Jamowska, R. Garcia-Valls, and M. Giamberini. *Eur. Polym. J.* Vol. 45, p. 1420, 2009.
101. E. Mathiowitz, and M.D. Cohen. *J. Membr. Sci.* Vol. 40, p. 43, 1989.
102. E. Mathiowitz, and M.D. Cohen. *J. Membr. Sci.* Vol. 40, p. 1, 1989.
103. E. Mathiowitz, and M.D. Cohen. *J. Membr. Sci.* Vol. 40, p. 27, 1989.

104. L.J.J.M. Janssen, and K. te Nijenhuis. *J. Membr. Sci.* Vol. 65, p. 69, 1992.
105. L.J.J.M. Janssen, and K. te Nijenhuis. *J. Membr. Sci.* Vol. 79, p. 11, 1993.
106. L. Danicher, P. Gramain, Y. Frère, and A. Le Calvé. *React. Funct. Polym.* Vol. 42, p. 111, 1999.
107. N. Yan, P. Ni, and M. Zhang. *J. Microencapsulation* Vol. 10, p. 375, 1993.
108. K. Hong, and S. Park. *Mater. Sci. Eng., A* Vol. 272, p. 418, 1999.
109. K. Hong, and S. Park. *Journal of Materials Science* Vol. 34, p. 3161, 1999.
110. K. Hong, and S. Park. *Mater. Chem. Phys.* Vol. 64, p. 20, 2000.
111. Y. Frère, L. Danicher, and P. Gramain. *Eur. Polym. J.* Vol. 34, p. 193, 1998.
112. B. Wang, Q. Tang, N. Hong, L. Song, L. Wang, Y. Shi, and Y. Hu. *ACS Appl Mater Interfaces* Vol. 3, p. 3754, 2011.
113. J.-S. Cho, A. Kwon, and C.-G. Cho. *Colloid & Polymer Science* Vol. 280, p. 260, 2002.
114. D. Saihi, I. Vroman, S. Giraud, and S. Bourbigot. *React. Funct. Polym.* Vol. 66, p. 1118, 2006.
115. E. Jabbari and M. Khakpour. *Biomaterials* Vol. 21, p. 2073, 2000.
116. F. Gaudin, and N. Sintes-Zydowicz. *Colloids Surf., A* Vol. 331, p. 133, 2008.
117. S.J. Wagh, S.S. Dhumal, and A.K. Suresh. *J. Membr. Sci.* Vol. 328, p. 246, 2009.
118. K. Bouchemal, S. Briançon, H. Fessi, Y. Chevalier, I. Bonnet, and E. Perrier. *Materials Science and Engineering: C* Vol. 26, p. 472, 2006.
119. K.Y. Choi, K.S. Min, and T. Chang. *Polymer (Korea)* Vol. 15, p. 548, 1991.
120. P. Siddhan, M. Jassal, and A.K. Agrawal. *J. Appl. Polym. Sci.* Vol. 106, p. 786, 2007.
121. J. Łukaszczyk, and P. Urba . *React. Funct. Polym.* Vol. 33, p. 233, 1997.
122. P. Persico, C. Carfagna, L. Danicher, and Y. Frère. *J. Microencapsulation* Vol. 22, p. 471, 2005.
123. K. Bouchemal, S. Briançon, E. Perrier, and H. Fessi. *Int. J. Pharm.* Vol. 280, p. 241, 2004.
124. I. Montasser, H. Fessi, S. Briançon, and J. Lieto. Method for preparing colloidal particles in the form of nanocapsules. Assigned 2003.
125. I. Montasser, H. Fessi, S. Briançon, and J. Lieto. *Polym. Bull.* Vol. 50, p. 169, 2003.
126. I. Montasser, S. Briançon, and H. Fessi. *Int. J. Pharm.* Vol. 335, p. 176, 2007.
127. F. Salaün, and I. Vroman. *Int. J. Chem. Reactor Eng.* Vol. 7, p. A55, 2009.
128. H.Y. Chao. Microencapsulation by in-situ polymerization of multifunctional epoxy resins. US Patent 4626471, assigned to Moore Business Forms, Inc., February 12, 1986.
129. K. Dietrich, H. Herma, R. Nastke, E. Bonatz, and W. Teige. *Acta Polym.* Vol. 40, p. 243, 1989.
130. K. Dietrich, E. Bonatz, H. Geistlinger, H. Herma, R. Nastke, H.-J. Purz, M. Schlawne, and W. Teige. *Acta Polym.* Vol. 40, p. 325, 1989.
131. E. Bonatz, K. Dietrich, H. Herma, R. Nastke, and M. Walter. *Acta Polym.* Vol. 40, p. 91, 1989.
132. K. Dietrich, E. Bonatz, R. Nastke, H. Herma, M. Walter, and W. Teige. *Acta Polym.* Vol. 41, p. 91, 1990.
133. K. Hong, and S. Park. *Mater. Chem. Phys.* Vol. 58, p. 128, 1999.
134. H.-Y. Lee, S.-J. Lee, W. Cheong, and J.-H. Kim. *J. Microencapsulation* Vol. 19, p. 559, 2002.

135. J.-S. Hwang, J.-N. Kim, Y.-J. Wee, H.-G. Jang, S.-H. Kim, and H.-W. Ryu. *Biotechnol. Bioprocess Eng.* Vol. 11, p. 391, 2006.
136. P.G. Shukla. Microencapsulation of liquid active agent. In *Functional coatings by polymer microencapsulation*, S.K. Ghosh, ed. Wiley-VCH, pp. 153–186, 2006.
137. B. Boh, I. Kosir, E. Knez, M. Kukovic, V. Skerlavaj, and A. Skvarc. *J. Microencapsulation* Vol. 16, p. 169, 1999.
138. F. Salaün, M. Lewandowski, I. Vroman, G. Bedek, and S. Bourbigot. *Polym. Degrad. Stab.* Vol. 96, p. 131, 2011.
139. C.A. Kim, M.J. Joung, S.D. Ahn, G.H. Kim, S.-Y. Kang, I.-K. You, J. Oh, H.J. Myoung, K.H. Baek, and K.S. Suh. *Synth. Met.* Vol. 151, p. 181, 2005.
140. B. Comiskey, J.D. Albert, H. Yoshizawa, and J. Jacobson. *Nature* Vol. 394, p. 253, 1998.
141. E.N. Brown, M.R. Kessler, N.R. Sottos, and S.R. White. *J. Microencapsulation* Vol. 20, p. 719, 2003.
142. G. Sun, and Z. Zhang. *J. Microencapsulation* Vol. 18, p. 593, 2001.
143. W.-J. Luo, W. Yang, S. Jiang, J.-M. Feng, and M.-B. Yang. *Polym. Degrad. Stab.* Vol. 92, p. 1359, 2007.
144. F. Salaün, and I. Vroman. *Eur. Polym. J.* Vol. 44, p. 849, 2008.
145. Q. Song, Y. Li, J. Xing, J.Y. Hu, and Y. Marcus. *Polymer* Vol. 48, p. 3317, 2007.
146. H. Zhang, and X. Wang. *Colloids Surf., A* Vol. 332, p. 129, 2009.
147. W. Li, X.-X. Zhang, X.-C. Wang, and J.-J. Niu. *Mater. Chem. Phys.* Vol. 106, p. 437, 2007.
148. B. Šumiga, E. Knez, M. Vrtačnik, V. F. Savec, M. Starešinič, and B. Boh. *Acta Chimica Slovenica* Vol. 58, p. 14, 2011.
149. K. Wu, Z. Wang, and H. Liang. *Polym. Compos.* Vol. 29, p. 854, 2008.
150. Z. Wang, K. Wu, and Y. Hu. *Polymer Engineering & Science* Vol. 48, p. 2426, 2008.
151. K. Wu, and Z. Wang. *Polymer-Plastics Technology and Engineering* Vol. 47, p. 247, 2008.
152. K. Wu, Z. Wang, and Y. Hu. *Polym. Adv. Technol.* Vol. 19, p. 1118, 2008.
153. K. Wu, L. Song, Z. Wang, and Y. Hu. *Polym. Adv. Technol.* Vol. 19, p. 1914, 2008.
154. K. Wu, L. Song, Z. Wang, Y. Hu, E. Kandare, and B.K. Kandola. *Journal of Macromolecular Science, Part A* Vol. 46, p. 837, 2009.
155. K. Wu, L. Song, Z. Wang, and Y. Hu. *J. Polym. Res.* Vol. 16, p. 283, 2009.
156. K. Wu, M.-M. Shen, and Y. Hu. *J. Polym. Res.* Vol. 18, p. 425, 2011.
157. S.-J. Park, Y.-S. Shin, and J.-R. Lee. *J. Colloid Interface Sci.* Vol. 241, p. 502, 2001.
158. S. Cosco, V. Ambrogi, P. Musto, and C. Carfagna. *J. Appl. Polym. Sci.* Vol. 105, p. 1400, 2007.
159. L. Yuan, G. Liang, J. Xie, L. Li, and J. Guo. *Polymer* Vol. 47, p. 5338, 2006.
160. C. Fan, and X. Zhou. *Colloids Surf., A* Vol. 363, p. 49, 2010.
161. A. Rochmadi, A. Prasetya, and W. Hasokowati. *American Journal of Applied Sciences* Vol. 7, p. 739, 2010.
162. H. Yoshizawa, E. Kamio, N. Hirabayashi, J. Jacobson, and Y. Kitamura. *J. Microencapsulation* Vol. 21, p. 241, 2004.
163. H. Zhang, X. Wang, and D. Wu. *J. Colloid Interface Sci.* Vol. 343, p. 246, 2010.
164. F.L. Sousa, S. Horta, M. Santos, S.M. Rocha, and T. Trindade. *Results in Pharma Sciences* Vol. 2, p. 52, 2012.

165. B.Y. Ahn, S.I. Seok, and I.C. Baek. *Materials Science and Engineering: C* Vol. 28, p. 1183, 2008.
166. J. Guo, W. Yang, Y. Deng, C. Wang, and S. Fu. *Small* Vol. 1, p. 737, 2005.
167. H. Zhang, S. Sun, X. Wang, and D. Wu. *Colloids Surf., A* Vol. 389, p. 104, 2011.
168. J.-X. Wang, Z.-H. Wang, J.-F. Chen, and J. Yun. *Mater. Res. Bull.* Vol. 43, p. 3374, 2008.
169. G. Fornasieri, S. Badaire, R. Backov, O. Mondain-Monval, C. Zakri, and P. Poulin. *Adv. Mater.* Vol. 16, p. 1094, 2004.
170. M.S. Kim, S.I. Seok, B.Y. Ahn, S.M. Koo, and S.U. Paik. *J. Sol-Gel Sci. Technol.* Vol. 27, p. 355, 2003.
171. S. Gouin. *Trends Food Sci. Technol.* Vol. 15, p. 330, 2004.

6

Encapsulation of Silica Particles by a Thin Shell of Poly(Methyl) Methacrylate

Isidora Freris and Alvise Benedetti

Department of Molecular Sciences and Nanosystems, Università Ca' Foscari Venezia, Venice, Italy

Abstract

The encapsulation of inorganic particles in a thin polymer shell generates core-shell hybrid materials. This chapter summarizes the main contributions from the literature for the preparation of a specific example of such hybrid materials, core-shell particles composed of an inner silica core and a poly(methyl methacrylate) outer shell. The spherical silica particles used in the examples have been obtained by sol-gel methods, most commonly via the Stöber synthesis and the reverse phase microemulsion method. Depending on the choice of method for their encapsulation, the surfaces of the silica particles have been modified to promote formation of poly(methyl methacrylate) at their surface. Surface modification methods may include the covalent attachment of a polymerizable organosilane which may co-polymerize with the monomer in conventional radical polymerization, or the covalent attachment of an initiator for controlled living radical polymerization. The methods presented in this chapter will include conventional *in situ* heterophase radical polymerization methods, namely emulsion, emulsifier-free emulsion, precipitation, dispersion, and vapor phase polymerization. We also provide several examples of surface initiated atom transfer radical polymerization for the controlled growth of poly(methyl methacrylate) brushes on silica particles.

Keywords: Encapsulation, inorganic nanoparticles, silica, core-shell, polymerization, poly(methyl) methacrylate

Vikas Mittal (ed.) Encapsulation Nanotechnologies, (175–202) © 2013 Scrivener Publishing LLC

6.1 Introduction

It is well established that the unique performance of an organic–inorganic hybrid material is strongly related to its structural features [1, 2]. For instance, polymer–inorganic materials can display extraordinary features which are derived from the synergism between the properties of an inorganic material, namely optical, electronic and magnetic properties, combined with those of polymers which include easy processing and good mechanical strength [3, 4]. The encapsulation of inorganic particles in a thin polymer shell generates core-shell hybrid materials that may display unique chemical and physical properties with respect to their individual components. The novel properties displayed by the combination of such chemically distinct organic and inorganic components are influenced by the physico-chemical interaction present at the hybrids' interface, and not only the sum of their individual contributions. The interface is of fundamental importance when designing materials with specific properties, as its physico-chemical nature determines a material's transparency, chemical homogeneity, and stability [5].

Encapsulation of inorganic particles with polymers is desirable in many applications, whereby the surface characteristics of the inorganic cores are modified by coating with a protective polymer layer [6, 7]. Polymer encapsulation may be applied to reduce particle toxicity, mask taste and odor, to enhance stability, and to improve dispersibility in organic media [2, 8, 9]. Accordingly, polymer encapsulated inorganic particles can offer interesting actual or potential properties for use within the biomedical or cosmetic fields, as novel textiles, paints, optics and electronics [9–11].

Prior to describing the methods that may be used for the generation of core-shell hybrids, and to avoid disambiguation with bulk inorganic-polymer composites, it is necessary to mention that not all composites derived from the inclusion of inorganic core particles in a polymer will posses core-shell morphology. For example, reinforced bulk polymers are routinely prepared by the uniform dispersion of inorganic nanoparticles within their matrix. Silica nanoparticles have been effectively used as inorganic fillers for thermoplastic polymers such as poly (methyl methacrylate) (PMMA) [12–16], whereby their inclusion in the bulk has been shown to improve the strength, abrasion resistance, friction and age-resistance of the polymer [15, 17]. In this context, nanosized inorganic nanoparticles, such as silica and titania, are exploited for both their rigid structure and large specific surface area which promotes greater interfacial bonding with the bulk polymer. Typically, these polymer composites are prepared by methods such as melt blending [16, 17], solution blending [16, 18, 19], single-screw extrusion [16, 20] and *in situ* polymerization [12, 16, 21, 22].

In this chapter we focus on methods for generating core-shell hybrid particles which differ from the aforementioned bulk polymer composites. The core-shell particles can be broadly defined as comprising an inner core material which is covered by an outer shell of a different material. The most common core-shell nanoparticles are spherical, however, other shapes are possible [23, 24]. The core and the shell may be composed of a variety of materials including polymers, inorganic solids, and metals which are chosen in accordance with their desired application.

In this chapter we will focus our attention on the preparation of core-shell particles containing a silica core, and provide reported methods for their encapsulation in a thin shell of PMMA. The silica core particles used in the encapsulation technologies described herein have been derived from sol-gel methods capable of producing spherical and monodisperse silica nanoparticles. Maintaining the particles well separated and achieving high encapsulation efficiency while limiting the growth of free polymer during the polymerization is by no means a trivial task, as will be evidenced in the methods described. Although obtaining this intricate architecture can be rather challenging to achieve, a diversity of preparative methods for their preparation have been demonstrated. The methods presented in this chapter will demonstrate the alternative approaches that can be used for this specific example.

We will firstly describe the common routes for yielding spherical silica particles followed by their surface modification to impart superficial hydrophobicity. The latter is often cited as a fundamental step in the PMMA encapsulation of silica, since it increases the compatibility of the seeds with the hydrophobic monomer to promote polymerization at their surface [25]. The encapsulation of silica particles with a thin shell of PMMA is divided into sections i) methods of *in situ* conventional heterophase radical polymerization, and ii) methods based on controlled living radical polymerization.

6.2 Synthesis of Silica (Nano)Particles and Their Surface Modification

Silica nanoparticles are widely used in the preparation of core–shell hybrid systems. They display excellent physical and chemical properties, which include high optical transparency, chemical inertness, ease of preparation and facile surface modification [26]. Their tunability in particle size, morphology and porosity renders them versatile for a variety of nanotechnological applications in both the industrial and biomedical fields. We have already mentioned their use as inorganic fillers, to impart strength, increase abrasion resistance and elevate thermal stability in polymer composites [17]. However, silica nanoparticles also find extensive use as host materials or carriers for biomedical applications. They are biocompatible and relatively transparent in the sense that they do not absorb light in the near-infrared, visible and ultra-violet regions. In addition, they do not interfere with magnetic fields which renders them ideal for imaging and theranostic applications [26, 27]. In their use as host materials or carriers, they may be loaded with catalysts, drugs, inorganic complexes or crystals, organic dyes, quantum dots and noble metals amongst others. These can either be physically entrapped inside the core by doping [27, 28], or covalently attached to the silica network during its synthesis [27–31].

6.2.1 Silica Synthesis

The sol–gel technique is a commonly used wet-chemical method for the synthesis of silica nanoparticles. It is an inorganic polymerization which involves the simultaneous hydrolysis and condensation of a metal alkoxide, resulting in the formation of a metal-oxo polymer [32, 33]. The most widely used metal alkoxides for the synthesis of silica nanoparticles in sol-gel processing are tetramethyl orthosilicate (TMOS) and tetraethyl orthosilicate (TEOS), which are relatively inexpensive and available commercially.

In 1956, Kolbe [34] first observed the formation of silica particles by reacting TEOS with water in alkali solution using certain bases. In 1968 this approach was expanded upon by Stöber *et al.*, who reported a simple method to produce monodisperse spherical silica particles by the controlled hydrolysis of TEOS in a dilute solution of ethanol catalyzed by ammonia [35]. It was found that uniform spheres with smooth surfaces were produced, and that their sizes could be tuned from 10 nm to 2μm (micrometer) by simple variation of the reactant concentrations. The formed particles are stabilized by electrostatic repulsion due to the ions in the ammonia solution. This simple method, which has since been improved by others [29, 36–43], remains the simplest and most effective route towards monodispersed silica spheres in solution.

The reverse phase microemulsion method can also be used to synthesize silica nanoparticles with a narrow size distribution and spherical shape, and is particularly important for the synthesis of particles with dimensions below 100 nm [44]. Reverse microemulsions (water-in-oil), are highly tunable systems that consist of nanometer-sized water droplets stabilized by a surfactant in the organic phase. The micelles of the microemulsion act as "nanoreactors" in which particle growth occurs, and the final size is controlled by the water to organic solvent ratio [44]. In 1990, Osseo-Asare and Arrigada [45] demonstrated that nanosized and monodisperse silica particles could be produced by controlled hydrolysis of TEOS in a reverse microemulsion using ammonia as catalyst. The synthesis of nanosized silica using the reverse microemulsion method has since been extended to include acid catalyzed systems [46–52].

Silica nanoparticles may also be prepared by aerosol or flame assisted methods [25], although these tend not to be cited as sources for the fabrication of core-shell hybrids. Powdered silica with dimensions in the range of 5–15 nm can be produced by the high temperature vapor hydrolysis of $SiCl_4$ in a flame of oxygen-hydrogen, although the process often leads to formation of larger-sized aggregates and agglomerates [25, 53].

Since the surface of silica nanoparticles is terminated with silanol and siloxane groups, they are hydrophilic in nature [54].

6.2.2 Surface Modification of Silica Particles

The hydrophilic surface of silica nanoparticles lowers their direct compatibility with hydrophobic monomers, such as methyl methacrylate (MMA). Nonetheless, an advantage of using silica nanoparticles in PMMA encapsulation is that the inherent incompatibility between the two components may be overcome by surface modification. It is possible to increase the surface hydrophobicity through covalent attachment of a suitable organosilane to the surface silanols [55]. Numerous organosilanes, also referred to as *silane coupling agents*, are commercially available, and a selection of common examples is given in Table 6.1 [25].

Table 6.1 Common examples of commercially available organosilanes.

Abbreviation	Name	Chemical structure
APMDES	aminopropyl methydiethoxysilane	$H_2N(CH_2)_3(CH_3)Si(OC_2H_5)_2$
APMDMOS	(3-acryloxypropyl) methydimethoxysilane	CH_2=$CHCOO(CH_2)_3(CH)_3Si(OCH_3)_2$
APTES (APTS, APTEOS, APrTEOS)	3-aminopropyltriethoxysilane	$H_2N(CH_2)_3Si(OC_2H_5)_3$
APTMS (APTMOS, APrTMOS)	3-aminopropyltrimethoxysilane	$H_2N(CH_2)_3Si(OCH_3)3$
APTMS (APTMOS)	(3-acryloxypropyl)trimethoxysilane	CH_2=$CHCOO(CH_2)_3Si(OCH_3)_3$
APTMS (APTMOS)	aminophenyltrimethoxysilane	$H_2NPhSi(OCH_3)_3$
TESPT	bis(trimethoxysilylpropyl)tetrasulfane	$(C_2H_5O)_3Si(CH_2)_3S_4(CH_2)_3Si(OC_2H_5)_3$
DDS	dimethyldichlorosilane	$(CH_3)_2SiCl_2$
GPS (GPTS, GOTMS, GPTMOS, KH560)	3-glycidoxypropyltrimethoxysilane, 3-glycidyloxypropyltrimethoxysilane	$CH_2(O)CHCH_2O(CH_2)_3Si(OCH_3)_3$
ICPTES	3-isocyanatopropyltriethoxysilane	$OCN(CH_2)_3Si(OC_2H_5)_3$
MMS	methacryloxymethyltriethoxysilane	CH_2=$C(CH_3)COOCH_2Si(OC_2H_5)_3$
MPS (MPTMS, MPTS, MAMSE, MATMS, MSMA, TPM, MEMO, KH570)	methacrylic acid 3-(trimethoxysilyl) propyl ester, 3-(trimethoxysilyl)propyl methacrylate, 3-methacryloxypropyltrimethoxysilane	CH_2=$C(CH_3)COO(CH_2)_3Si(OCH_3)3$
MPTES	methacryloxypropyltriethoxysilane	CH_2=$C(CH_3)COO(CH_2)_3Si(OC_2H_5)_3$
MPTS	mercaptopropyl triethoxysilane	$SH(CH_2)_3Si(OC_2H_5)_3$
MTES	methyltriethoxysilane	$CH_3Si(OC_2H_5)_3$
PTMS	phenyltrimethoxysilane	$PhSi(OCH_3)_3$
VTES	vinyltriethoxysilane	CH_2=$CHSi(OC_2H_5)_3$
VTS	vinyltrimethoxysilane	CH_2=$CHSi(OCH_3)_3$

Silane coupling agents are bifunctional molecules which have the general formula X-$(CH_2)_n$-$SiR_n(OR')_{3-n}$, where X represents the organofunctional headgroup, $(CH_2)_n$ is a flexible spacer, and $Si(OR)_n$ the hydrolyzable groups which can attach to free Si-OH surface groups by condensation. Typical hydrolyzable groups are chloro, ethoxy, or methoxy groups [56]. Surface modification is typically performed in organic solvents by the addition of 0.1 and 2.0% (w/v) of the coupling agent and a small amount of water to promote the hydrolysis [56, 57].

The organofunctional group may be characterized by a variety of terminal functionalities depending on the desired application. For example, methacryloxypropyltriethoxysilane (MPTES) has a terminal methacroyl moiety which may participate in polymerization reactions with the monomer phase via its double bond. This can lead to much stronger interfacial interaction in organo-inorganic hybrids derived from the co-polymerization of surface modified particles. The frequent use of MPTES as a surface modifier for silica particles encapsulated in PMMA will be shown throughout the chapter.

6.3 Encapsulation of Silica Particles in a Thin PMMA Shell

PMMA is an industrially important polymer which finds broad application because of its attractive chemical and physical properties. It is a synthetically produced resin made via the radical initiated polymerization of its monomer precursor, methyl methacrylate (MMA). Its properties, which include easy processing, high transparency and rigidity, render it highly applicable in a variety of areas [1]. Its toughness has led to its wide use as a glass substitute, which is also attributed to its almost perfect transmission of visible light. Other uses for PMMA include lighting fixtures, automobile components, signs, latex coatings, optical fibers, and medical applications such as soft-tissue augmentation [58–61]. Encapsulation of nanosized and submicron-sized silica particles to fabricate core-shell hybrids has been reported using a diversity of methods. Herein, we describe a selection of these methods that have been shown to yield a thin PMMA shell on the surface of individual silica particles, and examples for their application.

6.3.1 *In Situ* Conventional Heterophase Radical Polymerization

In situ heterophase radical polymerization is a widely used method for encapsulating inorganic particles, namely silica, titania and zirconia, within a polymer shell [25]. Generally speaking, *in situ* heterophase polymerization is a particle forming reaction which may also be performed in the presence of preformed inorganic particles, often referred to as seeds. The general method can be further divided into the following techniques: emulsion, emulsifier-free emulsion, miniemulsion, precipitation, dispersion and vapor deposition polymerization. The use of these methods for the coating of solid seeds can provide a great degree of morphogenetic control, as the solid and often spherical shape of the seeds act as internal templates for the polymer coating as it forms. The physical nature of the polymer coating, its uniformity and degree of surface coverage during the coating process depends on the surface preparation of the inorganic core, its effective dispersion and overall stability in the medium used for the ensuing polymerization. Obtaining individually encapsulated inorganic particles is a challenging feat, and is highly dependent on suitable processing conditions which prevent aggregation of the seeds during polymerization.

6.3.1.1 Emulsion Polymerization

Emulsion polymerization is widely used for the encapsulation of silica particles in polymers [62]. The technique is often referred to as seeded emulsion polymerization, in which the solid silica particles are used as seeds which are subsequently coated by the polymer during its *in situ* formation. Stabilization of the seed particles during polymerization is commonly achieved by the presence of an emulsifier or a mixture of emulsifiers, albeit not always required as will be demonstrated for the emulsifier-free processes in Section 6.3.1.2. The choice of emulsifier and its concentration, monomer/seed content ratio and its surface modification have all been reported as important parameters for limiting the growth of free polymer particles in the solution, and in promoting a high level of polymer coverage on the seed surface.

Luna-Xavier *et al.* used the seeded emulsion polymerization technique to encapsulate silica nanoparticles with PMMA [63]. They used a commercial sol of hydrophilic silica seeds with an average diameter of 68 nm and nonionic emulsifier, nonylphenol poly(oxyethylene) (NP_{30}) for the seeded emulsion polymerization. Their approach for forming a PMMA coating on the silica seeds was based on the use of the cationic initiator, 2,2′-azobis(2-amidinopropane) dihydrochloride (AIBA), which could electrostatically adsorb on the silica surface. They determined that the adsorption of AIBA molecules on the silica surface was strongly influenced by the pH of the system. Since AIBA is a strong base ($pK_a = 11$) and the silica surface is acidic, their interaction could be enhanced by raising the pH of the medium. By raising the pH to 9.8, they increased the silica surface charge density to give a negatively charged surface that strongly interacted with the cationic amidinium groups in the AIBA molecules. Their experimental findings indicated an AIBA adsorption of approximate 2 mg/g silica. The emulsion polymerization of MMA was conducted in the presence of the AIBA-adsorbed silica seeds at pH 9.8, and proceeded to give a PMMA coating on silica in addition to free PMMA latex particles. The coating they obtained was not a smooth encapsulating shell, but rather an aggregation of small PMMA particles strongly adhered to the silica surfaces. This aggregation of small PMMA particles at the silica surfaces is described as heterocoagulation, and has previously been observed for the coating of titania pigments by *in situ* formed PMMA following AIBA adsorption on the surface [64]. Although the silica-PMMA hybrid obtained was not strictly a core-shell structure, 65% of the PMMA particles that formed in the system were found to coat the silica particles, while 25% were present as free PMMA particles. The latter were stabilized as free PMMA particles by the high concentration of surfactant available in the continuous phase. For the coated silica particles, they found that 20% of the PMMA coating was strongly adhered to the silica surface and could not be extracted. Since the charge of the inorganic surface is opposite to that of the growing radicals at high pH, strong electrostatic interactions are expected to take place at the early stage of polymerization, as previously noted [65]. Hence, as the cationic oligomers are formed, they are thought to migrate towards the oppositely charged silica surface from which further growth takes place to form the eventual coating by PMMA particles. Dynamic light scattering measurements indicated that the average diameter of the silica-PMMA hybrid particles obtained was 239 nm.

A sequential study by Luna-Xavier *et al.* further examined the AIBA-silica surface initiated emulsion polymerization for silica particles obtained via the Stöber synthesis [66]. They prepared silica particles with average diameters of 230 nm and 340 nm, and compared their PMMA encapsulation with the commercial sol particles (previously 68 nm). The AIBA initiated emulsion polymerization of MMA in the presence of the Stöber silica led to the formation of silica-PMMA particles with a true core-shell architecture. A smooth shell of PMMA was observed to coat the individual silica particles as shown in TEM micrographs (Figure 6.1).

The different shell morphology they observed between the commercial sol and the Stöber particles was attributed to a greater interaction between the forming polymer and the Stöber silica seed in the early stages of polymerization. This was supported by zeta potential measurements, which indicated a higher surface charge density for the Stöber silica seeds than for the commercial silica sol. The Stöber silica seeds also demonstrated a higher adsorbed surfactant concentration and a greater carbon content (2%) that originated from the presence of residual unhydrolyxed ethoxy groups [10]. Hence, in addition to AIBA surface adsorption, greater electrostatic or hydrophobic interactions were also thought to promote polymer assembly at the silica surface earlier in the polymerization for the Stöber silica seeds, thus leading to an improved core-shell morphology.

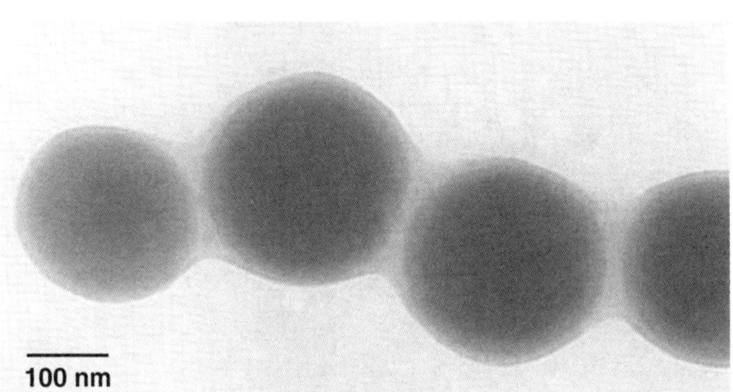

Figure 6.1 PMMA coating on Stöber silica beads (average diameter 230 nm) to give a core-shell morphology. Reproduced from [66] with permission from Elsevier.

Zhang *et al.* [67] used the seeded emulsion polymerization to prepare PMMA encapsulated silica particles with a core-shell architecture. Initially, Stöber silica particles ranging in size from 51 nm to 195 nm were organically modified by grafting the silane agent MPTES to their surface. The surface attachment of MPTES increases the surface hydrophobicity of the seeds for favorable adsorption of MMA. Furthermore, MPTES contains a methacroyl group with a terminal double bond which can co-polymerize with MMA during polymerization. It has been reported that grafting of polymerizable silane agents such as MPTES ensures the formation of covalent bonds between the silica particles and the polymer shell [68]. The MPTES-silica seeds were subsequently encapsulated by PMMA during emulsion polymerization of MMA in an aqueous-ethanolic medium [67]. In their experiments, water soluble potassium persulfate (KPS) was used as the radical initiator, sodium dodecyl benzene sulfonate (SDBS) as emulsifier and 4,4′-isopropylidenediphenol bimethacrylate (BVA) was used as crosslinker. Polymerizations were performed in a nitrogen atmosphere at 80°C for 10 hours, followed by centrifugation to remove any empty PMMA particles. The authors gave evidence for co-polymerization between the MPTES terminal double bond and the free MMA in the medium, while their attempts to extract the PMMA shell from the inorganic core were only minimally successful. Their extraction attempts decreased the PMMA weight proportion by 32%, suggesting that a significant amount of the PMMA chains formed were linked to the silica surface and could not be removed. This was in contrast to their similarly prepared poly(stryrene) (PS) encapsulated silica particles, obtained by emulsion polymerization of styrene in the presence of MPTES-silica [69], for which 79% of the PS could be removed by extraction. The higher removal of PS in the latter core-shell particles was attributed to a different coating mechanism, namely physical crosslinking and surface adsorption. The different polymer formation mechanisms were also supported by the different morphologies observed in TEM micrographs (Figure 6.2).

The silica-PMMA particles displayed higher symmetry with the cores being well centered in their respective polymer shells (Figure 6.2a). The lower symmetry in the silica-PS particles (Figure 6.2b) gave further evidence for the adsorption of twisted PS chains on the seed surface, as would be expected to arise from the shearing stress caused during agitation.

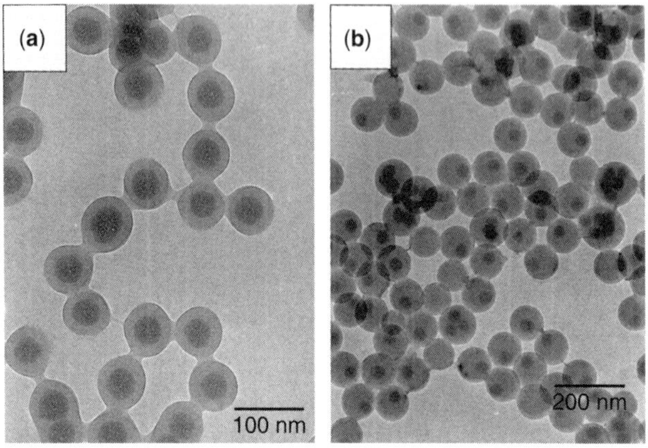

Figure 6.2 (a) TEM images of Silica-PMMA core-shell particles, and (b) silica-PS core-shell particles. Reproduced from [67] with permission from Elsevier.

The authors further established the importance of emulsifier concentration and its role in the PMMA encapsulation process. When the emulsifier (SDBS) concentration was increased from 0.0002 to 0.0018 g/mL, two important observations were noted: a decrease in PMMA shell thickness from 30 to 9 nm was observed, and a greater quantity of empty PMMA spheres would form. The high solubility of MMA in the system was thought to lead to its rapid polymerization towards formation of PMMA oligomers, stabilized as empty spheres when the emulsifier concentration was high. This consequently lowered the concentration of MMA available for co-polymerization with the surface bound methacroyl group on the silica seed. The variation of emulsifier concentration in the system described could be used as a tool for the tuning of PMMA shell thickness.

Changing the dimensions of the silica core particles also influenced the thickness of the shell when emulsifier concentration, seed and monomer content were kept constant. The TEM images in Figure 6.3 show the differently sized core-shell particles they obtained as the core size was increased. The PMMA shells increasingly became thinner with increasing silica core size. In the micrographs depicted, the silica cores of 51, 126, 165 and 195 nm, were visibly encapsulated with the average thickness of the shells being 40, 19, 17 and 15 nm, respectively. Since the particle surface area is greater when their dimensions are smaller, the

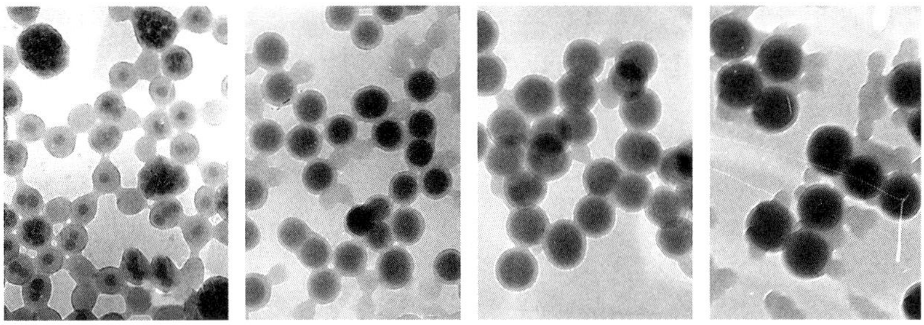

Figure 6.3 TEM images of the silica-PMMA core-shell particles where the size of silica is 51, 126, 165, 195 nm, respectively (from left to right). Reproduced from [67] with permission from Elsevier.

availability of MPTES would also be higher in the smaller particles. Consequently, this provided a greater number of sites for the nucleation of PMMA and is consistent with the thinner PMMA shell encapsulating the larger seeds. As a result, the increased availability of MMA in solution also led to a greater quantity of empty PMMA particles being formed.

The utility of this emulsion polymerization method [67] was further demonstrated for the fabrication of hollow PMMA spheres containing Ag nanoparticles [70]. Encapsulation of MPTES modified Ag-embedded silica particles led to the formation of colloidal hybrid particles, comprising Ag-embedded silica cores and smooth PMMA shells. The silica core was subsequently removed from within the shell by etching to yield the hollow Ag nanoparticle containing spheres.

The following two examples also demonstrate the utility of emulsion polymeriziation for encapsulating silica particles which are host carriers. The encapsulation polymerization of a dye containing silica core with PMMA to yield fluorescent core-shell particles was described by Ribeiro *et al.* [71]. Their overall objective was to prepare hybrid materials with potential application in photoactive high performance coatings. The authors applied the emulsion polymerization technique to obtain the core-shell hybrids, which they further used to construct thin films that were transparent, flexible and fluorescent. In order to prepare hybrid films, a water dispersion of core-shell particles is usually cast onto a substrate and dried [71].

A triethoxysilyl derivative of the fluorescent dye perylenediimide was used to prepare the fluorescent silica particles, through co-condensation with TEOS in an adaptation of the Stöber process. Restricting the movement of the dye in the matrix by covalent attachment is desirable in optical applications as it contributes to reduced fluorescence quenching. The fluorescent silica particles were prepared with a particle size range of 270–440 nm, and were modified in a successive step by the surface grafting of MPTES to increase their hydrophobicity and promote adsorption of MMA in the polymemerization step. The semicontinuous emulsion polymerization was used to provide a steady growth of the PMMA coating on the silica seeds and limit the formation of free latex PMMA particles in the system. In their polymerizations of MMA, the water soluble radical initiator potassium persulfate (KPS) and emulsifier sodium dodecyl sulfate (SDS) were used in the presence of the crosslinking agent, ethylene glycol dimethacrylate. The authors were not able to visually examine the core-shell morphology of the particles using TEM, as the PMMA coating would undergo fluidification under the beam. However, they were able to establish a 100% monomer conversion which was calculated from the mass balance. Additionally, with the presence of a PMMA coating on the fluorescent seeds the core-shell hybrid particles were successfully cast into thin films. Aqueous solutions of the core-shell particles were evaporated and then annealed at 90°C for 1 hour. Upon heating, the PMMA shells undergo interdiffusion in the void space between particles, which subsequently leads to the formation of transparent and flexible films containing homogeneously dispersed fluorescent silica. Their successful fabrication of transparent and photoactive films verifies that well dispersed core-shell particles were formed during the emulsion polymerization.

Chen *et al.* [72] have successfully shown a valuable biological application that utilizes PMMA encapsulated magnetic silica particles that could be used in proteomics research. Their motivation for coating the particles with PMMA was based on the finding that PMMA can be used as a powerful absorbent for the enrichment of peptides and proteins [73–77]. They prepared iron-oxide-embedded silica particles and modified their surface by grafting MPTES [38]. Subsequently, the hydrophobic MPTES modified silica particles were suspended in droplets of MMA which were stabilized in the aqueous phase with the aid of the anionic emulsifier, sodium lauryl benzenesulfate. Following the polymerization reaction, the PMMA-coated silica beads were magnetically separated from the reaction medium and purified by exploitation of their magnetic properties. They observed PMMA-coated particles in TEM micrographs, composed of a thin polymeric coating which fully encased the magnetic-silica particles.

6.3.1.2 *Emulsifier-Free Emulsion Polymerization*

Percy and Armes [78] demonstrated that silica-PMMA core-shell particles could be prepared via emulsion polymerization in the absence of emulsifiers when conducted within an aqueous-alcoholic medium. The utility of their polymer encapsulation method was later extended to include monomers styrene and alkyl-acrylates [79]. In their simple PMMA encapsulation process, they used commercial silica sols containing 14 nm average-sized particles in isopropyl alcohol (IPA). The polymerization of MMA was performed in an aqueous-IPA silica sol under mild conditions at 25°C for up to 24 hours by introducing solutions of the initiator ammonium persulfate and *N,N,N′,N′*-tetramethylethylenediamine (TEMED). The latter was required to catalyze the decomposition of the initiator at 25°C. Stable colloidal dispersions of the PMMA-coated particles were obtained over a range of reaction conditions. They varied the MMA concentration while keeping the silica content fixed to examine the changes, and found that lowering the MMA concentration produced particles of higher silica content. TEM and dynamic light scattering (DLS) measurements also indicated a trend of decreasing silica-PMMA particle size with decreasing MMA concentration as would be expected. The silica-PMMA particle sizes ranged from 424 nm to 134 nm, indicating the presence of multiple silica seeds within the PMMA coating. Although the multicore particles are not strictly core-shell hybrids, variation of the reaction conditions can be used to vary their silica content. The authors demonstrated that it was possible to effectively produce submicron-sized monodisperse PMMA particles which were colloidally stable in the absence of any added surfactants, by replacing the aqueous medium with an alcohol containing system.

6.3.1.3 *Precipitation Polymerization*

In contrast to the aforementioned methods, the precipitation polymerization is performed in a continuous phase system in which the monomer and radical initiator are homogeneously dissolved [80]. The continuous phase is selected accordingly to be a nonsolvent for the forming polymer, which undergoes precipitation from the medium as polymerization proceeds.

The use of precipitation polymerization as a method for encapsulating Stöber silica particles with a thin shell of PMMA was shown by Freris *et al.* [81]. In this system the hydrophobic MMA was completely solubilized and homogeneously dispersed in the medium. It was therefore crucial to enhance the affinity of MMA with the otherwise hydrophilic silica seeds prior to polymerization. Surface grafting of MPTES was chosen to impart hydrophobicity of the silica seeds, provide a polymerizable group on their surface and increase their dispersibility in the organic phase medium used for the polymerization. The negatively charged silanols on the Stöber particles (approximately 180 nm diameter) were modified *in situ* with MPTES by direct addition of the silane agent in the ammonium containing aqueous-ethanolic medium used for their synthesis. They were subsequently washed with ethanol to remove any physisorbed silane.

The solvent used for the polymerization of MMA with the MPTES-silica seeds was tetraethyl orthosilicate (TEOS), which is traditionally used as a precursor for silica synthesis. In this context it was selected as a solvent medium on the basis of a previously reported precipitation polymerization for which a stabilized PMMA latex was formed [82]. In the synthesis of PMMA latex particles it was thought to act as a surface stabilizer during the polymer bead growth, which led to the formation of stable colloids comprising monodisperse spheres.

While the presence of MPTES on the silica particles was evidenced by IR, their ready dispersibility and stability in the hydrophobic MMA/TEOS (1:2 volume ratio) provided further support for their surface hydrophobization. The encapsulation polymerization of MPTES-silica (0.1% w/v to MMA) was thermally initiated using benzoyl peroxide (BPO) (1% w/v to MMA) as radical initiator, and conducted under static conditions for 10 minutes. Although complete monomer conversion could not be obtained in 10 minutes, longer reaction times would lead to flocculation and sedimentation of the particles. The encapsulation obtained is visible in TEM micrographs which show silica cores coated by smooth PMMA shells (Figure 6.4). They observed that PMMA shell thickness varied throughout the sample, ranging between 2 nm and 10 nm.

The presence of empty PMMA beads was not observed, indicating that polymer growth was favored entirely on the seed surface, thought to arise through co-polymerization of the attached

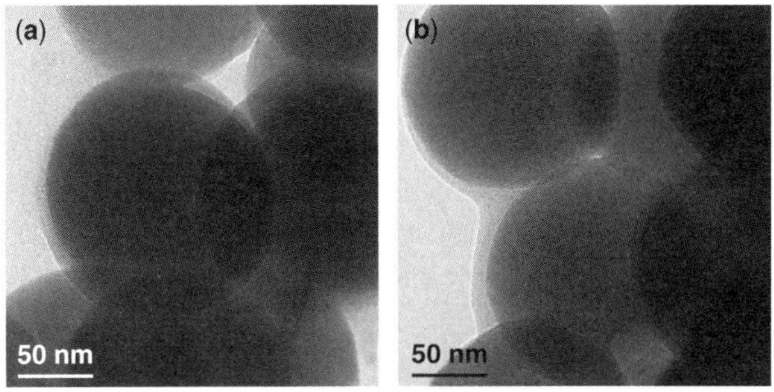

Figure 6.4 TEM micrographs of silica–PMMA hybrid demonstrating the presence of a thin film of PMMA encapsulating silica core particles. Reproduced from [81] with permission from Elsevier.

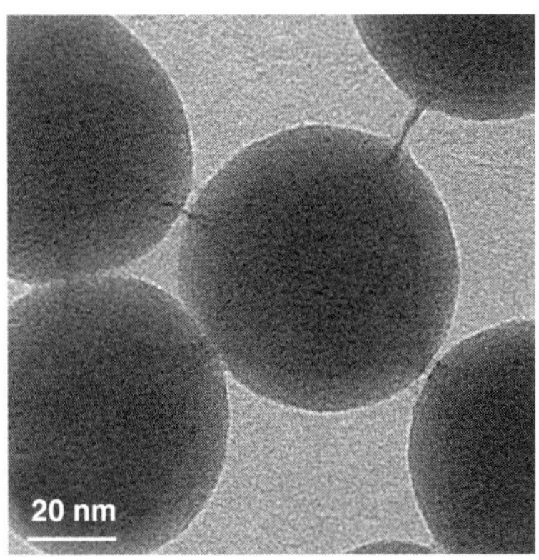

Figure 6.5 TEM micrographs of silica–PMMA hybrid obtained under stirred conditions evidences string-like PMMA links.

methacrylate group on the silica. The importance of using static conditions to obtain core-shell morphology was demonstrated by conducting the same polymerization with stirring. Figure 6.5 evidences the formation of string-type linkages amongst particles, thought to be coiled PMMA. While encapsulation by PMMA shells was not obtained under stirred conditions, it did provide further evidence that PMMA growth was promoted at the silica seed surface.

In a sequential study of the materials by solid state nuclear magnetic resonance (SSNMR) [83], it was found that not all the MPTES was covalently attached to the silica surface, but also present as adsorbed self-condensed oligomers. SSNR showed that in the polymer encapsulated particles a lower quantity of MPTES oligomers was detected when compared to the original MPTES-silica seeds, suggesting their removal during the encapsulation process. Additionally, post extraction of the polymer from the core-shell hybrid would result in removal of MPTES. It is likely that in the latter case the MPTES molecules were covalently attached to the PMMA rather than the silica surface. This indicated that although the PMMA shell was not entirely bound to the silica surface through covalent attachment, its nucleation and growth occurred at the surface through hydrophobic attraction. Interestingly, the extractive removal of the surface adsorbed MPTES oligomers prior to conducting the polymerization would lower the encapsulation efficiency, leading to formation of thinner shells. Hence, the authors established that the physically adsorbed oligomers play a crucial role in increasing the compatibility with MMA and promoting PMMA nucleation at the surface.

6.3.1.4 Dispersion Polymerization

Dispersion polymerization may be defined as a type of precipitation polymerization in which the polymerization of a monomer is conducted in the presence of a suitable polymeric stabilizer or dispersant. The solvent selected as the reaction medium must solubilize the monomer and the steric stabilizer, yet act as a nonsolvent for the polymer being formed. Hence, dispersion polymerization involves a homogeneous solution of monomer, initiator and dispersant, in which sterically stabilized polymer particles are formed by the precipitation of the resulting polymer [84].

The use of supercritical CO_2 ($scCO_2$) in a dispersion polymerization was first presented as a viable alternative to the conventional organic solvent-based methods by Desimone *et al.* [85, 86]. They showed that the supercritical solvent medium could be used for the formation of stabilized micrometer-sized PMMA latex particles, with a narrow size distribution and a high degree of polymerization.

Park *et al.* [87] prepared PMMA encapsulated silica particles by dispersion polymerization in $scCO_2$ with the aid of block copolymer poly(dimethyl siloxane)-poly[alkyl(meth)acrylic acid] (PDMS-*b*-PMMA) [88] as stabilizer. In their study they used a commercial source of silica nanoparticles with an average diameter of 107 nm. Similar to the aforementioned polymerizations, the hydrophilic silica was modified by surface grafting of MPTES to provide a polymerizable group on the surface. The surface grafting of MPTES also served to increase the stability of the silica containing suspension in $scCO_2$, which is promoted by the favorable interaction that exists between MPTES molecules and CO_2 [89].

In their polymerizations they used the radical initiator 2,2-azobisisobutyronitrile (AIBN) with a 2% w/w ratio to MMA, 20% MMA (v/v to CO_2), 5 wt% of MPTES-silica (w/w to MMA), and varied the amount of PDMS-*b*-PMMA. They examined the product morphology as a function of stabilizer content, by testing 5%, 10% and 15% PDMS-*b*-PMMA (w/w to MMA). The polymerizations proceeded to give monomer conversions > 95% after 12 hours, and a trend of decreasing particle size from 1.87 µm to 300 nm when the PDMS-*b*-PMMA amount was increased from 5 to 15% (w/w to MMA). This decreasing trend in particle size with increasing stabilizer content has previously been noted in $scCO_2$ dispersion polymerizations [90]. They obtained particles with a true core-shell morphology in all experiments with 5–15% PDMS-*b*-PMMA, whereby individual silica seeds were fully encapsulated by the PMMA shell. They found that the uniformity of the overall particle shape improved with increasing stabilizer content to provide a spherical morphology when 15% stabilizer was used. Slight aggregation between core-shell particles was observed by TEM analyses, although similar aggregation between polymer latex particles derived in $ScCO_2$ dispersion polymerizations with silicone-based stabilizers has previously been noted [91]. The necessity for a stabilizer was confirmed when a polymerization attempt conducted in the absence of PDMS-*b*-PMMA produced a hard and aggregated material.

6.3.1.5 *Vapor Phase Polymerization*

The vapor phase deposition (VPD) technique can be used for the gradual coating of inorganic particles with a polymeric shell, allowing good control over core-shell architecture. Jang and Li demonstrated the method by the gradual coating of both silica and titania particles with thin shells of PMMA and polydivinylbenzene (PDVB) [92]. The vapor phase method is capable of producing smooth and uniform polymer layers, and allows for control over shell thickness since the polymer is applied via gradual deposition steps on the particle surface. In the example reported [92], spherical silica particles with two different sizes (200 nm and 25 nm) were used as the core materials, following their surface modification with chlorodimethylvinylsilane (CDV). As for the previously described encapsulation methods, the surface was modified to improve affinity for the organic monomers in the polymerization step. The polymerization was performed in a reactor comprising two chambers. The inorganic particles and initiator contained in one chamber were evacuated to 10^{-1} torr at room temperature, and then closed off by a valve to maintain a static vacuum. The second chamber was used to introduce the liquid monomer via injection, which was subsequently vaporized by heating to 70°C. At this point, polymerization is activated by thermal decomposition of the radical initiator and the valve is opened to allow monomer vapor into the chamber where the inorganic particles are maintained under constant stirring. Stirring was established as necessary to circumvent the aggregation of particles during the polymer encapsulation.

The vapor phase polymerization led to the formation of individual silica core-PMMA shell particles characterized by smooth surfaces and an overall spherical shape. The thin shell of PMMA displayed an approximate thickness of 8 nm and fully encapsulated the silica core particles. The method as described did not lead to the formation of empty PMMA particles, and the core-shell hybrids obtained were well separated. The shell thickness could be tuned by varying the MMA/SiO_2 weight ratio. For example, a shell thickness of approximately 25 nm was obtained with a ratio of 0.75, while increasing the ratio to 1.5 resulted in a shell thickness of approximately 40 nm. The method consistently produced a smooth PMMA coating, even when the MMA/SiO_2 weight ratio was incremented to increase the thickness of the shell.

The formation of highly-uniform PMMA shells was attributed to the nature of the VPD combined with the large specific surface of the particles being encapsulated. The vast surface area of the nano-sized particles provides a favorable surface for which the monomers may adsorb from the vapor phase. This process of exclusive surface adsorption prior to polymerization was supported by the absence of empty PMMA particles, whereby the polymerization proceeded from growing polymer radicals confined in the adsorbed layers. Upon completion of the polymerization, the core-shell hybrid particles are ready to be separated by venting any residual monomer vapor from the chamber.

6.3.2 Controlled Living Radical Polymerization

The methods described thus far for the PMMA encapsulation of silica have been based on conventional free radical polymerization. Although the preparation of silica-PMMA hybrids with core-shell morphologies was possible, precise control over the polymers' properties was absent. Typically, such polymerizations are characterized by broad molecular weight distributions, and give limited control of the molecular weight and chain end functionality [93].

Alternatively, surface initiated controlled living radical polymerization (CLRP) has proven to be a useful technique for the growth of organic polymers with tailored architectures on the surface of silica particles [94–100]. By using this approach, it has been possible to tailor the structure of the polymer coating, by careful selection and control of the reaction parameters. Specifically, the life-time of the growing radical is controlled, resulting in the synthesis of polymers with a precision over molecular weight, molecular weight distribution, its structure and terminal functionality.

Atom transfer radical polymerization (ATRP) is among the most effective and most widely used methods of CLRP, and has been used for the growth of well-defined polymer brushes from the surface of silica particles [100]. Herein we present some examples where it has been used to grow well-defined PMMA brushes on the surface of silica particles, and its utility for the fabrication of ordered structures.

6.3.2.1 Atom Transfer Radical Polymerization

Patten and von Werne reported one of the first examples for controlled growth of styrene and PMMA by ATRP on nanosized silica particles [96]. The approach consisted of synthesis and covalent immobilization of the initiator molecule on the surface of spherical silica particles with 75 nm and 300 nm dimensions. Tandem ATRP initiators/organosiloxanes were prepared by hydrosilation of allyl ester group-containing ATRP initiators with dimethylethoxysilane. This produced initiators with a singly hydrolyzable monosiloxane group, offering single site attachment to the nanoparticle surface with its superficial silanol groups. For the surface-initiated polymerization of MMA they grafted the initiator (3-(2-bromoisobutyryl)propyl)dimethylethoxysilane (BIDS) on the silica particles. The successive polymerizations using the nanoparticles as seed macroinitiators were conducted by heating with MMA, copper(I) bromide, ligand, and solvent. This led to the surface initiated growth of densely grafted PMMA chains directly from the silica nanoparticles. In the surface-initiated polymerization from the smaller 75 nm particles, they established that growth of PMMA chains would proceed in a controlled/living manner with good molecular weight control when a small amount of "sacrificial" free initiator, ethyl 2-bromoisobutryate (2-(EiB)Br), was also added to the system. In contrast, the polymerization of MMA from the 300 nm silica nanoparticles did not exhibit molecular weight control. The difference in behavior between polymerizations employing smaller versus larger initiator-modified nanoparticles was correlated to their surface area, and specifically the amount of initiator present per unit mass of initiator. The 75 nm particles contained approximately 0.1-0.3 mmol of initiator sites per gram of silica. Hence a polymerization with 1 g of sample in a 65% monomer solution provided an initial monomer/initiator ratio of 200-300, which is typical of ATRP experiments that provide good molecular weight control. In contrast, the 300 nm-sized particles were covered with approximately 0.07-0.09 mmol of initiator sites per gram of silica. The corresponding monomer/initiator ratio for a polymerization using 1 g in a 65% monomer solution is approximately 500–800, which would exceed the limit for good molecular weight control in ATRP.

The overall dimensions of the core-shell particles could be tuned through progressive growth of the PMMA brush on the surface. They demonstrated a linear relationship for molecular weight (M_n) growth with monomer conversion, an increase in overall hydrodynamic diameter with monomer conversion, and obtained narrow molecular weight distributions (M_w/M_n) as the surface initiated polymerization of MMA proceeded under their experimental conditions.

Ohno *et al.* [97] similarly employed the surface-initiated ATRP method for controlled growth of PMMA brushes on silica nanoparticles. They synthesized the surface initiator, (2-bromo-2-methyl)propionyloxyhexyltriethoxysilanetriethoxysilyl, via a two-step process. This initiator being a triethyl silyl derivative, could be readily grafted to the silica particles by ammonium catalyzed hydrolysis and condensation as is routinely performed with commonly used silane coupling agents. They used silica nanoparticles with an average diameter of 130 nm, which they subsequently coated with a closely-packed monolayer of the initiator to obtain a graft density of approximately 2 initiator molecules/nm^2. The initiator-coated particles were used in the copper-mediated ATRP of MMA which led to the growth of PMMA chains with a graft density approximately equal to 0.65 chains/nm^2. The authors found that the following parameters were essential for successful grafting of PMMA. The initiator-coated silica particles should never be dried and should be maintained in solvent until their use. These could then be transferred to the monomer containing polymerization solution by solvent exchange. Additionally, the presence of "sacrificial" free initiator 2-(EiB)Br was essential to accumulate an appropriate amount of Cu(II) species via the termination of polymer radicals, and to control the polymerization by the so-called persistent radical effect. They characterized the bare and coated particles by dynamic light scattering and observed an increasing hydrodynamic particle diameter from 145 nm for the bare silica particles to 495 nm for the PMMA grafted particles.

The controlled and uniform growth of PMMA chains on silica spheres obtained by ATRP is finding application in the fabrication of ordered two-dimensional (2D) arrays [97, 99]. Core-shell particles featuring a narrow size distribution can self-assemble to generate highly ordered structures, such as 2D colloidal crystals, provided they are well dispersed with suitable interparticle separation. Since ATRP provides a high level of control in the polymer graft density it is a viable tool in the construction of colloidal crystals. This was shown by Ohno *et al.* in a sequential study, where they demonstrated the effective assembly of PMMA-grafted silica particles to form an ordered 2D hexagonal array [99].

The authors applied the PMMA grafting method for 55 nm-sized silica particles that were obtained via the reverse micelle method. The silica particles were surface grafted with the initiator, (2-bromo-2-methyl)propionyloxyhexyltriethoxysilanetriethoxysilyl, and subsequently subjected to the copper-mediated ATRP of MMA as per their previous method [97]. They obtained silica-PMMA hybrid particles that comprised the 55 nm-sized core and a shell of PMMA grafted chains with a molecular weight (M_n) of 122 000 and a surface graft density of 0.8 chains/nm^2. The silica-PMMA core-shell particles were prepared as a 6.14 vol% suspension in a mixture of chlorobenzene/1,2-dichloroethane (volume ratio 66/34) and used to fabricate thin films of colloidal crystals. Because of their exceptionally high uniformity, the core-shell particles formed an ordered array by arranging in a hexagonally close-packed monolayer upon solvent evaporation. The mean nearest neighbor center-to-center interparticle distance was found to be 350 nm.

6.4 Summary

The recent developments for the preparation of core-shell particles composed of an inner silica core and a poly(methyl methacrylate) outer shell have been reviewed. As widely reported in the literature, the choice of the method for the encapsulation of silica particles, their preparation methods and their surface modification influence their interaction with the monomer during polymer formation. Furthermore, the degree of dispersion for the silica particles in the polymer is strongly influenced by the interfacial interaction that exists between the two, which plays an important role in enhancing or limiting the overall properties of the system.

In particular, this chapter reports:

a. the common routes for yielding spherical silica particles, namely sol-gel methods such as the Stöber synthesis and the reverse phase microemulsion method;
b. their surface modification to impart superficial hydrophobicity and/or promote monomer polymerization at the surface. These methods include the covalent attachment of a polymerizable organosilane which may co-polymerize with the monomer in conventional radical polymerization, or the covalent attachment of an initiator for controlled living radical polymerization;
c. the encapsulation of silica particles with a thin shell of PMMA by conventional *in situ* heterophase radical polymerization methods, with examples given for emulsion, emulsifier-free emulsion, precipitation, dispersion, and vapor phase polymerization techniques. Additionally, some examples of surface initiated atom transfer radical polymerization, for the controlled growth of poly(methyl methacrylate) brushes on silica particles were also provided.

References

1. S. Gross, D. Camozzo, V. Di Noto, L. Armelao, E. Tondello. *European Polymer Journal* Vol. 43, p. 673, 2007.
2. I. Sondi, T.H. Fedynyshyn, R. Sinta, E. Matijevic. *Langmuir* Vol. 16, p. 9031, 2000.
3. P. Gómez-Romero, C. Sanchez. *Functional hybrid materials*. Weinheim, Wiley–VCH, 2004.
4. G. Kickelbick. *Hybrid materials. Synthesis, characterization, and applications.* Weinheim, Wiley–VCH, 2007.
5. P. Judeinstein, C. Sañchez. *Journal of Materials Chemistry* Vol. 6, p. 511, 1996.
6. M. Ohmori, E. Matijevic. *Journal of Colloid and Interface Science* Vol. 160, p. 288, 1993.
7. D.V. Goia, E. Matijevic. *New Journal of Chemistry* Vol. 22, p. 1203, 1998.
8. T. Sato, R. Ruch. *Stabilization of colloidal dispersions by polymer adsorption.* New York, Dekker, 1980.
9. F. Caruso. *Advanced Materials* Vol. 13, p. 11, 2001.
10. E. Bourgeat-Lami, J. Lang. *Journal of Colloid and Interface Science* Vol. 197, p. 293, 1998.
11. R.A. Caruso, M. Antonietti. *Chemistry of Materials* Vol. 13, p. 3272, 2001.
12. F. Yang, G.L. Nelson. *Journal of Applied Polymer Science* Vol. 91, p. 3844, 2004.
13. H. Wang, P. Xu, W. Zhong, L. Shen, Q. Du. *Polymer Degradation and Stability* Vol. 87, p. 319, 2005.
14. H. Wang, P. Xu, S. Meng, W. Zhong, W. Du, Q. Du. *Polymer Degradation and Stability* Vol. 91, p. 1455, 2006.
15. N. Katsikis, F. Zahradnik, A. Helmschrott, H. Münstedt, A. Vital. *Polymer Degradation and Stability* Vol. 92, p. 1966, 2007.
16. H. Althues, J. Henle, S. Kaskel. *Chemical Society Reviews* Vol. 36, p. 1454, 2007.
17. M.L. Saladino, T.E. Motaung, A.S. Luyt, A. Spinella, G. Nasillo, E. Caponetti. *Polymer Degradation and Stability* Vol. 97, p. 452, 2012.
18. D.Q. Zou, H. Yoshida. *Journal of Thermal Analysis and Calorimetry* Vol. 99, p. 21, 2010.
19. N. García, T. Corrales, J. Guzmán, P. Tiemblo. *Polymer Degradation and Stability* Vol. 92, p. 635, 2007.
20. F. Yang, G.L. Nelson. *Polymers for Advanced Technologies* Vol. 17, p. 320, 2006.
21. T. Kashiwagi, A.B. Morgan, J.M. Antonucci, M.R. VanLandingham, R.H. Harris, W.H. Awad, J.R. Shields. *Journal of Applied Polymer Science* Vol. 89, p. 2072, 2003.
22. Y.H. Hu, C.Y. Chen, C.C. Wang. *Polymer Degradation and Stability* Vol. 84, p. 545, 2004.
23. M.S. Fleming, T.K. Mandal, D.R. Walt. *Chemistry of Materials* Vol. 13, p. 2210, 2001.
24. R.G. Chaudhu, S. Paria. *Chemical Reviews* Vol. 112, p. 2373, 2012.
25. H. Zou, S. Wu, J. Shen. *Chemical Reviews* Vol. 108, p. 3893, 2008.
26. J.L. Vivero-Escoto, R.C. Huxford-Phillips, W. Lin. *Chemical Society Reviews* Vol. 41, p. 2673, 2012.
27. W. Schärtl. *Nanoscale* Vol. 2, p. 829, 2010.

28. R.P. Bagwe, C. Yang, L.R. Hilliard, W. Tan. *Langmuir* Vol. 20, p. 8336, 2004.
29. A. van Blaaderen, A. Vrij. *Langmuir* Vol. 8, p. 2921, 1992.
30. N.A.M. Verhaegh, A. van Blaaderen. *Langmuir* Vol. 10, p. 1427, 1994.
31. H. Ow, D.R. Larson, M. Srivastava, B.A. Baird, W.W. Webb, U. Wiesner. *Nano Letters* Vol. 5, p. 113, 2005.
32. L.L. Hench, J.K. West. *Chemistry Reviews* Vol. 90, p. 13, 1991.
33. C.J. Brinker, G. Scherrer. *Sol-gel science; The physics and chemistry of sol-gel processing*. San Diego, Academic Press, 1989.
34. G. Kolbe. Ph.D. Thesis, Friedrich-Schiller-Universität Jena, Germany,1956.
35. W. Stöber, A. Fink, E. Bohn. *Journal of Colloid and Interface Science* Vol. 26, p. 62, 1968.
36. A.K. van Helden, J.W. Jansen, A. Vrij. *Journal of Colloid and Interface Science* Vol. 81, p. 354, 1981.
37. A.P. Philipse. *Colloid and Polymer Science* Vol. 266, p. 1174, 1988.
38. A.P. Philipse. A. Vrij. *Journal of Colloid and Interface Science* Vol. 128, p. 121, 1989.
39. G.H. Bogush, M.A. Tracy, C.F. Zukoski. *IV Journal of Non–Crystalline Solids* Vol. 104, p. 95, 1988.
40. G.H. Bogush, C.F. Zukoski. *IV Journal of Non–Crystalline Solids* Vol. 142, p. 1, 1991.
41. G.H. Bogush, C.F. Zukoski. *IV Journal of Non–Crystalline Solids* Vol. 142, p. 19, 1991.
42. A. van Blaaderen , J. van Geest, A. Vrij. *Journal of Colloid and Interface Science* Vol. 154, p. 481, 1992.
43. A. van Blaaderen, A. Vrij. *Journal of Colloid and Interface Science* Vol. 156, p. 1, 1993.
44. J.L. Vivero-Escoto, Y.-T. Huang. *International Journal of Molecular Sciences* Vol. 12, p. 3888, 2011.
45. K. Osseo-Asare, F.J. Arriagada. *Colloids and Surfaces* Vol. 50, p. 321, 1990.
46. F.J. Arriagada, and K. Osseo-Asare. *Colloids and Surfaces* Vol. 69, p. 105, 1992.
47. F.J. Arriagada, and K. Osseo-Asare. *Journal of Dispersion Science and Technology* Vol. 15, p. 59, 1994.
48. F.J. Arriagada, and K. Osseo-Asare. *Journal of Colloid and Interface Science* Vol. 211, p. 210, 1999.
49. K.S. Finnie, J.R. Bartlett, C.J.A. Barbé, L. Kong. *Langmuir* Vol. 23, p. 3017, 2007.
50. P. Riello, M. Mattiazzi, J.S. Pedersen, A. Benedetti. *Langmuir* Vol. 24, p. 5225, 2008.
51. F. Asaro, A. Benedetti, N. Savko, G. Pellizer. *Langmuir* Vol. 25, p. 3224, 2009.
52. F. Asaro, A. Benedetti, I. Freris, P. Riello, N. Savko. *Langmuir* Vol. 26, p. 12917, 2010.
53. A. Camenzinda, W.R. Caserib, S.E. Pratsinis. *Nano Today* Vol. 5, p. 48, 2010.
54. E.A. Wovchko, J.C. Camp, J.A. Glass, Jr., J.T. Yates, Jr. *Langmuir* Vol. 11, p. 2592, 1995.
55. G. Gellermann, W. Storch, H. Wolter. *Journal of Sol-Gel Science and Technology* Vol. 8, p. 173, 1997.
56. F.D. Blum. Silane coupling agents. In *Encyclopedia of polymer science and technology*. New York, John Wiley & Sons, 2003.
57. I.J. Bruce, T. Sen. *Langmuir* Vol. 21, p. 7029, 2005.

58. J.P. Davim, C. Oliveira, N. Barricas, M. Conceição. *The International Journal of Advanced Manufacturing Technology* Vol. 35, p. 875, 2008.
59. K. Kuriki, Y. Koike, Y. Okamoto. *Chemical Reviews* Vol. 102, p. 2347, 2002.
60. Q.J. Zhang, P. Wang, X.F. Sun, Y. Zhai, P. Dai, B. Yang, M. Hai, J.P. Xie. *Applied Physics Letters* Vol. 72, p. 407, 1998.
61. G. Lemperle, V. Morhenn, U. Charrier. *Aesthetic Plastic Surgery* Vol. 27, p. 354, 2003.
62. E. Bourgeat-Lami, M. Lansalot. *Advances in Polymer Science* Vol. 233, p. 53, 2011.
63. J.-L. Luna-Xavier, E. Bourgeat-Lami, A. Guyot. *Colloid and Polymer Science* Vol. 279, p. 947, 2001.
64. Y. Haga, T. Watanabe, R. Yosomiya. *Angewandte Makromolekulare Chemie* Vol. 189, p. 23, 1991.
65. K. Yoshinaga, T. Yokoyama, Y. Sugawa, H. Karakawa, N. Enomoto, H. Nishida, M. Komatzu. *Polymer Bulletin* Vol. 28, p. 663, 1992.
66. J.-L. Luna-Xavier, A. Guyot, E. Bourgeat-Lami. *Journal of Colloid and Interface Science* Vol. 250, p. 82, 2002.
67. K. Zhang, L. Zheng, X. Zhang, X. Chen, B. Yang. *Colloids and Surfaces A: Physicochemical and Engineering Aspects* Vol. 277, p. 145, 2006.
68. S. Zhang, S. Zhou, Y. Weng, L. Wu. *Langmuir* Vol. 21, p. 2124, 2005.
69. K. Zhang, H. Chen, X. Chen, Z. Chen, Z. Cui, B. Yang. *Macromolular Materials and Engineering* Vol. 288, p. 380, 2003.
70. Z. Chen, T. Gang, K. Zhang, J. Zhang, X. Chen, Z. Sun, B. Yang. *Colloids and Surfaces A: Physicochemical and Engineering Aspects* Vol. 272, p. 151, 2006.
71. T. Ribeiro, C. Baleizão, J.P.S. Farinha. *Journal of Physical Chemistry, C* Vol. 113, p. 18082, 2009.
72. H. Chen, C. Deng, X. Zhang. *Angewandte Chemie International Edition* Vol. 49, p. 607, 2010.
73. W. Jia, X. Chen, H. Lu, P. Yang. *Angewandte Chemie* Vol. 118, p. 3423, 2006.
74. W. Jia, X. Chen, H. Lu, P. Yang. *Angewandte Chemie International Edition* Vol. 45, p. 3345, 2006.
75. W. Shen, H. Xiong, Y. Xu, S. Cai, H. Lu, P. Yang. *Analytical Chemistry* Vol. 80, p. 6758, 2008.
76. H. Xiong, X. Guan, L. Jin, W. Shen, H. Lu, Y. Xia. *Angewandte Chemie* Vol. 120, p. 4272, 2008.
77. H. Xiong, X. Guan, L. Jin, W. Shen, H. Lu, Y. Xia *Angewandte Chemie International Edition* Vol. 47, p. 4204, 2008.
78. M.J. Percy, S.P. Armes. *Langmuir* Vol. 18, p. 4562, 2002.
79. M.J. Percy, J.I. Amalvy, D.P. Randall, S.P. Armes, S.J. Greaves, J.F. Watts. *Langmuir* Vol. 20, p. 2184, 2004.
80. S. Slomkowski, J.V. Alemán, R.G. Gilbert, M. Hess, K. Horie, R.G. Jones, P. Kubisa, I. Meisel, W. Mormann, S. Penczek, R.F.T. Stepto. *Pure and Applied Chemistry* Vol. 83, p. 2229, 2011.
81. I. Freris, D. Cristofori, P. Riello, A. Benedetti. *Journal of Colloid and Interface Science* Vol. 331, p. 351, 2009.
82. D. Wang, Q. Luo, X. Li, X. Wang, H. Yong, Z. Zhen, X. Liu, D. Jia. *Colloid and Polymer Science* Vol. 282, p. 48, 2003.

83. U.P. Sudhakaran, I. Freris, M. Geppi, S. Borsacchi, D. Cristofori, P. Riello, A. Benedetti. *Colloids and Surfaces A: Physicochemical and Engineering Aspects*, Vol. 369, p. 191, 2010.
84. S. Kawaguchi, K. Ito. *Advanced Polymer Science* Vol. 175, p. 299, 2005.
85. J.M. DeSimone, E.E. Maury, Y.Z. Menceloglu, J.B. McClain, T.J. Romack, J.R. Combes. *Science* Vol. 265, p. 356, 1994.
86. D.A. Canelas, D.E. Betts, J.M. DeSimone. *Macromolecules* Vol. 29, p. 2818, 1996.
87. E.J. Park, W.S. Kim, H.S. Hwang, C. Park, K.T. Lim. *Macromolecular Symposia* Vol. 249–250, p. 196, 2007.
88. K.T. Lim, S.E. Webber, K.P. Johnston. *Macromolecules* Vol. 32, p. 2811, 1999.
89. B. Yue, J. Yang, C.Y. Huang, R. Dave, R. Pfeffer. *Macromolecular Rapid Communications* Vol. 26, p. 1406, 2005.
90. H. Shiho, J.M. DeSimone. *Macromolecules* Vol. 34, p. 1198, 2001.
91. M.Z. Yates, G. Li, J.J. Shim, S. Maniar, K.P. Johnston, K.T. Lim, S. Webber. *Macromolecules* Vol. 32, p. 1018, 1999.
92. J. Jang, B. Lim. *Angewandte Chemie International Edition* Vol. 42, p. 5600, 2003.
93. B. Radhakrishnan, R. Ranjan, W.J. Brittain. *Soft Matter* Vol. 2, p. 386, 2006.
94. C. Perruchot, M.A. Khan, A. Kamitsi, S.P. Armes, T. von Werne, T.E. Patten. *Langmuir* Vol. 17, p. 4479, 2001.
95. T. von Werne, T.E. Patten. *Journal of the American Chemical Society* Vol. 121, p. 7409, 1999.
96. T. von Werne, T.E. Patten. *Journal of the American Chemical Society* Vol. 123, p. 7497, 2001.
97. K. Ohno, T. Morinaga, K. Koh, Y. Tsujii, T. Fukuda. *Macromolecules* Vol. 38, p. 2137, 2005.
98. T. Morinaga, M. Ohkura, K. Ohno, Y. Tsujii, T. Fukuda. *Macromolecules* Vol. 40, P. 1159, 2007.
99. K. Ohno, T. Akashi, Y. Huang, Y. Tsujii. *Macromolecules* Vol. 43, p. 8805, 2010.
100. K. Matyjaszewski. *Macromolecules* Vol. 45, p. 4015, 2012.

7

Organic Thin-Film Transistors with Solution-Processed Encapsulation

Feng-Yu Tsai and Yu Fu

Department of Materials Science and Engineering, National Taiwan University, Taipei, Taiwan, ROC

Abstract

Organic thin-film transistors (OTFT) are susceptible to air- or environment-induced degradations and therefore must be effectively encapsulated to achieve sufficient stability for practical applications. A successful encapsulation method must be designed with the specific degradation mechanisms of the device materials in mind, so as to minimize both environment-induced and encapsulation-induced degradations. This chapter reviews recent progress in the development of OTFT encapsulation techniques, covering topics including mechanisms of environment-induced degradations, mechanisms of encapsulation-induced degradations, and results of OTFT encapsulation employing various encapsulation approaches. Focus is placed on OTFT based on the two most prevalent organic semiconductors: poly-3-hexylthiophene (P3HT) and pentacene, with attention paid to solution-processed encapsulation methods.

Keywords: Organic field-effect transistors, organic semiconductors, gas-permeation barriers, passivation, flexible electronics, thin-film encapsulation

7.1 Introduction

Organic thin-film transistors (OTFT) offer many advantages, such as processability and mechanical flexibility, over inorganic technologies [1–3] and have been developed for potential uses in a wide range of applications including displays [4, 5], sensors [6, 7], and

Vikas Mittal (ed.) Encapsulation Nanotechnologies, (203–224) © 2013 Scrivener Publishing LLC

radio frequency identification [8, 9]. Through the intensive research efforts of recent years, reasonably high device performance as well as manufacture-enabling processing techniques have been demonstrated for OTFTs [10, 11]. Despite the remarkable progress in OTFT technology, actual commercialization of OTFTs has been hindered by their susceptibility to environment-induced degradations. Therefore, an effective encapsulation method is paramount to the development of OTFT technology. For the general TFT device structures shown in Figure 7.1, encapsulation involves depositing a barrier film on top of the device, forming a hermetic seal to insulate the device from the environment. This encapsulation approach is referred to as "thin-film encapsulation," as opposed to more traditional encapsulation methods such as those using a glass or metal lid and glue. The substrate beneath the TFT device is typically adequate in blocking out degradation-inducing agents from the surroundings, but in the case of flexible OTFTs based on plastic substrates, an additional barrier film may be needed between the device and the substrate due to the high permeability of many plastic substrates.

Success of an encapsulation method for OTFTs is determined by a myriad of factors, chief among which include 1) effectiveness of the encapsulating film in blocking out degradation-inducing agents from the environment, mainly oxygen and moisture;

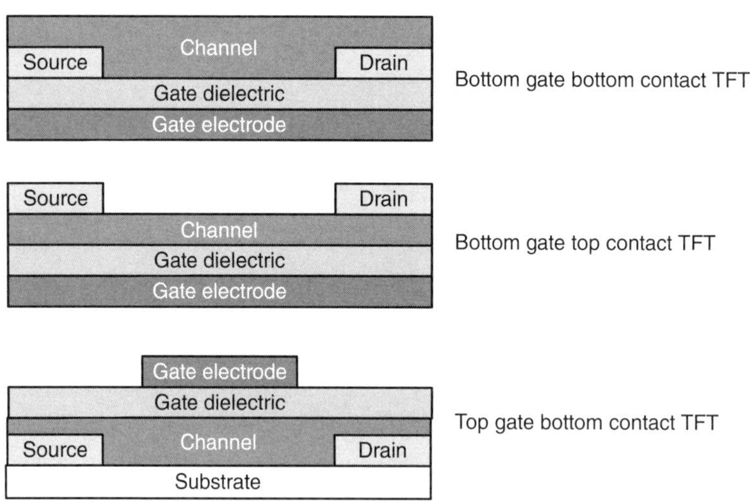

Figure 7.1 General device structures of thin-film transistors.

2) compatibility with the to-be-encapsulated OTFT device, so as to not compromise the device performance upon application of the encapsulating layer; 3) compatibility with any subsequent process which the encapsulated OTFT device may undergo; 4) processability and cost. A variety of approaches have been pursued in developing encapsulation methods for OTFTs, with various degrees of success in terms of the above-mentioned factors. This review will provide an overview to recent processes in encapsulation technologies for OTFTs. General mechanisms of environment-induced degradation to OTFTs will first be reviewed, and the general requirements of encapsulation will be discussed. Case studies on the encapsulation of OTFTs will then be reviewed, with the main focus on two of the most widely-used organic semiconductors: pentacene and poly-3-hexylthiophene (P3HT), as well as their respective derivatives. Vacuum- as well as solution-processed encapsulation methods will both be covered, but emphasis will be placed on the latter for its advantages in processability and cost.

7.2 Environment-Induced Degradations of OTFTs

The susceptibility of OTFTs to environment-induced degradations originates mainly from the high HOMO and low LUMO of organic semiconductors, which readily enable electron transfer between the organic semiconductors and environmental species that come into contact with them, causing the electrical characteristics of the OTFTs to change accordingly. Such degradation-inducing environmental species can include a wide variety of substances, but for practical purposes, those from the ambient air are the most important. Air-induced degradations to OTFTs have been found to be mainly caused by moisture, oxygen, and light; and the effects typically include reduced on current, reduced field-effect mobility, increased off current, lowered on/off ratio, positively shifted threshold voltage (V_{th}), and hysteresis. The degradation behavior varies among different organic semiconductors, but the mechanisms are similar. The following sections will review previous studies on air-induced degradations of OTFT made from the two types of organic semiconductors that are the most widely used: pentacene and polythiophenes.

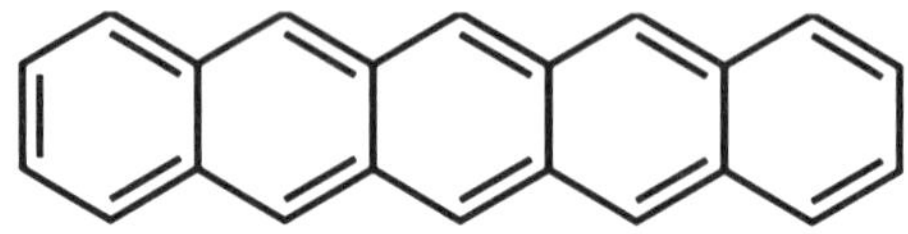

Figure 7.2 Chemical structure of pentacene.

7.2.1 Pentacene-Based OTFTs

Pentacene (structure in Figure 7.2) has been a popular choice of active material for OTFTs because of its high mobility and on/off ratio as p-type semiconductor for field-effect transistors [12]. Air-induced degradation of pentacene-based OTFTs has combined contributions from mechanisms including photo-oxidation, oxygen doping, charge trapping by moisture, and moisture-induced doping. Details of these mechanisms are described as follows:

1. Photo-oxidation
   Pentacene has been shown to photo-oxidize in the presence of oxygen and light, with transannular endoperoxide and dimeric peroxide as the oxidation products [13–16]. The mechanism of photo-oxidation has been suggested to be via sensitization of singlet oxygen by the triplet excitation state of pentacene, whose energy is raised by thermal activation to the necessary level for the sensitization during its rather long lifetime (~110 μs) [17, 18]. Photo-oxidation of pentacene has been found to be far less severe in films than in solution; the better photo-oxidation resistance of pentacene films has been attributed to the characteristically high crystallinity of pentacene films, which may impede permeation of oxygen into a film and also shorten the lifetime of the excited state of pentacene [19].

   In terms of the effects of photo-oxidation on the electrical characteristics of pentacene OTFTs, there has not been explicit disclosure in the literature. It is to be expected that photo-oxidation will lower the charge carrier mobility of pentacene and thus lead to lower on current of TFT devices. However, previous studies examining electrical properties of pentacene after exposure to oxygen and light have observed little of such effects [20, 21], inferring that photo-oxidation may not be a major contributing factor to the degradation of pentacene OTFTs.

2. Oxygen doping
   A more pronounced effect of oxygen on the electrical properties of pentacene has been observed to be oxygen doping, which occurs as a result of absorbed oxygen extracting electrons from pentacene, generating holes [21]. Oxygen doping is greatly enhanced in the presence of light. The effects of oxygen doping include increased conductivity, increased on and off current of TFT devices, and positively shifted V_{th} [20, 21].
3. Charge trapping by moisture
   Pentacene OTFTs have been found to show reduced on current and charge carrier mobility with hysteresis in the device characteristics in the presence of moisture, and the effects worsen with increasing humidity [22–29]. The reduction of charge carrier mobility and hysteresis have been attributed to charge trapping by water molecules residing at the grain boundaries through dissolution and diffusion from the environment, which can attract holes through charge-dipole interactions, increase energy barrier for inter-grain charge transport, and screen the electric field at the channel to reduce gate-induced carriers [22, 24, 27]. The magnitude of degradation is dependent upon the structure of TFT device, being the largest for devices with bottom contact and short channel lengths, as a result of a greater number of grain boundaries on top of the bottom contacts and larger influence of grain boundaries in the case of short channel lengths [27]. Charge trapping is also observed in single-crystal pentacene, where water molecules are found to be incorporated into crystal lattices [21].
4. Moisture-induced doping
   Besides impeding charge transport and trapping charges, the strong dipoles of the polar water molecule can also induce holes in pentacene, causing the off current to increase and V_{th} to shift toward a larger positive value [20, 27–29]. The combination of increased off current by doping and reduced on current by charge trapping results in significant lowering of the on/off ratio of pentacene OTFTs upon exposure to moisture. The effects of moisture, charge trapping or doping, have been found to be independent of light [21].

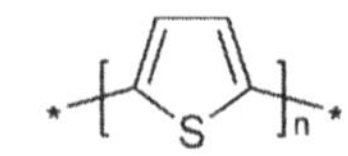

Figure 7.3 Chemical structure of polythiophene.

7.2.2 Polythiophenes-Based OTFTs

Polythiophenes (structure in Figure 7.3) are a desirable alternative to pentacene owing to their solution processability and reasonably high carrier mobility. In terms of resistance against air-induced degradations, however, polythiophenes are usually far inferior to pentacene. The aforementioned four mechanisms of air-induced degradation of pentacene OTFTs are also applicable to polythiophene OTFTs, and therefore the description below of the degradation mechanisms will be brief unless notable differences or exceptions exist.

Photo-oxidation of polythiophenes has been shown to occur in the presence of oxygen and light via 1,4 Diels-Alder addition of singlet oxygen which is formed through sensitization by photo-excited polythiophenes [30]. The resultant shortened conjugation length of polythiophenes reduces the on current and charge carrier mobility of OTFT devices [31, 32]. Oxygen by itself without light has been found to cause no detectable degradation to polythiophene OTFTs [32].

Both oxygen and moisture induce p-type doping in polythiophenes [32–34]. Oxygen doping has been found to noticeably occur only in the presence of light, while moisture doping is independent of light, and both effects are fully recoverable upon complete removal of oxygen and moisture through evacuation [32]. Charge trapping by moisture is likely similar to the case of pentacene OTFTs, but its effects—lowered on current and mobility—have not been directly observed, probably as a result of the strong moisture doping effect, which raises both the on and off currents drastically, masking the reduction in the on current caused by charge trapping [32].

7.2.3 Requirements of Encapsulation

Given the susceptibility of OTFTs to air-induced degradation as described above, an encapsulating film that is capable of insulating an OTFT device from oxygen, moisture, and light is crucial in obtaining air-stability from the device. The effectiveness of an encapsulating film in preventing ingression of oxygen and moisture is quantified by its oxygen transmission rate (OTR) and water vapor transmission rate (WVTR), respectively. Organic electronic devices generally require an encapsulating film with very low OTR and WVTR because of their highly reactive constituent materials; e.g., for organic light-emitting diodes (OLED), the OTR and WVTR of an adequate encapsulating film have to be below 10^{-5}–10^{-3} cc/m^2 day and 10^{-6} g/m^2 day, respectively [35]. The requirements in OTR and WVTR differ among different types of devices as well as among different materials selected for a given type of device; for OTFTs, the required OTR and WVTR values are typically much higher than those for OLEDs owing to the better air-stability of common OTFT materials. Specifically, for poly-3-hexylthiophene (P3HT) OTFTs, it has been shown that encapsulating films with OTR and WVTR as high as 10^1–10^2 cc (g) /m^2 day can be adequate, provided that the encapsulated OTFTs are shielded from light [32].

In addition to meeting the upper limits on oxygen and moisture transmission rates, a good encapsulation method must also avoid causing degradation during the encapsulation process. This requires low processing temperature, use of solvents compatible with the underlying OTFT device (in the case of solution-processed encapsulation), use of encapsulating materials that do not adversely interact with the underlying OTFT materials, etc. Such degradation-avoiding measures can be determined through systematically studying the response of OTFTs to various aspects of a given encapsulation process, as exemplified in some of the works reviewed in the following section.

7.3 Encapsulation of OTFTs

7.3.1 Polythiophene-Based OTFTs

7.3.1.1 Vacuum-Processed Encapsulation

Earlier attempts on encapsulating polythiophene OTFTs have logically employed vacuum-deposited inorganic films as encapsulating films, taking advantages of the low OTR and WVTR of such films (typically orders of magnitude lower than those of organic films) [35], and the cleanliness of the vacuum process. Due to the low thermal resistance of the organic active materials in OTFTs, the selection of vacuum deposition processes has been limited to those with low deposition temperatures.

Ferrari *et al.* utilized atomic layer deposition (ALD) to apply a 50 nm Al_2O_3 encapsulating film to P3HT OTFTs with a bottom gate/bottom contact layout (see Figure 7.1) [36]. The technique of ALD has been demonstrated to produce exceptionally effective barrier films at low deposition temperatures; e.g., 25 nm ALD Al_2O_3 films deposited on plastic substrates at 120°C have been shown to exhibit a WVTR value in the 10^{-6} g/m^2 day range, meeting the requirement of OLEDs [37]. On P3HT OTFTs, however, the ALD Al_2O_3 film caused severe deterioration to the device characteristics. The deterioration was attributed to the interaction between P3HT and the ALD precursors—trimethylaluminum (TMA) and water, whose vapors repeatedly imbue the P3HT layer during the cyclic steps of the ALD process. The strong electron-withdrawing tendency of TMA caused holes to be generated in P3HT, raising the on and off currents and positively shifting V_{th}, similar to the effects of moisture. The ALD-induced degradation could be modestly alleviated by applying a poly(vinyl phenol) (PVP) film as a buffer layer between the device and the encapsulating ALD Al_2O_3 film, but the resultant degradation was still significant, likely as a consequence of the polar interaction between PVP and P3HT or inadequate blocking of the ALD precursors by the PVP buffer layer. Despite the large encapsulation-induced degradation, the encapsulated OTFTs remained stable in air for 30 days owing to the excellent barrier performance of the ALD encapsulating film. To better prevent the ALD precursors from damaging P3HT, Fumagalli *et al.* added a crosslinked PVP layer on top of a PVP/ALD Al_2O_3 stack, and the results confirmed that such a 3-layer encapsulating film satisfactorily eliminated encapsulation-induced degradation and enabled the P3HT OTFTs to obtain long lifetime [38].

P3HT OTFTs have also been encapsulated with a silicon nitride film deposited by hot-wired chemical vapor deposition (HWCVD) at a deposition temperature of 60°C [39]. The encapsulation process did not result in noticeable device degradation, but the encapsulated devices, despite being much more air-stable than the unencapsulated control devices, still showed substantial increase (by a factor of ~4) in the off current after 170 h in air.

Ong *et al.* adopted an approach where a silver–indium zinc oxide (Ag–IZO) encapsulating film was deposited on a polyethylene naphthalate (PEN) film by DC and RF sputtering, and the

Ag-IZO-coated PEN film was then glued onto a P3HT OTFT using a UV-curable epoxy sealant [40]. This approach avoided exposure of OTFT devices to the energetic environment of the sputtering process, thereby avoiding encapsulation-induced degradation to the devices. Thanks to the good gas-barrier performance of the Ag-IZO film, with WVTR down to 1.6 x10^{-4} g/day m^2, the encapsulated OTFTs maintained stable electrical characteristics for 3600 h in air.

7.3.1.2 Solution-Processed Encapsulation

Although the vacuum-deposition-based encapsulation methods have achieved a certain degree of success with polythiophene OTFTs, encapsulation methods that are solution-processable remain far more attractive for their potential advantages of low cost, ease to scale up (to large-area substrates), ease of process integration with the solution-processable polythiophene OTFTs, and compatibility to roll-to-roll processing. Solution-processed encapsulation, however, presents additional challenges: 1) the process involves bringing solvents into contact with the underlying OTFT device, which may dissolve the layers constituting the device or change their morphology or properties; 2) the processing temperature has to be compatible with the OTFT device, which limits the selection of encapsulating material to mostly organics, whose gas-barrier capability is far inferior to that of inorganic materials and therefore may not be adequate for encapsulating OTFTs.

The challenges in developing solution-processed encapsulation were addressed in the authors' own study on solution-processed encapsulation of P3HT OTFTs [32]. The possible solvent-induced degradation to the OTFTs was examined by characterizing bottom gate/bottom contact OTFT devices soaked in a variety of solvents which were orthogonal to P3HT. The selection of orthogonal solvents was to minimize dissolution or swelling of the underlying OTFT layers. It was found that the solvents caused varying degrees of p-type doping (i.e., increased off current and positively shifted Vth) and charge trapping effects (i.e., reduced on current) depending upon the polarity of each given solvent, as shown in Figure 7.4. The solvents with higher-polarity functional groups, i.e., water and benzonitrile, caused strong p-type doping and charge trapping effects, while those with lower-polarity functional groups showed only charge trapping effects without detectable p-type doping.

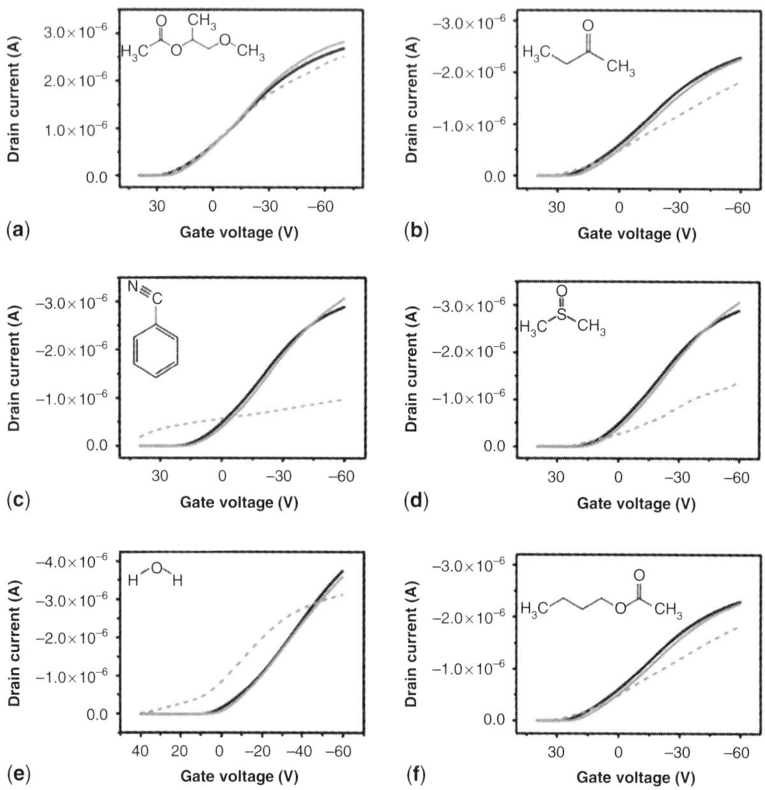

Figure 7.4 Transfer characteristics of P3HT OTFTs before (dark line) and after (dotted line) soaking in and after evacuation (grey line) of (a) propylene glycol monomethyl ether acetate (PGMEA), (b) methyl ethyl ketone, (c) benzonitrile, (d) dimethyl solphoxide, (e) water, and (f) butyl acetate. Insets show the chemical structures of the solvents. The source-drain bias was 60V.

Importantly, the effects of the solvents were fully reversible upon the complete removal of the solvents by evacuation or baking. This indicated that by using an orthogonal solvent to cast the encapsulating film followed by thorough drying, effects of the solvent on the device characteristics can be prevented.

Besides the solvent for the encapsulating film, the encapsulating film itself was also found to cause device degradation, with the extent of degradation dependent upon the chemical structure of the encapsulating material. Figures 7.5 and 7.6 show the changes in device characteristics of P3HT OTFTs encapsulated with a film of one of the following 10 polymers: poly(vinylidene

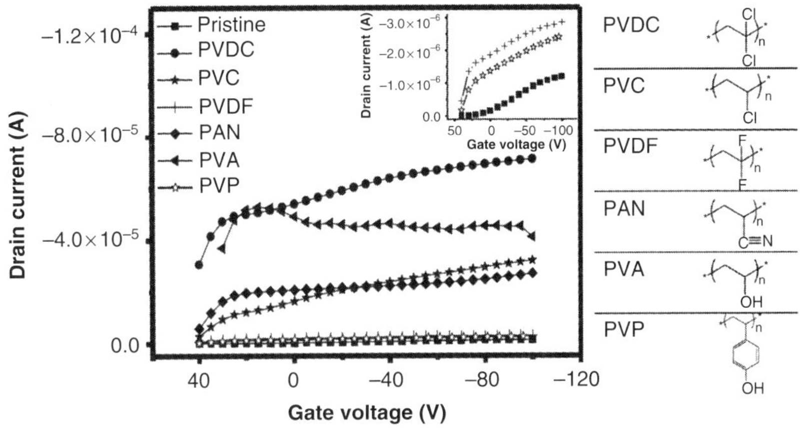

Figure 7.5 Transfer characteristics of OTFTs before and after being encapsulated with PVDC-co-PVC, PVC, PVDF, PAN, PVA, and PVP. Inset shows the device characteristics with PVDF and PVP in smaller drain current range. The chemical structures of the polymers are also provided. The source-to-drain bias was 60V.

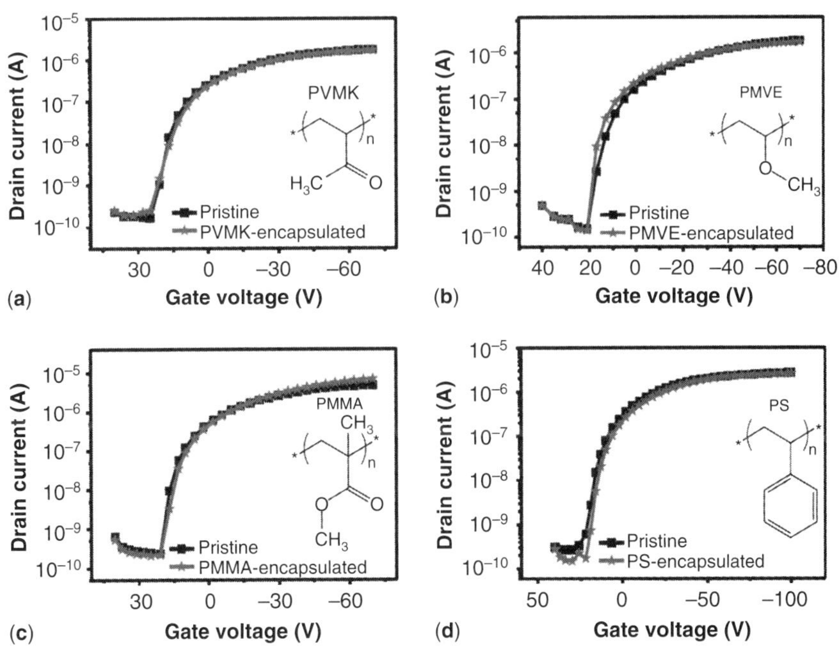

Figure 7.6 Transfer characteristics of OTFTs before and after being encapsulated with (a) PVMK, (b) PMVE, (c) PMMA, and (d) PS. Insets show the chemical structures of the polymers. The source-to-drain bias was 60V.

chloride-co-vinyl chloride) (PVDC-co-PVC) (solvent: dimethyl sulfoxide), poly(vinyl chloride) (PVC) (solvent: dimethyl sulfoxide), poly(vinylidene fluoride) (PVDF) (solvent: dimethyl sulfoxide), polyacrylonitride (PAN) (solvent: dimethyl sulfoxide), poly(vinyl alcohol) (PVA) (solvent: water), poly(vinyl phenol) (PVP) (solvent: propylene glycol monomethyl ether acetate), poly(vinyl methyl ketone) (PVMK) (solvent: methyl ethyl ketone), poly(methyl vinyl ether) (PMVE) (solvent: water) , poly(methyl methacrylate) (PMMA) (solvent: methyl ethyl ketone), and polystyrene (PS) (solvent: methyl ethyl ketone). The polymers with strong electron-withdrawing side groups (those shown in Figure 7.5) induced substantial p-type doping, while those with lower-polarity side groups (in Figure 7.6) did not cause noticeable device degradation. Among the p-doping-inducing polymers, the magnitude of the doping effects correlated with the number, strength, and steric hindrance of the electron-withdrawing side groups, as can be seen in the following comparisons of the p-doping effect: 1) PVDC-co-PVC >> PVC, which was attributable to the greater number of Cl atoms on PVDC (two per repeating unit) than on PVC (one per repeating unit); 2) PVDC-co-PVC >> PVDF, which was due to the stronger dipole moment, thus stronger polar interaction with P3HT, of the C-Cl bond than C-F; 3) PVA >> PVP, which was attributable to PVP's greater steric hindrance (by the phenyl ring) against the –OH/P3HT interactions.

The knowledge of the mechanisms of air-induced degradation to polythiophene OTFTs (as discussed in Section 7.2.2) in conjunction with the understanding of the effects of solvents and encapsulating polymers (as described above), allows optimization of solution-processed encapsulation methods to minimize encapsulation-induced degradation and achieve high air-stability from encapsulated OTFTs. On this front, the authors' own group demonstrated that by using a combination of a low-polarity encapsulating polymer—polystyrene—and a light-blocking black dye to encapsulate P3HT OTFTs, encapsulation-induced degradation was avoided and long lifetime from encapsulated devices was achieved, as shown in Figures 7.7 and 7.8 [32]. The low polarity of the encapsulating polymer prevented encapsulation-induced degradation, and also blocked the permeation of moisture to avoid the effects of p-type doping and charge trapping of moisture. Meanwhile, the light-blocking dye prevented the occurrence of photo-oxidation, thereby removing the

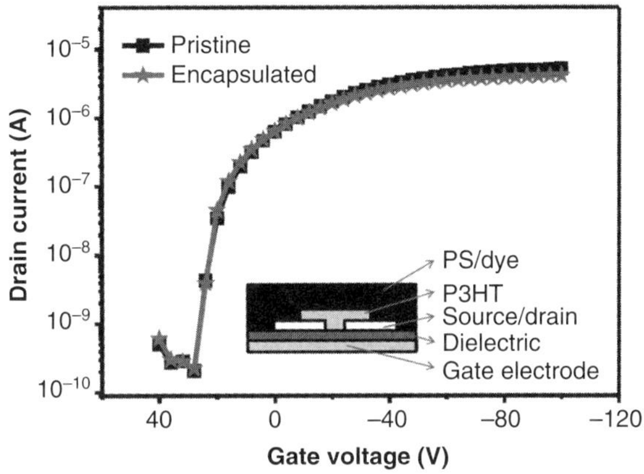

Figure 7.7 Transfer characteristics of OTFTs before and after being encapsulated with the PS/dye approach. Inset shows a schematic drawing of the encapsulation approach. The source-to-drain bias was 60V.

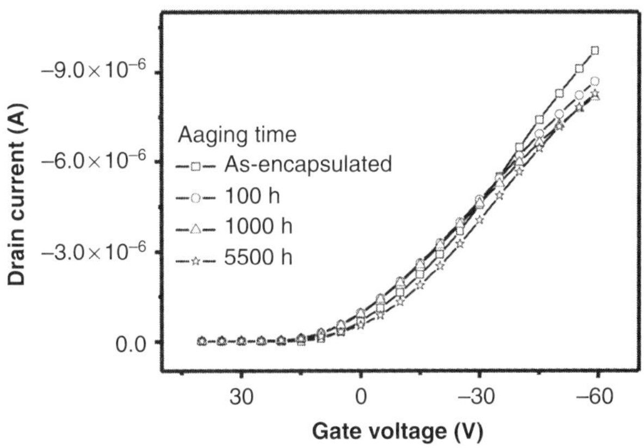

Figure 7.8 Transfer characteristics of the PS/dye-encapsulated devices as a function of aging time in air at room temperature. The source-to-drain bias in (a) was 60V.

need for an O_2 barrier and allowing the high-OTR polystyrene film (OTR ~200–500 cc/m^2 day) to be an adequate encapsulating film. The encapsulated devices showed nearly identical device characteristics before and after encapsulation, and they remained stable through > 5500 h of storage in air at room temperature.

Although the low-polarity polymer/dye approach was effective, its application is likely limited to cases where the substrate is not transparent and where optical transparency of the device is not required. For applications that require optical transparency and use transparent substrates, the encapsulating polymer film must be good oxygen barrier in addition to having low polarity, which may be difficult to obtain as polymers with low polarity are generally poor oxygen barriers. Composites of polymer and inorganic material may be one possible solution to this dilemma [41, 42].

Alternatively, solution-processed inorganic oxides can offer substantial improvement in gas-barrier performance over organic polymers, but they generally require high processing temperatures, which render them unsuitable for OTFT encapsulation. On this front, Nam *et al.* demonstrated a promising approach: a SiO_2-based, titania-containing organic–inorganic hybrid encapsulating material that could be wet-cast in a solventless process and cured at 90°C [43]. The hybrid encapsulating material was synthesized from organosilicon compounds—3-Glycidoxypropyltrimethoxysilane (GPTMS), tetraethyl orthosilicate (TEOS), and diphenylsilanediol (DPSD)—with barium hydroxide monohydrate [$Ba(OH)_2{\cdot}H_2O$] as catalysts and titania as both reinforcement and catalyst; the synthesis was through a nonhydrolytic sol-gel process, which does not require solvents as alcohol or water, does not cause significant volume shrinkage, and can be carried out at low temperatures. The hybrid encapsulating material showed a low WVTR of 0.434 g/m^2 day. When the hybrid material was applied to bottom-gate/top-contact poly[9,9-dioctylfluorenyl- 2,7-diyl]-co-(bithiophene)] OTFTs, the devices showed no encapsulation-induced degradation and maintained stable device characteristics for 48 days.

7.3.2 Pentacene-Based OTFTs

7.3.2.1 Vacuum-Processed Encapsulation

Pentacene OTFTs are fabricated with vacuum deposition processes except for special cases where pentacene derivatives that are specifically designed for solution process are used in place of pentacene. The vacuum-deposition fabrication process of pentacene OTFTs renders it readily integrable with vacuum-processed encapsulation methods, and therefore many attempts at encapsulating pentacene OTFTs have utilized vacuum-deposited films.

Several types of vacuum-deposited organics/polymer have been used as encapsulating films for pentacene OTFTs, including parylenes [44–46], polyimide [47], and polyolefins and fluorinated polyolefins [48–51]. The results with these encapsulating polymers are summarized as follows:

1. Parylenes
   Parylenes can be deposited by chemical vapor deposition (CVD) at room temperatures, and therefore are ideal for avoiding thermal damage to the underlying OTFTs. Moreover, the low polarity of parylenes also helps reduce doping-inducing interactions between the encapsulating film and the underlying OTFTs. Previous studies on parylene encapsulation of pentacene OTFTs have confirmed that device degradation induced by parylene encapsulation was indeed minimal [44–46]. Kymissis *et al.* showed that a parylene encapsulating layer could also adequately serve as a protecting layer during a photolithographic process which patterned the underlying bottom-gate/bottom-contact device [44]. Sekitani *et al.* demonstrated that parylene-encapsulated bottom-gate/top-contact OTFTs based on a plastic substrate achieved excellent flexibility, with critical bending radius down to 0.5 mm [45].

   The ability of parylenes to insulate OTFT devices from air-induced degradations, however, has been found unsatisfactory. Simeone *et al.* observed that parylene-encapsulated bottom-gate/bottom-contact OTFTs still showed significant hysteresis in their transfer characteristics, which was a symptom of moisture-induced charge trapping [46]. They also found that the addition of a spin-cast polyacrylate film on top of the parylene encapsulating film was still unable to prevent device hysteresis, whose elimination was found to require another addition of a thermally evaporated aluminum film.
2. Polyimide
   Hyung *et al.* used a polyimide film deposited by vapor deposition polymerization to encapsulate pentacene OTFTs with a bottom-gate/top-contact configuration [47]. The polyimide film was deposited by co-evaporating hexafluoropropane dianhydride (6FDA) and 4,40- oxydianiline (ODA) at 150°C in high vacuum, followed by thermal curing at 190°C. The polyimide

encapsulating film did not cause noticeable degradation to the OTFT devices, and the encapsulated devices showed a lifetime of 360 h as opposed to $<$ 24 h of unencapsulated control devices. The achieved lifetime, however, was rather short compared with that obtained with inorganic encapsulating films (see below), indicating that the barrier performance of the polyimide film was not adequate.

3. Polyolefins and fluorinated polyolefins
   Jung *et al.* used a 200 nm thermally evaporated tetratetracontane (n-$C_{44}H_{90}$) film to encapsulate bottom-gate/top-contact pentacene OTFTs and reported observing only slight encapsulation-induced degradation [48]. The encapsulated devices were able to remain stable for 50 days in air. Rapisarda *et al.* reported encapsulation of pentacene OTFTs with a PTFE-like polymer film deposited by plasma-enhanced CVD with a CHF_3/Ar gas mixture as the precursor [50]. The PTFE-like film significantly increased the off current of the OTFT devices due to its poor interface with the pentacene layer and plasma damage incurred during the deposition process. The encapsulation-induced degradation was fully recoverable after annealing at 110°C, which repaired the plasma damage and interface defects. The PTFE-like film was found able to protect the OTFT devices from oxygen but not moisture, which still caused large hysteresis in the encapsulated devices. Seo *et al.* encapsulated bottom-gate/top-contact pentacene OTFTs with a thermally evaporated fluorinated ethylene propylene (FEP) polymer film. The FEP film slightly shifted the Vth of the devices, from -14.7 to 12.5 V, but did not change the on and off currents. The FEP film alone was unable to insulate the devices from air-induced degradation, but with the addition of a solution-cast polymer stack of [poly(methylmethacrylate) (PMMA)/poly (urethaneacrylate) (PUA)/poly (ethylene terephthalate) (PET)], the devices exhibited air-stability for over a week.

The ineffectiveness of vacuum-deposited polymer films as gas barriers as described above has led some researchers to develop vacuum-deposited inorganic films as the sole encapsulating layers or as reinforcements to organic films. Kim *et al.* encapsulated bottom-gate/top-contact pentacene OTFTs with a SnO_2 film deposited by ion-beam-assisted deposition (IBAD) at room temperature, and observed moderate encapsulation-induced degradation as well as moderate air-induced degradation over 100 days of storage in air [52, 53]. Kim *et al.* later improved their approach by adding a spin-coated poly(vinyl alcohol) layer on pentacene OTFTs before the deposition of the IBAD SnO_2 film [54]. The PVA layer protected the devices from ion-beam damages during the IBAD process, thus eliminating the encapsulation-induced degradation. Moreover, the PVA layer planarized the pentacene surface to allow for a more complete coverage of the overcoated SnO_2 film and also contributed to the barrier function of the overall encapsulation stack, thereby enabling the devices to achieve good air stability.

Atomic-layer-deposited (ALD) oxide films have also been used to encapsulate pentacene OTFTs with good results. Kim *et al.* encapsulated bottom-gate/top-contact pentacene OTFTs with a thermally evaporated SiO_x film followed by an plasma-enhanced ALD AlO_x film and obtained air stability from the devices over 100 days of air storage without encapsulation-induced degradation [55]. They also found that similar results could be otained by using a spin-coated CYTOP™ polymer layer in place of the ALD AlO_x film. Seol *et al.* used an alternating ALD Al_2O_3 and plasma-polymerized methylcyclohexane (MCH) stack as encapsulating film for bottom-gate/top-contact pentacene OTFTs, which were observed to exhibit stability against bending to a 10 mm radius in air [56].

7.3.2.2 Solution-Processed Encapsulation

Different from P3HT OTFTs, where many solvents cause negligible damage if removed completely as described in Section 7.3.1.2, pentacene OTFTs have been found to suffer sustained damage after exposure to organic solvents. Gundlach *et al.* observed that the mobility of pentacene OTFTs dropped by an order of magnitude upon exposure to several types of solvent, as a result of a change in the crystal structure of pentacene from a thin-film phase to a bulk-like phase [57]. In light of this adverse effect of solvents, subsequent efforts to develop solution-processed encapsulation methods for pentacene OTFTs have utilized water as solvent, which does not induce crystal-structure change owing to its low affinity to (i.e. low solubility in) pentacene. Although water can cause p-type doping and charge trapping, such effects are reversible upon its complete removal [58]. Sheraw *et al.* encapsulated bottom-gate/bottom-contact pentacene OTFTs with a PVA film spin-coated from an aqueous solution [59]. The devices showed some degradations after encapsulation in lowered on current and shifted V_{th}, likely as a result of residual water or polar interactions between pentacene and the PVA layer. However, the PVA layer successfully protected the devices in subsequent processes for fabricating liquid-crystal displays, enabling demonstration of OTFT-driven flexible liquid-crystal displays. Also using a water-based PVA encapsulating film with the addition of a UV-cured polyacrylate top layer, Han *et al.* achieved 11000 h of lifetime from bottom-gate/bottom-contact pentacene OTFTs with a slight decrease in the field-effect mobility upon encapsulation [60]. Ahn *et al.* demonstrated that the lifetime of PVA-encapsulated pentacene OTFTs can be doubled by blending hydrophilic layered silicates (HLS) into the PVA film [61]. HLS are gas-impermeable platelets with very high diameter/thickness ratios, e.g., 200–300 nm/1 nm, and can create long tortuous path for the permeants through the polymer matrix, thereby substantially improve the barrier performance of the polymer matrix, as schematically illustrated in Figure 7.9.

In addition to using water-based PVA as an encapsulating material to minimize solvent-induced degradation to pentacene OTFTs, Qiu *et al.* demonstrated another approach which utilized a solventless UV-curable resin as the encapsulating film [62]. The encapsulated devices showed constant electrical characteristics over 100 h of storage in air.

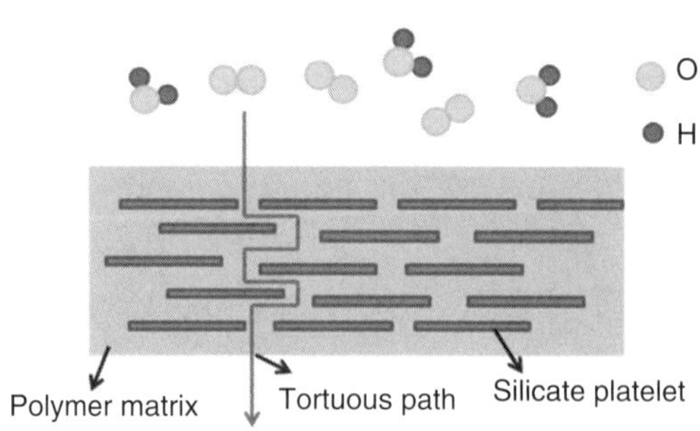

Figure 7.9 Illustration of moisture and oxygen permeations through a HIS-reinforced polymer matrix.

7.4 Summary and Outlook

Encapsulation of OTFTs to obtain air-stability has been a relatively new subject of research and development where continuing efforts are required to establish manufacturing-worthy technologies. Previous studies have determined mechanisms of air-induced degradations to major classes of organic semiconductors, effects of solvents, and effects of encapsulating materials. Based on these findings, solution- and vacuum-processed encapsulation methods have been demonstrated with various degrees of success. Further progress toward commercial applications will require improvement in the barrier property of solution-processed organic materials, through approaches such as incorporating inorganic additives or developing novel synthesis routes for organic/inorganic hybrids, and development of organic semiconductors with better air-stability and chemical resistance.

References

1. S.R. Forrest. *Nature* 2004, **428**, 6986
2. G.H. Gelinck, H. Edzer, A. Huitema, E. van Veenendaal, E. Cantatore, L. Schrijnemakers, J.B.P.H. van der Putten, T.C. Geuns, T.M. Beenhakkers, J.B. Giesbers, B. Huisman, E.J. Meijer, E.M. Benito, F.J. Touwslager, A.W. Marsman, B.J.E. van Rens, D.M. de Leeuw. *Nat. Mater.* 2004, 3, 106.
3. A.C. Arias, S.E. Ready, R. Lujan, W.S. Wong, K.E. Paul, A. Salleo, M.L. Chabinyc, R. Apte, R.A. Street, Y. Wu, P. Liu, B. Ong. *Appl. Phys. Lett.* 2004, **85,** 3304
4. H. Sirringhaus, N. Tessler, R.H. Friend. Science 1998, 280, 1741
5. L. Zhou, A. Wanga, S.-C. Wu, J. Sun, S. Park, T.N. Jackson. *Appl. Phys. Lett.* 2006, 88, 083502.
6. J.W. Jeong, Y.D. Lee, Y.M. Kim, Y.W. Park, J.H. Choi, T.H. Park, C.D. Soo, S.M. Won, I.K. Han, B.K. Ju. *Sens. Actuators B* 2010, 146, 40.
7. J. Huang, J. Miragliotta, A. Becknell, H.E. Katz. *J. Am. Chem. Soc.* 2007, **129,** 9366
8. E. Cantatore, T.C.T. Geuns, G.H. Gelinck, E. van Veenendaal, A.F.A. Gruijthuijsen, L. Schrijnemakers, S. Drews, D.M. de Leeuw. *IEEE J. Solid-State Circuits* 2007, 42, 84
9. K. Myny, S. Steudel, P. Vicca, M.J. Beenhakkers, N.A.J.M. van Aerle, G.H. Gelinck, J. Genoe, W. Dehaene, P. Heremans. Solid-State Electron. 2009, 53, 1220.
10. C.D. Dimitrakopoulos, P.R.L. Malenfant. *Adv. Mater.* 2002, 14, 99
11. B.S. Ong, Y. Wu, Y. Li, P. Liu, H. Pan. *Chem. Eur. J.* 2008, 14, 4766

12. D.J. Gundlach, Y.Y. Lin, T.N. Jackson, S.F. Nelson, D.G. Schlom. *IEEE Electron Device Lett.* 1997, 18, 87
13. J. Birks, J. Appleyard, R. Pope. *Photochem. Photobiol.* 1963, 2, 493.
14. I. Lewis, L. Singer. *J. Phys. Chem.* 1981, 85, 354.
15. M. Yamada, I. Ikemoto, H. Kuroda. *Bull. Chem. Soc. Jpn.* 1988, 61, 1057.
16. E. Clar. *Polycyclic aromatic hydrocarbons.* Academic Press: London, 1964; Vol. 1.
17. B. Stevens, S. Perez, J. Ors. *J. Am. Chem. Soc.* 1974, 96, 6846.
18. S. Murov, I. Carmichael, G. Hug. *Handbook of photochemistry.* 2nd ed. Marcel Dekker: New York, 1993.
19. A. Maliakal, K. Raghavachari, H. Katz, E. Chandross, T. Siegrist. *Chem. Mater.* 2004, 16, 4980.
20. R. Yea, M. Baba, K. Suzuki, Y. Ohishi, K. Mori. *Thin Solid Films* 2004, 464–465, 437.
21. O.D. Jurchescu, J. Baas, T.T.M. Palstra. *Appl. Phys. Lett.* 2005, 87, 052102
22. D.J. Gundlach, T.N.D. Jackson, G. Schlon, S.F. Nelson. *Appl. Phys. Lett.* 1999, 74, 3302
23. J.H. Schön, B. Batlogg. *Appl. Phys. Lett.* 1999, 74, 260
24. D.H. Dunlap, P.E. Parris, V.M. Kenkre. *Phys. Rev. Lett.* 1996, 77, 542
25. S.V. Novikov, D.H. Dunlap, V.M. Kenkre, P.E. Parris, A.V. Vannikov. *Phys. Rev. Lett.* 1998, 81, 4472.
26. Z.T. Zhu, J.T. Mason, R. Dieckmann, G.G. Malliaras. *Appl. Phys. Lett.* 2002, 81, 24.
27. D. Li, E.-J. Borkent, R. Nortrup, H. Moon, H. Katz, Z. Bao. *Appl. Phys. Lett.* 2005, 86, 042105.
28. G. Gu, M.G. Kane. *Appl. Phys. Lett.* 2008, 92, 053305.
29. Y. Qiu, Y. Hu, G. Dong, L. Wang, J. Xie, Y. Ma. *Appl. Phys. Lett.* 2003, 83, 1644.
30. M.S.A. Abdou, S. Holdcroft. *Macromolecules* 1993, 26, 2954.
31. J. Ficker, H. von Seggern, H. Rost, W. Fix, W. Clemens, I. McCulloch. *Appl. Phys. Lett.* 2004, 85, 1377.
32. Y. Fu, F.-Y. Tsai. *Org. Electron.* 2011, 12, 179.
33. J.-M. Zhuo, L.-H. Zhao, R.-Q. Png, L.-Y. Wong, P.-J. Chia, J.-C. Tang, S. Sivaramakrishnan, M. Zhou, E.C.-W. Ou, S.-J. Chua, W.-S. Sim, L.-L. Chua, P.K.-H. Ho. *Adv. Mater.* 2009, 21, 4747.
34. S. Hoshino, M. Yoshida, S. Uemura, T. Kodzasa, N. Takada, T. Kamata, K. Yase. *J. Appl. Phys. Lett.* 2004, 95, 5088.
35. J.S. Lewis, M.S. Weaver. *IEEE J. Sel. Top. Quant. Electron* 2004, 10, 45.
36. S. Ferrari, F. Perissinotti, E. Peron, L. Fumagalli, D. Natali, M. Sampietro. *Org. Electron.* 2007, 8, 407.
37. P.F. Carcia, R.S. McLean, M.H. Reilly, M.D. Groner, S.M. George. *Appl. Phys. Lett.* 2006, 89, 031915.
38. L. Fumagalli, M. Binda, I.S. Lopez, D. Natali, M. Sampietrol, S. Ferrari, L. Lamagna, M. Fanciulli. *Org. Electron.* 2009, 10, 692.
39. S.P. Tiwaria , P. Srinivasa, S. Shrirama, N.S. Kalea, S.G. Mhaisalkarb, V.R. Raoa. *Thin Solid Films* 2008, 516, 770.
40. K.S. Ong, R.G.C. Ruey, E. Ou, Z. Zheng, D.L.M. Ying. *Org. Electron.* 2010, 11, 463.
41. W.S. Jang, I. Rawson, and J.C. Grunlan. *Thin Solid Films* 516, 2008, 4819–4825.
42. M.A. Priolo, D. Gamboa, K.M. Holder, J.C. Grunlan. *Nano Lett.* 2010, 10, 4970.
43. S. Nam, J. Jang, K. Kim, W.M. Yun, D.S. Chung, J. Hwang, O.K. Kwon, T. Chang, C.E. Park. *J. Mater. Chem.* 2011, 21, 775.

44. I. Kymissis, C.D. Dimitrakopoulos, S. Purushothaman. *J. Vac. Sci. Technol. B* 2002, 20, 956.
45. T. Sekitani, S. Iba, Y. Kato, Y. Noguchi, T. Sakurai, T. Someya. *J. Non-Cryst. Solids* 2006, 352, 1769.
46. D. Simeone, S. Cipolloni, L. Mariucci, M. Rapisarda, A. Minotti, A. Pecora, M. Cuscunà, L. Maiolo, G. Fortunato. *Thin Solid Films* 2009, 517, 6283.
47. G.W. Hyung, J. Park, J.H. Kim, J.R. Koo, Y.K. Kim. *Sol.-Stat. Elec.* 2010, 54, 439.
48. H. Jung, T. Lim, Y. Choi, M. Yi, J. Won, S. Pyo. *Appl. Phys. Lett.* 2008, 92, 163504.
49. M. Scharnberg, V. Zaporojtchenko, R. Adelung, F. Faupel, C. Pannemann, T. Diekmann, U. Hilleringmann. *Appl. Phys. Lett.* 2007, 90, 013501.
50. M. Rapisarda, D. Simeone, G. Fortunato, A. Valletta, L. Mariucci. *Org. Electron.* 2011, 12, 119.
51. S.-M. Seo, C.-H. Jang, J.-H. Park. *Org. Electron.* 2008, 9, 899.
52. W.J. Kim, W.H. Koo, S.J. Jo, C.S. Kim, H.K. Baik, J. Lee, S. Im. *Jpn. J. Appl. Phys.* 2005, 44, 37.
53. W.J. Kim, W.H. Koo, S.J. Jo, C.S. Kim, H.K. Baik, J. Lee, S. Im. *Appl. Surf. Sci.* 2005, 252, 1332.
54. W.J. Kim, C.S. Kim, S.J. Jo, H.S. Hwang, S.Y. Ryu, H.K. Baik. *Semicond. Sci. Technol.* 2008, 23, 075034.
55. S.H. Kim, W.M. Yoon, M. Jang, H. Yang, J.-J. Park, C.E. Park. *J. Mater. Chem.* 2012, 22, 7731.
56. Y.G. Seol, W. Heo, J.S. Park, N.-E. Lee, D.K. Lee, Y.J. Kim. *J. Electrochem. Soc.* 2011, 158, H931.
57. D.J. Gundlach, T.N. Jackson, D.G. Schlom, S.F. Nelson. *Appl. Phys. Lett.* 1999, 74, 3302.
58. H.N. Lee, Y.G. Lee, I.H. Ko, E.C. Hwang, S.K. Kang. *Curr. Appl. Phys.* 2008, 8, 626.
59. C.D. Sheraw, L. Zhou, J.R. Huang, D.J. Gundlach, and T.N. Jackson, M.G. Kane, I.G. Hill, M.S. Hammond, J. Campi, B.K. Greening, J. Francl, J. West. *Appl. Phys. Lett.* 2002, 80, 1088.
60. S.H. Han, J.H. Kim, J. Jang, S.M. Cho, M.H. Oh, S.H. Lee, D.J. Choo. *Appl. Phys. Lett.* 2006, 88, 073519.
61. T. Ahn, H.J. Suk, J. Won, M.H. Yi. *Microelectron. Eng.* 2009, 86, 41.
62. Y. Qiu, Y. Hu, G. Dong, L. Wang, J. Xie, Y. Ma. *Appl. Phys. Lett.* 2003, 83, 1644.

8

Tunable Encapsulation Property of Amphiphilic Polymer Based on Hyperbranched Polyethylenimine

Decheng Wan[1] and Toshifumi Satoh[2]

[1]Institute of Functional Polymers, College of Materials Science and Engineering, Tongji University, Shanghai, China
[2]Division of Biotechnology and Macromolecular Chemistry, Faculty of Engineering, Hokkaido University, Sapporo, Hokkaido 0608628, Japan

Abstract

A highly specific supramolecular entrapment is traditionally and exclusively promoted by specific noncovalent interactions. This strategy is limited to two aspects: the guest species are limited to those which are topologically or electronically featured; and the hosts have to be meticulously tailored in terms of size, morphology and electronic motif. Therefore, the host synthesis is tedious and challenging, and the spectrum of well-recognizable guest species is narrow. In this chapter, it is shown that the derivatives of a hyperbranched polymer (mainly hyperbranched polyethylenimine (PEI)) can encapsulate a variety of guest species, and the encapsulating system shows a rather high guest selectivity in which a specific interaction is absent or very weak. It is known that a complex system tends to deviate from linearity. The nonlinear property of a supramolecular system implies that the appropriate combination of nonspecific elementary interactions possibly results in a high guest selectivity. Experiments have shown that with the electronic engineering of a PEI-based nanocapsule, its guest affinity can be switched, the guest selectivity can be improved, and the guest releasing behavior becomes adjustable. It was found that 100% charge selective separation could be a general case, and effective separation of many anionic mixtures was also possible. These features of PEI-based nanocapsules have been employed for mixture separation and controlled guest release. The unimolecularity of a nanocapsule can also be enhanced by core engineering.

Vikas Mittal (ed.) Encapsulation Nanotechnologies, (225–254) © 2013 Scrivener Publishing LLC

Keywords: Encapsulation, separation, supramolecular chemistry, polyethylenimine

8.1 Introduction

A hyperbranched polymer [1–3] is a dendritic polymer as well as a dendrimer, the former roughly resembles the latter in multifunctionality and three-dimensional morphology. The solubility of these sphere-like macromolecules is mainly determined by the surface groups. A dendrimer features dense peripheral groups which offer a versatile platform for chemical tuning, and thus may be soluble in a wide spectrum of media. Meanwhile, a dendrimer can possess a fundamentally different core from the shell, which acts as a function available only for small molecular species due to the topological selectivity of the congested periphery [4–7]. As a consequence, a dendrimer and its derivatives possess a special supramolecular property. For example, it can act as a phase transfer agent and may mimic certain functions of a protein or an enzyme. In contrast to a dendrimer, a hyperbranched polymer is less congested in the periphery and the core of a conventional hyperbranched polymer is more open than a high generation dendrimer, thus rarely showing a topological selectivity. Therefore, the supramolecular host–guest property of a hyperbranched polymer mainly stems from the electronic complement to a guest rather than from a topological complement. However, unlike a dendrimer in which the functional groups are exclusively and regularly arrayed on the periphery, the functional groups of a hyperbranched polymer are randomly distributed throughout the entire polymer. This structural feature renders the interior electronic environment of a hyperbranched polymer relatively homogeneous and chemically designable. In recent years, it has been shown that for a core–shell amphiphilic macromolecule (CAM) based on a hyperbranched polyethylenimine (PEI-CAM), the electronic property of the core is conveniently modulated in a chemical manner, and this modulation can lead to a switchable guest affinity, significantly improved guest selectivity and a controllable guest release [8–14].

Traditionally, highly selective entrapment of a guest molecule in a host–guest system is exclusively promoted by one or several specific interactions, such as multiple hydrogen–bonds, metal–ligand interaction, topological trapping and π–π stacking, in which the selectivity stems from the directionality, saturability, and specificity of a specific interaction. Such a strategy is limited to two aspects, one is that the host has to be rigorously tailored in terms of size, morphology and electronic motif so that a strict complementary host–guest interaction is realizable, rendering the synthesis of such a host tedious and challenging; the other is that only the molecules, which are either topologically or electronically featured, can be well recognized. The effective recognition of a common molecule by an artificial host has remained a general challenge up to now.

Some artificial dendrimers or nanoscale molecular devices have been shown to possess a good topological selectivity during guest encapsulation [5, 6]. Since the pioneering work of Vogtle, Newkome and Tomalia [15–18], guest selectivity remains a central concern. Meijer *et al.* [5] and Okamoto *et al.* [6] experimentally proved that for high generation dendrimers, topological selectivity was feasible. Later, Haag and Zimmerman [19] and Rzayev *et al.* [20] showed that even a derivative of a hyperbranched polymer or a nanotube derived from a block copolymer, if carefully controlled during shell crosslinking, could conduct a high topological selectivity as well, in which the shell congestion played a critical role in the topological selectivity. For the most common micelles, topological selectivity is poorly available.

CAM derived from hyperbranched polymers are readily available due to their cost-effective production, wide structural availability, multifunctionality and morphological features of hyperbranched polymers [1, 3]. The CAM is stable due to its covalent structure, and thus can be used under rigorous conditions, and can replace a physical micelle in many fields. In a common host–guest system composed of CAM and a guest, a nonspecific interaction usually plays a dominant role, and along with the irregular cavities, a CAM is generally known for wide guest affinities and low guest selectivities. In a supramolecular system in which a nonspecific interaction is dominant, the host–guest interaction is dynamic and multisite statistical. As a result, high selectivity was rarely reported. Vogtle *et al.* [21] noticed that their dendrimer-based CAMs could highly differentiate the topologically similar rose Bengal and eosin Y (both belong to the xanthene family), and thus attributed the encapsulating selectivity to an electronic host–guest complement. Recent efforts by Wan *et al.* [8, 10, 12] further showed that tailoring the electronic property (termed core engineering) of the CAMs could lead to switching of the guest affinity and significantly improved guest selectivity. The mechanism is related to the nonlinearity of a complex system [22]. A host–guest system can be regarded as a complex system if nonspecific, multisite statistical interactions are predominant. The nonlinearity of a complex system implies that core engineering of a CAM is possible to amplify the difference in the complementary strength between a CAM and the competitive guest species which leads to its selectivity. The experimental facts and mechanism will be presented in this chapter.

A CAM based on a dendritic molecule can conduct guest release in a manner fundamentally different from a microcapsule. A microcapsule has a permeable wall and hollow interior space with a nanometer or scores of nanometer dimension, guest molecules with a subnanometer size can be loaded in the hollow core and the resulting material can be used as a reservoir for controlled release. This release mode is mainly based on kinetic inhibition of the guest diffusion. Because diffusion is usually related to a number of factors such as wall thickness and wall porosity of the microcapsule, the release reproducibility is relatively poor. In contrast, for a dendritic molecule, the core is a network with subnanometer cavities, and a small guest molecule is usually thermodynamically confined in the CAM rather than kinetically confined, and the thermodynamically controlled release is more stable and of higher reproducibility. However, when the guest molecule is relatively large or rigid, the release is also likely to be kinetically controlled. For a thermodynamic process, the electronic host–guest complementary strength is adjustable by core engineering of the host and the desired releasing rate is thus accessible. The stimuli-responsive release will also be mentioned in this chapter.

This chapter mainly focuses on the encapsulation and release of small organic dyes by a CAM, and the CAMs are mainly limited to PEI-CAMs. It is known that a PEI or a PEI-CAM can also serve as a template or a carrier of inorganic species, inorganic particles, and as well-known gene transfect vectors, but will not be described in this chapter.

8.2 Synthesis of PEI-CAMs

The synthesis of PEI-CAM has been reported by a number of research groups, Figure 8.1 shows several main routes. Although an amine is well-known as an active group in organic chemistry,

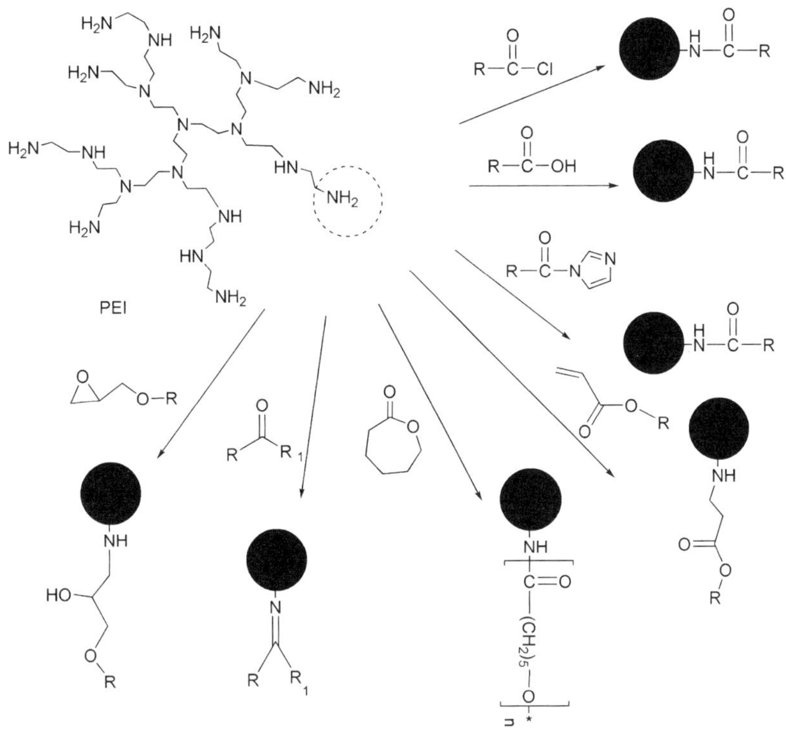

Figure 8.1 Several routes for the synthesis of PEI-CAMs.

sufficient functionalization of the amino groups of a PEI is usually difficult. The challenge mainly arises from the very poor solubility of the PEI upon exposure to acidic substances and tedious purification of an incomplete reaction. Amidation of a PEI by acid chloride is generally effective in the presence of an acid-absorbing agent such as pyridine [24–26]. If fatty acids are used in the place of the acid chloride, the degree of functionalization is limited at normal temperature, and additional purification is necessary to remove the alkylammonium salt. However, if the acid was activated by carbodiimidazole prior to exposure to PEI, the degree of functionalization could be increased to 90% [27]. Acrylate with a PEO pendent could be attached to the PEI via the very effective Michael addition [28], and the resulting product was stable at low temperature. A pH sensitive CAM is also available by the addition reaction between an aldehyde (or ketone) and the PEI via the formation of a Schiff base bond, which is cleavable in a weakly acidic environment with pH 5–6 [25, 29]. The reaction of oxirane with PEI is mild and quantitative and usually needs no additional purification, and the resulting CAMs are stable under rigorous acidic or basic conditions [12–14]. This reaction leads to alkylation of amino groups with the additional introduction of hydroxyls. Chen and others reported that a PEI could act as a multisite initiator for the ring-opening polymerization of monomers such as a lactide and caprolactone, leading to a degradable, multiarm star-like polymer micelle, with a high initiating efficiency, and the primary amine is more effective than the secondary amine [30–32]. The poly(amino acid) of such a monomer as γ-benzyl-L-glutamate-N-carboxyanhydride was also introduced as a shell of PEI [33]. Jiang and Yin [34–36] reported the synthesis and property of a hyperbranched polymer somewhat like PEI, namely poly(ether amine). This polymer is like PEI regarding the polyamine structure, but is also known for its additional response to pH, temperature and ionic strength.

8.3 Unimolecularity versus Aggregate of PEI-CAMs

In the pioneering era, it was found that an amphiphilic dendritic architecture could exist as a unimolecular micelle [17, 18]. Later, it was found by many research groups [12–14, 37–39] that a large fraction of the amphiphilic dendritic architectures tended to aggregate, just like most amphiphilic block copolymers, which should be mainly ascribed to their amphiphilic nature. Employing this property, Yan's groups have synthesized many interesting self-assembled structures [37–39]. However, unimolecularity is also highly desired in many cases. The concept of a critical micelle concentration (CMC) was also used to describe the aggregation of CAMs. Dynamic light scattering (DLS) is a tool to measure the absolute size of a particle in a solution or dispersion. When the size of a CAM is monitored as a function of its concentration, a deviation from a stable size may mean a CMC. However, if the CMC value is very low, and the size of a CAM is not large (within several nanometers), the scattering intensity may be too weak to detect. Small angle X-ray scattering can be a powerful tool in this case. Indirect measurement techniques are also used to detect the CMC. Hawker *et al.* [40] suggested monitoring the encapsulating capacity as a function of the concentration of a CAM, and a deviation from linearity suggested a CMC.

For water-soluble CAMs, pyrene and Nile red are frequently used as a fluorescent probe to detect the CMC because the fluorescent spectra of these probes are sensitive to the hydrophobicity of their surroundings.

The unimolecularity is adjustable by core engineering of the CAM. Some molecular parameters of a CAM were found to influence the unimolecularity and were employed to access the unimolecularity. Satoh *et al.* [41–43] found that for a hyperbranched polyether polyol, a higher degree of functionalization was favorable for the unimolecularity. Wan *et al.* [13] similarly found that for a PEI-CAM, a higher degree of functionalization enhanced the unimolecularity, and a thicker hydrophobic shell was also beneficial to the unimolecularity of the reverse-micelle-like CAM. Moreover, introduction of ionic charges into the core favored the unimolecularity due to ionic repulsion among the CAMs [11].

8.4 Host–Guest Chemistry of PEI-CAMs

Maciejewski [44] first predicted molecular encapsulation by a dendrimer. Tomalia [16] and Newkome [17, 18] were among the first to find that a molecule with subnanometer dimensions could be entrapped by a dendrimer. On the debit side, synthesis of a dendrimer is multistep and tedious, which limits its large-scale application. Fortunately, the cost-effective hyperbranched polymer can be a substitute of a dendrimer. Phase transfer extraction by a derivative of a hyperbranched polymer was possible and could be used for mixture separation and purification. It was found that a nonionic derivative of a hyperbranched polyglycerol was able to transfer an ionic organic dye into an aploar medium [45]. This supramolecular property was partly attributed to the three-dimension topological feature of the parent hyperbranched polymer because a linear counterpart could hardly transfer the same solute [46]. PEI is a commercially available hyperbranched polymer. Mecking *et al.* [24] and Haag *et al.* [25] were among the first to explore the dye-encapsulating property of a PEI-CAM. Stiriba *et al.* [26] later pointed out that the globular shape of the PEI-CAMs was critical to the supramolecular encapsulation, as compared with the poor encapsulating property of a linear analogue. Besides the topological factor, they pointed out that the polarity factor influenced the encapsulating capacity as well [26]. Haag *et al.* [23] synthesized similar PEI-CAMs and evaluated their guest entrapping property, and found that anionic groups, such as sulfonate, carboxylate, phosphorate or phenol groups of an organic guest, favored encapsulation. Since a PEI is labile to protonation by water below pH 12 and exists as a cationic polyelectrolyte, the encapsulation of an anionic guest is understandable from an electrostatic complement viewpoint. Haag *et al.* [23] also found that certain types of neutral molecules were also able to be encapsulated by their PEI-CAMs, which suggested that an elementary interaction other than the electrostatic complement was also important for the encapsulation. In fact, Frey's group [45] and Satoh's group [41–43, 47] found that CAMs derived from nonionic, polyol hyperbranched polymers could encapsulate anionic dyes, indicating that an electrostatic complement is favorable, but not necessary for the encapsulation. Haag *et al.* [30] and Chen *et al.* [31–32, 48–49] found that either NH_2 or NH could initiate the ring-opening polymerization of a lactide and ε-caprolactone so that the PEI could be formed into a spheroid-like PEI-CAM with a biodegradable polyester shell, and the resulting PEI-CAM could encapsulate ionic, water-soluble dyes. Biocompatible polyethylene oxide (PEO) was also introduced to the PEI via an amido or acetal bond to form the widely soluble PEI@PEO, and its aggregate showed a guest encapsulating property [29]. There are other studies related to PEI-CAMs for guest encapsulation and release [50–54], and pertinent reviews are available [55, 56].

The simultaneous entrapment of distinctly different guests, such as polar and apolar guests, by physical or covalent micelles were reported in recent years [56–59]. PEI-CAMs were similarly explored. Chen *et al.* [60] synthesized an amphiphilic calix[4]arene molecule bearing four apolar aliphatic chains and four phenol groups. Upon mixing with a PEI in certain media, a physical micelle was formed, which could host both an anionic guest and cationic guest in a site-isolated state. Haag *et al.* [61] synthesized a multishell micelle with a PEI core and a shell consisting of an apolar aliphatic middle layer and a PEO outer layer. The multishell micelle usually existed as an aggregate and could entrap both apolar and polar guests. Liang *et al.* [62] synthesized a covalent micelle with PEI as the core and polystyrene (PS) and PEO as the hybrid shell. This covalent micelle could simultaneously host an apolar pyrene and ionic RB, moreover, this micelle is soluble in a wide spectrum of solvents and is medium-responsive.

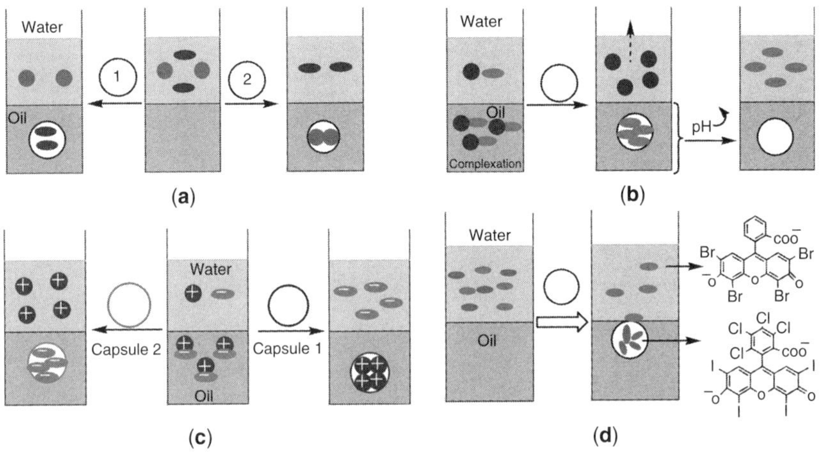

Figure 8.2 Selective phase transfer extraction by PEI-CAMs for separation of a variety of water-soluble organic dyes. (A) CAMs with different cores showed different guest affinities; (B) the anionic–cationic complex could be separated and pH-sensitive recycling of the host CAM was possible; (C) charge selective encapsulation of either cationic component or anionic component led to complete separation; (D) even very similar guest species could be efficiently separated.

The guest selectivity of a hosting micelle is evoking increasing interest. Wan *et al.* [8–14] studied in detail the core structure–encapsulating property of PEI-CAMs and found that the electronic property of the core was critical to the guest selectivity. This property could be employed for mixture separation, as shown in Figure 8.2. The details of the guest selectivity versus host structure will be discussed in the next subsection.

8.5 Charge Selective Encapsulation and Separation

8.5.1 Charge Selective Encapsulation for Separation of Oppositely Charged Dyes

Wan *et al.* [12–14] prepared PEI-CAMs in a quantitative manner by the reaction between oxirane and PEI, in which the functional degree could be well controlled up to 90%. The resulting PEI-CAMs (Figure 8.3) were oil-soluble due to the hydrophobic shell, but the polar core could interact with a hydrophilic guest.

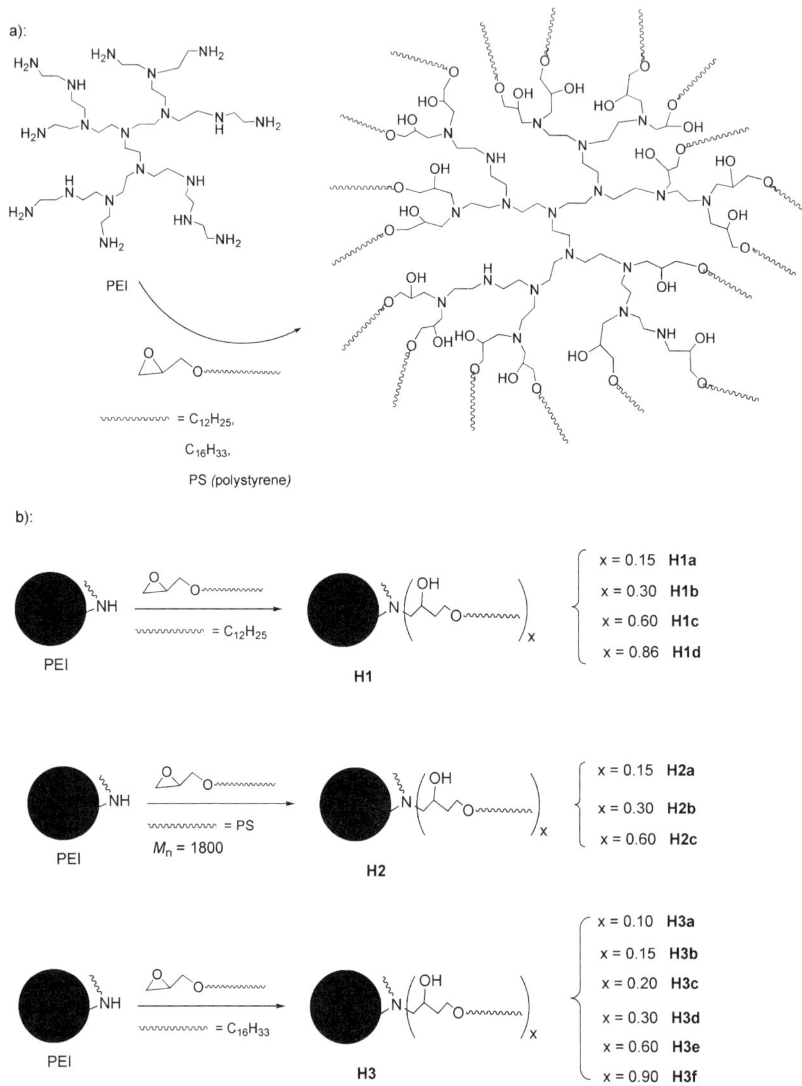

Figure 8.3 Outline of the synthesis of several PEI-CAMs (PEI has 232 repeat units on average, but only several are shown here for clarity).

One can find that the modification of a PEI not only introduces an apolar shell, but also introduces free hydroxyl groups into the core. This multifunctional core provided a platform for core engineering, as will be discussed later. In an oil/water biphasic system, organic aqueous solutes could be transferred into an otherwise insoluble apolar phase. Moreover, due to the supramolecular selectivity, the

CAMs were successfully used for mixture separation based on the ionic nature of the components [64]. A variety of water-soluble dyes (Figure 8.4) were tested and it was found that the positively charged dyes could not be entrapped by the CAM, while the negatively charged species could be (Figure 8.5). It is known that the

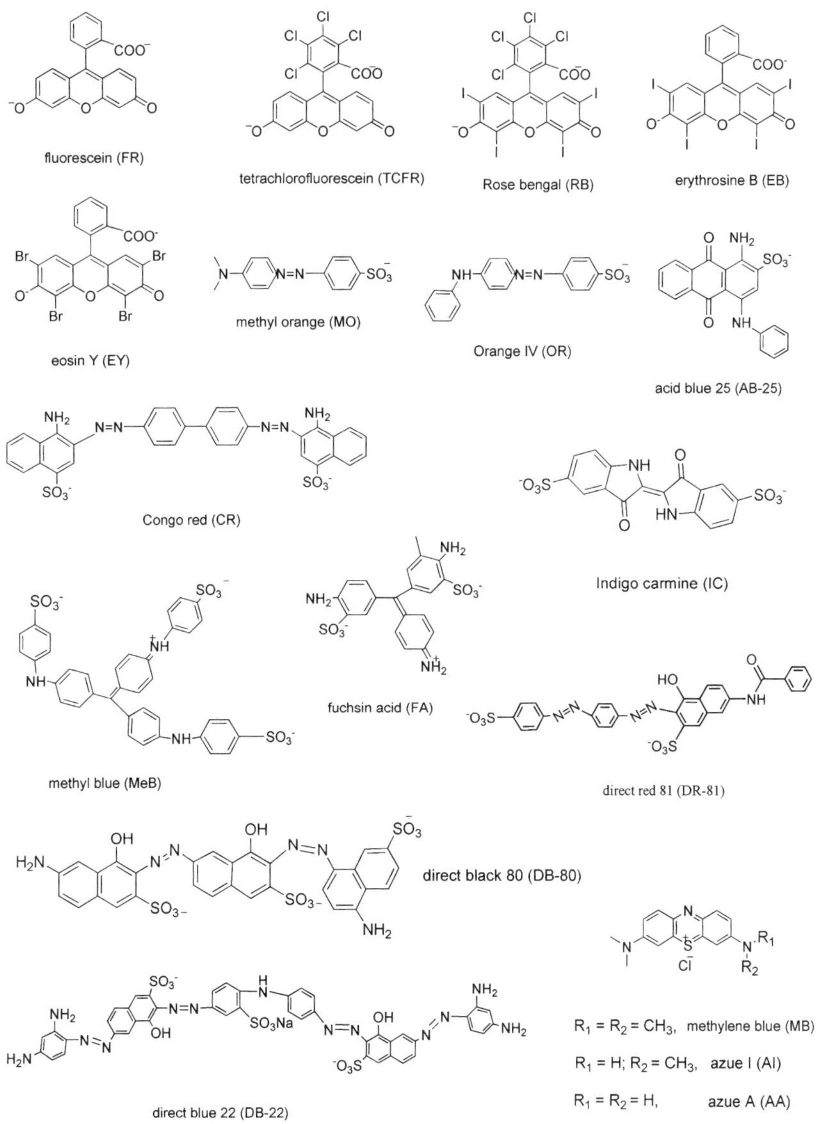

Figure 8.4 Chemical structures of water-soluble dyes.

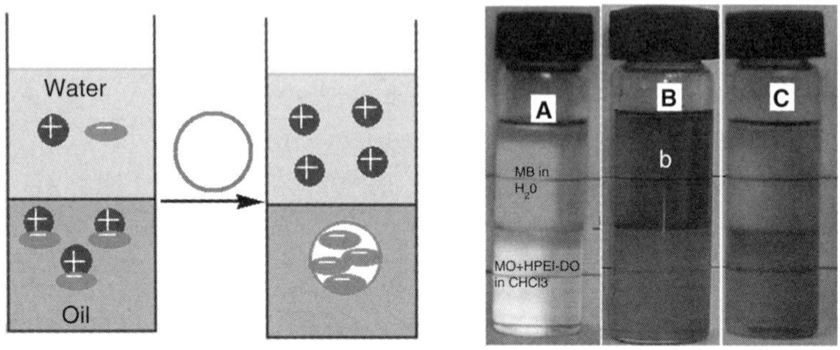

Figure 8.5 (Left) Schematic representation of the separation of anionic–cationic mixture by a CAM; (Right) a PEI-CAM could exclusively transfer the anionic MO (A), RB (B) and CR (C) from the upper aqueous layer to the bottom oil layer while the cationic MB remained intact in the upper aqueous phase.

PEI is a polyamine polymer and is labile to protonation (complete deprotonation occurs at pH > 11), thus the PEI-CAM is a weak cationic electrolyte and tends to entrap anionic dyes. This charge selective separation is advantageous in the following several aspects: 1) 100% separation is widely available; 2) it can be applied to many cationic–anionic binary mixtures of small molecules with a few exceptions; 3) the separation is convenient; excess CAM exerts no influence on the separation efficiency; and 4) in many cases, the encapsulation is pH-reversible, thus the PEI-CAM is recyclable.

One can find that a PEI-CAM can exclusively entrap anionic species, while in some cases it is desired that the cationic species be entrapped and separated. For this purpose a reverse-micelle-like assembly with dense carboxylic functionalities as the core and oil-soluble polystyrene as the shell (Figure 8.6) was also synthesized [63] and evaluated [64].

The unimer is amphiphilic and can form an aqueous micelle in water or form a reverse micelle in an apolar organic medium. In the latter case, the polyacrylic acid (PAA) block formed the core and the polystyrene block formed the shell. Due to the anionic core of the reverse micelle, cationic dyes were exclusively extracted from the anionic dyes (Figure 8.7). The encapsulation was also pH-reversible, but the reversibility depended on the guest species.

The pK_a of COOH is typically 3~4, not far from pH 7, favorable for the facile recycling of the host nanocapsule. Huang *et al.* [20] also reported that an organic nanotube with dense carboxylic functionalities in the interior surface could undergo a charge selective

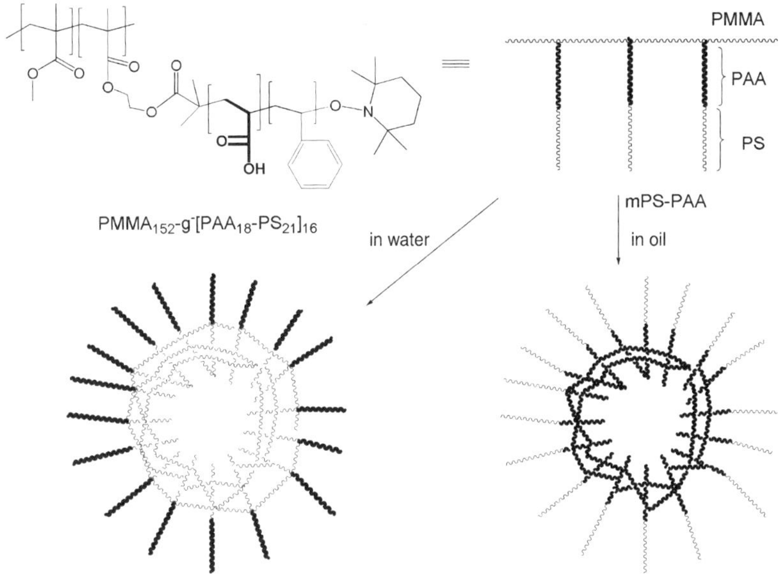

Figure 8.6 The PMMA-g-(PAA-b-PS) can form an oil-soluble or water-soluble assembly.

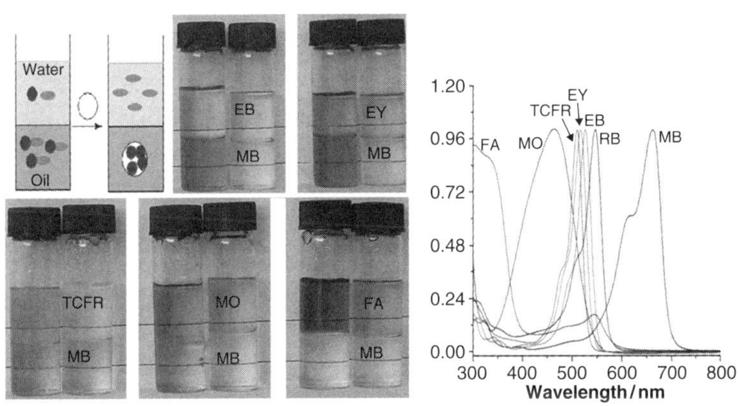

Figure 8.7 An aqueous soluble anionic–cationic mixture became oil-soluble due to the formation of an anionic–cationic complex, but charge selective encapsulation could lead to complete separation of the mixture. The top left scheme shows the process and the digital images show the separation of a variety of mixtures. The host nanocapsule was mPS-PAA, with the anionic PAA as the core and polystyrene as the shell (Figure 8.6); the mixture consisted of the cationic MB and a variety of anionic dyes. Conditions: the upper layer was water and the bottom layer was chloroform. Attention: in each pair of the vials, a nanocapsule was absent in the left vial but present in the right vial. The ionic dye species was completely separated, as detected by UV-vis spectra (Right spectra) [64].

encapsulation, and they further showed that with an appropriate shell crosslinking, a topologically selective encapsulation was also feasible.

8.5.2 Switchable Charge Selectivity and pH Recycle of the Host

For practical separation applications, recycling of the host material is important. As already mentioned, either PEI or PAA can be reversibly protonated, thus the pH response is feasible, but the guest releasing property of the PEI- and PAA-based nanocapsule is not always ideal, depending on the guest species. For example, at a high pH, the small guest molecule of MO could be quickly and completely released from a PEI-CAM, but the larger RB could slowly and partly be released, while the still larger and rigid CR could hardly be released even after several days. In a detailed study, it was found that both thermodynamic and kinetic factors contributed to the pH-reversibility [64]. For MO, at a high pH, the PEI was deprotonated and the host–guest interaction strength became weak, thus the hydrophilic MO was released due to the competition of the bulk water, namely, a thermodynamic factor played a dominant role in the process. For CR, encapsulation at pH = 7 was observable in several days. When the pH was improved to above 11, release of the entrapped CR was not observed within several days. On the other hand, no encapsulation of CR was observed at pH = 11 within one week. These facts indicated that the encapsulation and release of CR was a kinetic process. This is understandable because CR is large, rigid and rod-like, so its encapsulation or release requires considerable conformational adjustment of the host CAM. To enhance the recyclability of a host nanocapsule, a nanocapsule with a zwitterionic core was synthesized and evaluated (Figure 8.8) [64].

When a large number of carboxylic acids was introduced into the PEI core, a zwitterion would be formed. This is because the pK_a of COOH is around 3–4, while pK_a of protonated primary amine, secondary amine and tertiary amine are 9.64, 8.59 and 7.50, respectively. When $pH < 3$, the core is cationic, when $pH > 10$, the core is anionic, and when $3 < pH < 10$, the core is zwitterionic. Experiments showed that the zwitterionic host showed a good pH reversibility. The zwitterionic host is very useful for a single species transfer because either the anionic or cationic guest can be entrapped by only adjustment of the pH value, and the pH response of this CAM is outstanding. For example, at a high pH, the CAM switched from zwitterionic to anionic, and the electrostatic repulsion would promote the release of

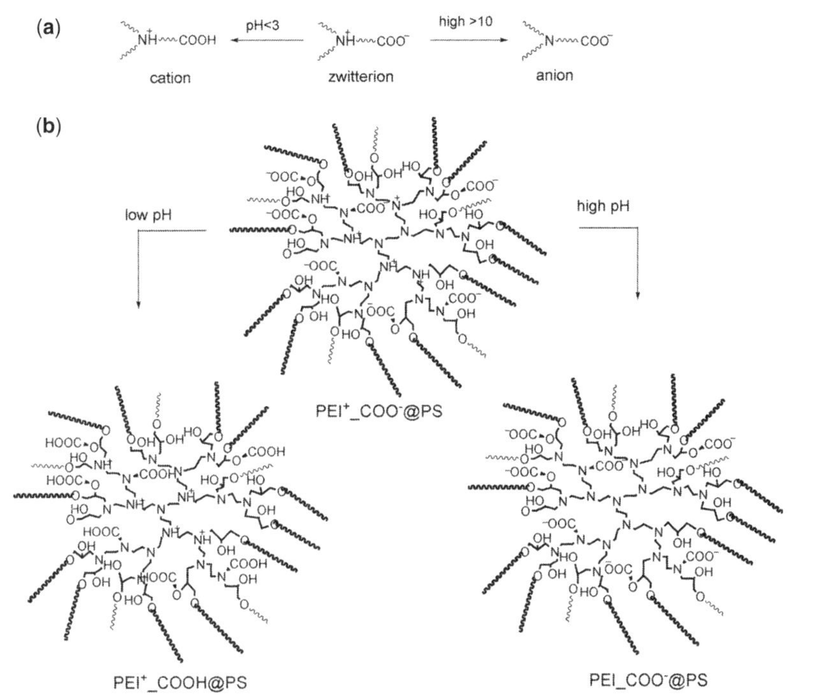

Figure 8.8 CAMs with pH-switchable zwitterionic cores.

an anionic guest. For the guest of RB, only 38.7% could be released by a PEI-CAM, but this value was improved to 91% when the host was replaced by the zwitterionic CAM. With the combination of the ion discriminating nature and pH-sensitive property of the above host CAMs, a wider spectrum of ionic mixtures could be well separated, and better recycling of the host was available. Charge selective encapsulation was also shown by other polymeric devices [20, 65].

8.6 Recognition and Separation of Anionic–Anionic Mixtures by Core Engineering of a CAM

8.6.1 The Core Structure–Guest Selectivity Relationship

It was found that a PEI-CAM could distinguish not only a cationic–anionic binary mixture of dyes, but also many anionic–anionic dyes, and this selectivity was dependent on the core structure of the PEI-CAM. It was experimentally found that with core engineering of a

PEI-CAM, many anionic mixtures could be effectively separated. As shown in Figure 8.9, there are still many amino protons in the core of PEI-CAM **H3d**; these residual amines can be further treated with propylene oxide, glycidol, succinic anhydride, or methyl iodide,

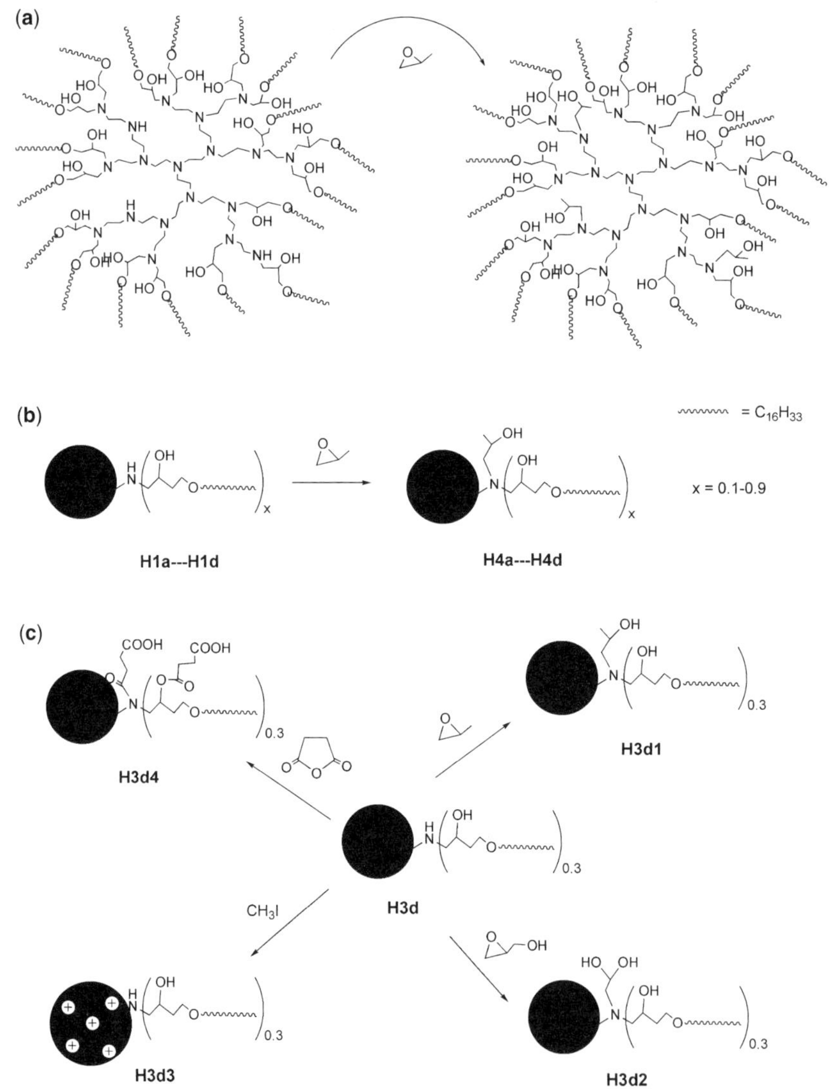

Figure 8.9 (a) core engineering of PEI-CAM by alkylation of the residual amines with propylene oxide; b) core engineering of H1a–H1d resulting in H4a–H4d; (c) outline of the synthesis of H3d1–H3d4 by the core engineering of H3d [12]. For the structures of H1a–H1d and H3d, see Figure 8.3.

leading to **H3d1–H3d4**, respectively (Figure 8.9) [12]. The separation based on molecular recognition was similarly carried out in an oil/water biphasic system. Typically, the binary anionic dyes of MO/RB were charged in a water phase, and with a limited amount of oil-soluble **H3d1** added to the system while shaking, the anionic species of RB was preferentially transferred to the oil layer, indicating that the PEI-CAM could differentiate the anionic species of MO/RB. It was found that for some binary anionic species, even in the case when an excess PEI-CAM was added, 100% separation was possible because one of the species was reluctant to be encapsulated; while for other mixtures, the dose of PEI-CAM was critical to the separation efficiency. It was found that the separation efficiency was very dependent on the core structure of the PEI-CAM. For all the anionic species (Figure 8.4) tested, **H4a–H4d** showed a better ability to differentiate anionic mixtures than **H1a–H1d** [12], suggesting that the tertiary amines or the hydroxyls or both are favorable for the recognition of anionic dyes. Furthermore, it was found that **H3d** could not efficiently distinguish the binary mixture of MO/RB, while **H3d1** could; **H3d2** showed a poorer affinity to RB than did **H3d1**, showing that the polar hydroxyl groups were unfavorable for the accommodation of RB. **H3d3** showed the highest encapsulating capacity to RB due to electrostatic complement, but showed a much poorer ability to differentiate MO/RB than **H3d1** and **H3d2**; **H3d4** showed the poorest encapsulating capacity and a poor ability to differentiate MO/RB. These facts indicated that the electronic property of a PEI-CAM is important for guest affinity, and by the core engineering of a PEI-CAM, the complementary interaction strength to different guest species varies in different degrees.

That some guests could not be encapsulated regardless of the core engineering of a PEI-CAM can be attributed to several factors listed below [9]. One is a topological factor; for example, the fact that DB-80 could hardly be encapsulated [9] can be attributed to its large and rigid structure, and encapsulation of such a guest requires a tremendous conformational change which a PEI-CAM can hardly offer. Another factor is the strong hydrophilicity of a guest; for example, MeB is highly hydrophilic and can be encapsulated only when the PEI-CAM is sufficiently quaternized [9]. IC is smaller than MeB, but cannot be encapsulated due to its high hydrophilicity [9].

To evaluate the role of the hydroxyls during guest differentiation, **H3e1–H3e3** (Figure 8.10) were synthesized and evaluated [10]. One can find that **H3e1–H3e3** bear the same shell, but the cores are

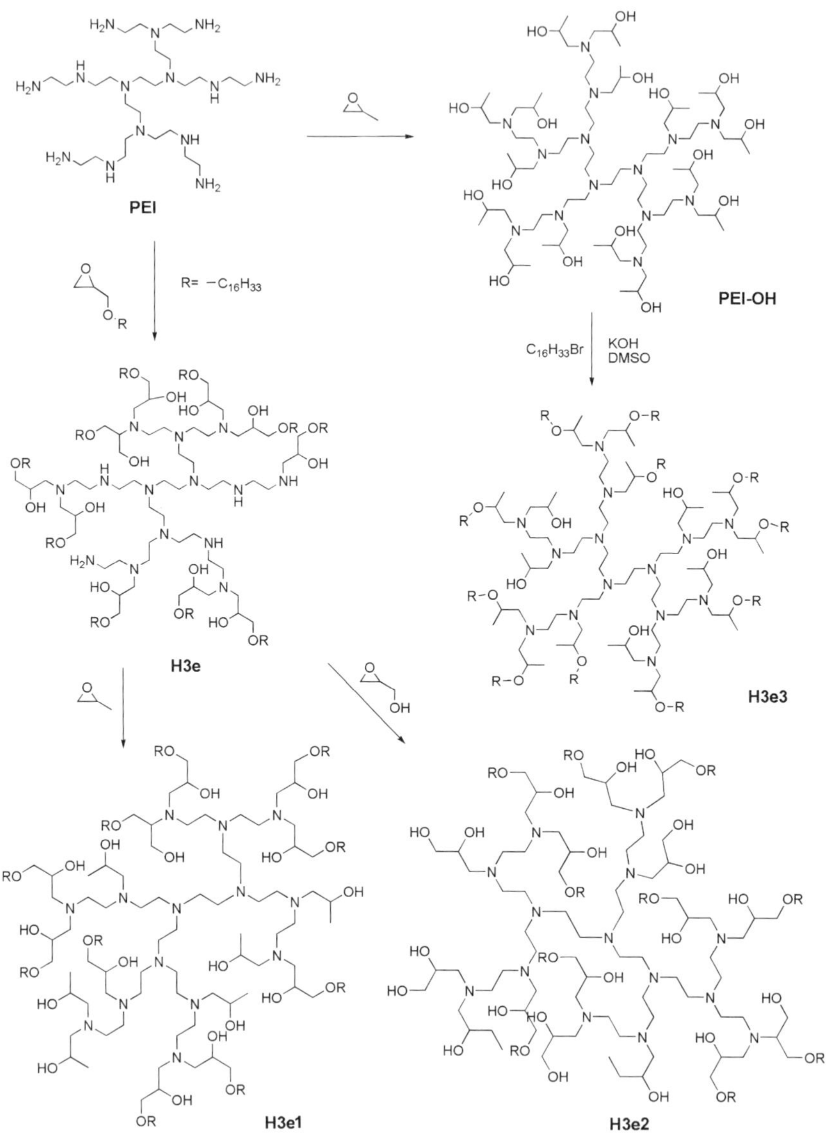

Figure 8.10 Outline of the synthesis of H3e1–H3e3 which had similar tertiary amines but different hydroxyl groups [10].

different in terms of the OH groups in the following order: **H3e1** > **H3e2** > **H3e3**. For the separation of FR/RB, the efficiency was in the following order: **H3e3** > **H3e2** > **H3e1**, indicating the polar OH groups were more unfavorable to RB than to FR. Meanwhile, it was noticed that **H3d1** also showed a better ability to differentiate FR/RB than **H3d**. Since the former bears more tertiary amine and more OH groups than the latter, and OH groups were found to be unfavorable for the recognition of FR/RB, it could be concluded that the tertiary amines should be very critical to the recognition of FR/RB. One can find that both FR and RB belong to the xanthene family, but RB is more hydrophobic and acidic than FR, so the rational combination of its hydrophobic and basic environment can sufficiently differentiate RB from FR.

8.6.2 Recognition of Similar Guest Molecules in a Mixture

The recognition and separation of similar molecules remains a current challenge in the scientific and industrial community. However, it was recently found that in a host–guest system in which nonspecific interactions were dominant, the separation of similar molecules was successfully carried out [8, 10]. For example, the FR/TCFR and RB/EB [Figure 8.4]) are very similar guest pairs, and their separation is a challenge. For FR/TCFR, the structural frameworks are similar, but TCFR is slightly more hydrophobic and acidic than FR. If a host CAM is rationally designed in a hydrophobic and basic environment, recognition of FR/TCFR is possible. Wan *et al.* [8] synthesized **H3d5**, **H3d6**, **H3f1** and **H3f2** (Figure 8.11) and evaluated their ability to recognize FR/TCFR and RB/EB. One can find that **H3d5** and **H3d6** share a similar shell but different core; in the case of **H3d6**, the OH groups were transformed into less polar ester groups but the tertiary aliphatic amines are the same, while for **H3d5**, partial amines were transformed into amido groups, meaning that **H3d5** is less basic than **H3d6**. The more basic **H3d6** was found to show a much better ability to differentiate RB/EB or FR/TCFR. **H3f1** shared a different shell density from **H3d6** but their cores were similar, and their ability to recognize these guest species was similar, indicating that it was the core that determined the guest affinity. **H3f2** showed a better ability to differentiate these guest mixtures than **H3f1** because of its higher hydrophobicity. Their ability to differentiate RB/EB and FR/TCFR is shown in Figures 8.12 and 8.13. In both cases, the host nanocapsule could extract almost a pure component from the excess mixtures. It was concluded from these facts that a rational combination of a hydrophobic interaction with an electrostatic interaction (acid–base interaction) could lead to the

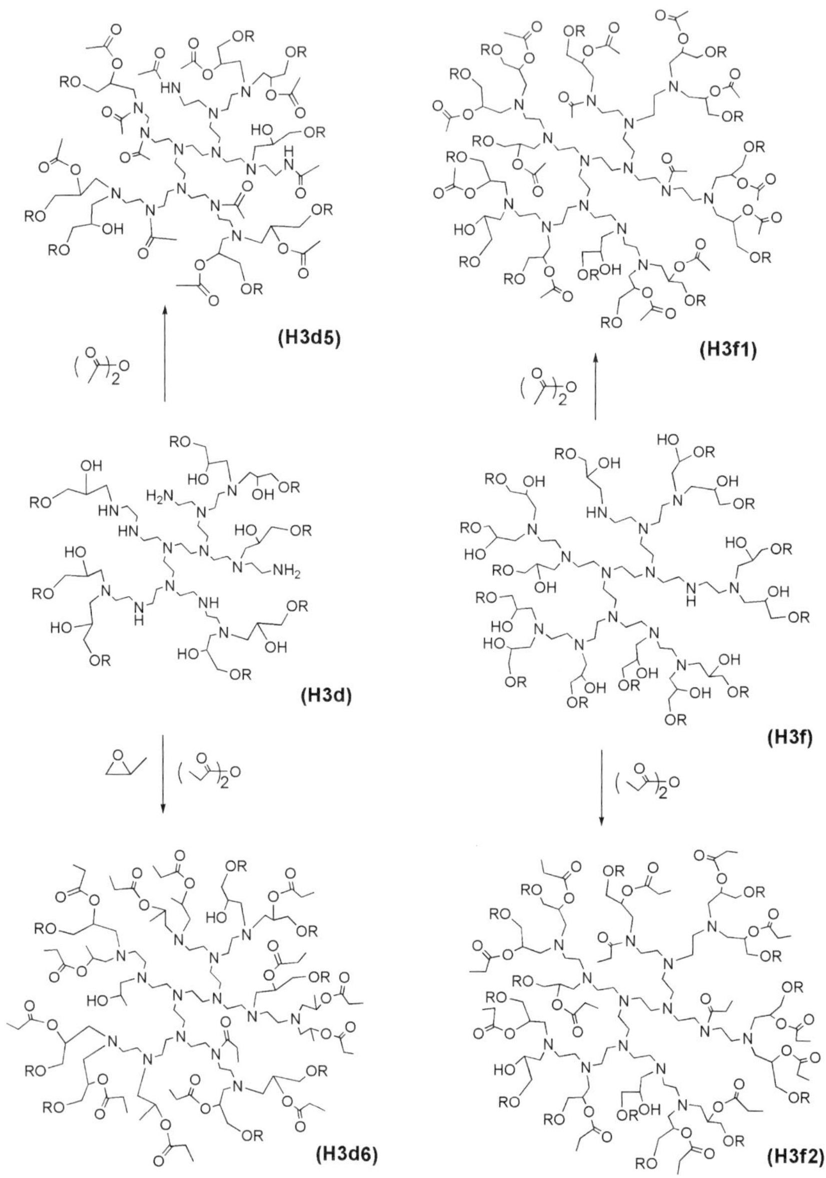

Figure 8.11 Outline of the synthesis of H3d5, H3d6, H3f1 and H3f2 [8].

effective recognition of similar guest pairs such as FR/TCFR and RB/EB. In these experiments, that a CAM prefers TCFR to FR (and prefers RB to EB) is understandable because either more halogen substituents or larger halogen atoms can enhance the dispersion force between the host and the guest. However, the high selectivity

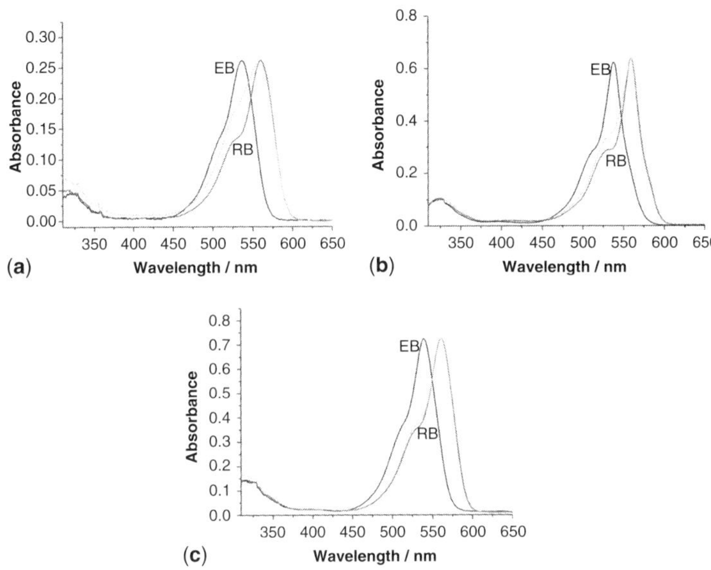

Figure 8.12 Recognition of the very similar RB/EB with H3f (A), H3f1 (B) and H3f2 (C) as host. Either EB (black line) or RB (red line) alone could be transferred to the organic layer, but a certain amount of PEI-CAM preferentially entrapped RB to the EB (dashed line) in water. The dash line is normalized with the red line at their maximum absorbance. Conditions: [CAM] = 10^{-6} M; [RB] = [EB] = 10^{-4} M; pH 7.4 (PBS buffer) [8].

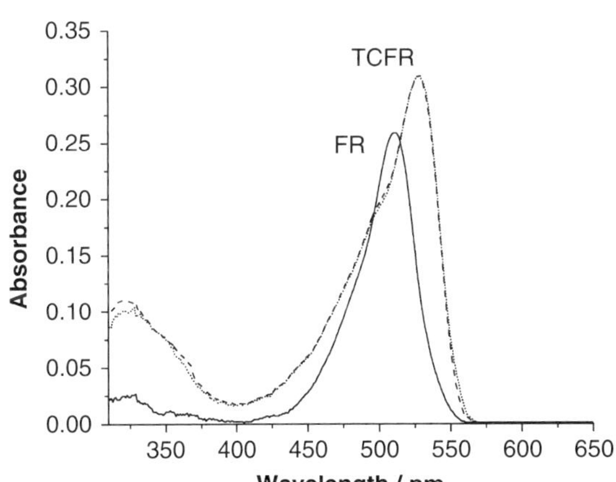

Figure 8.13 Recognition of FR/TCFR with H3f2. Either FR (black line) or TCFR (dotted line) could be transferred to the organic layer, but a certain amount of H3f2 preferentially trapped TCFR to the FR (dashed line) in water, as detected by the UV/vis spectra. The dash line and the dot line of the UV/vis spectra were normalized at their maximum absorbance. Conditions: [H3f2] = 5×10^{-5} M; [TCFR] = [FR] = 10^{-4} M; pH 7.4 (PBS buffer) [8].

seems amazing. Additionally, the experimental facts suggest that only a rational combination of the hydrophobicity and basicity of a CAM can lead to a high selectivity. These facts may suggest that certain synergic effects exist between the hydrophobic complement and electrostatic complement.

8.6.3 The Mechanism of Guest Selectivity in Encapsulation

Why can an appropriate combination of nonspecific elementary interactions between a host and competitive guests lead to a significantly improved selectivity? Generally speaking, the host CAMs employed above cannot undergo a specific encapsulation due to the irregular cavities and featureless electronic environment of the flexible CAMs. The host–guest interactions in a CAM-based system are of various natures, and each interaction style contributes more or less to the encapsulation. For example, in the PEI-CAM/RB system, it is certain that an electrostatic interaction contributes to the host–guest complement, but it was found that at a high pH when the PEI was completely deprotonated, some RBs still couldn't be released, indicating that the hydrophobic interaction contributed to the host–guest complement as well. Additionally, ion–dipole, dipole–dipole, and even hydrogen-bonding interactions should also contribute to the host–guest complement. The guest–guest interaction could also influence the encapsulation, resulting in a parallel, competitive, and synergic encapsulation [66] of different guest species. Regardless of these facts, mixture separation based on molecular recognition is theoretically possible for a CAM. As was recently pointed out [22], a complex system was characterized by incompleteness, imprecision, a time-varying property and nonlinearity. Wan *et al.* [10] suggested that this principle could be applied to a supramolecular system. The nonlinearity of a complex host–guest system means that for a series of components in a mixture, the affinity of each component to the host will change nonlinearly with the change in the host structure and a certain host structure can sufficiently differentiate the components, thus leading to molecular recognition. This mechanism was termed supramolecular fuzzy recognition [8, 10], and it seems that it is the only effective means for the recognition of a common molecule that is featureless in topology and electronic environment.

8.7 Modulation of the Guest Release of a CAM

The solution and guest release behavior of a delivery micelle during degradation has been little studied. How does the degradation influence the unimolecularity of the micelle? How is the guest release behavior dependent on the shell degradation? To address these issues, Wan and Satoh [67] synthesized a physical micelle with a PEI core and a sheddable" PEO shell, in which the core and shell are connected by DAD-ADA (D and A represent the hydrogen bonding donor and acceptor, respectively) complementary hydrogen-bonds, as shown in Figure 8.14. In this strategy, the shell layer is well adjustable and thus can somewhat mimic the shell degradation. It was found that the transition from a "unimolecular micelle" to aggregate occurred with a certain degree of shell shedding; similarly, a quick guest release suddenly occurred when certain shell shedding was reached; the host–guest complementary strength influenced the guest release, and in the case of CR, reduction of the basicity of the host was beneficial to the release of the acidic CR; certain small molecules bearing ADA hydrogen-bonding sites could replace the shell and led to guest release, namely, the micelle was chemically responsive.

The stimuli-responsive CAM was also explored. The stimuli source includes common factors, such as temperature, pH, ionic strength, optics and a specific factor such as chemicals. However, a quantitative response is rarely reported. Wan and Satoh [68] synthesized a covalent micelle of PEI@PEO (Figure 8.15), which retained a good water-solubility and unimolecularity and could encapsulate anionic species. When cyclodextrins were covalently

introduced into the core, the micelle remained unimolecular with a good water-solubility. Additionally, apolar pyrenes could also be encapsulated due to the presence of cyclodextrin moieties in the core. What was special about this micelle was that the host nanocapsule could undergo a quantitative stimuli-responsive release of pyrene under the trigger of certain anionic species (Figure 8.16). It was found that either MO or RB could enter the nanocapsule and trigger the release of pyrene, while MB and MeB could not enter the nanocapsule, and therefore were not able to trigger the release of pyrene. It was postulated that the triggered release should be related to the partly naked pyrene from its shuttle of cyclodextrin. A further study showed that the pH could also very effectively trigger the release of pyrene, which should also be related to the partly

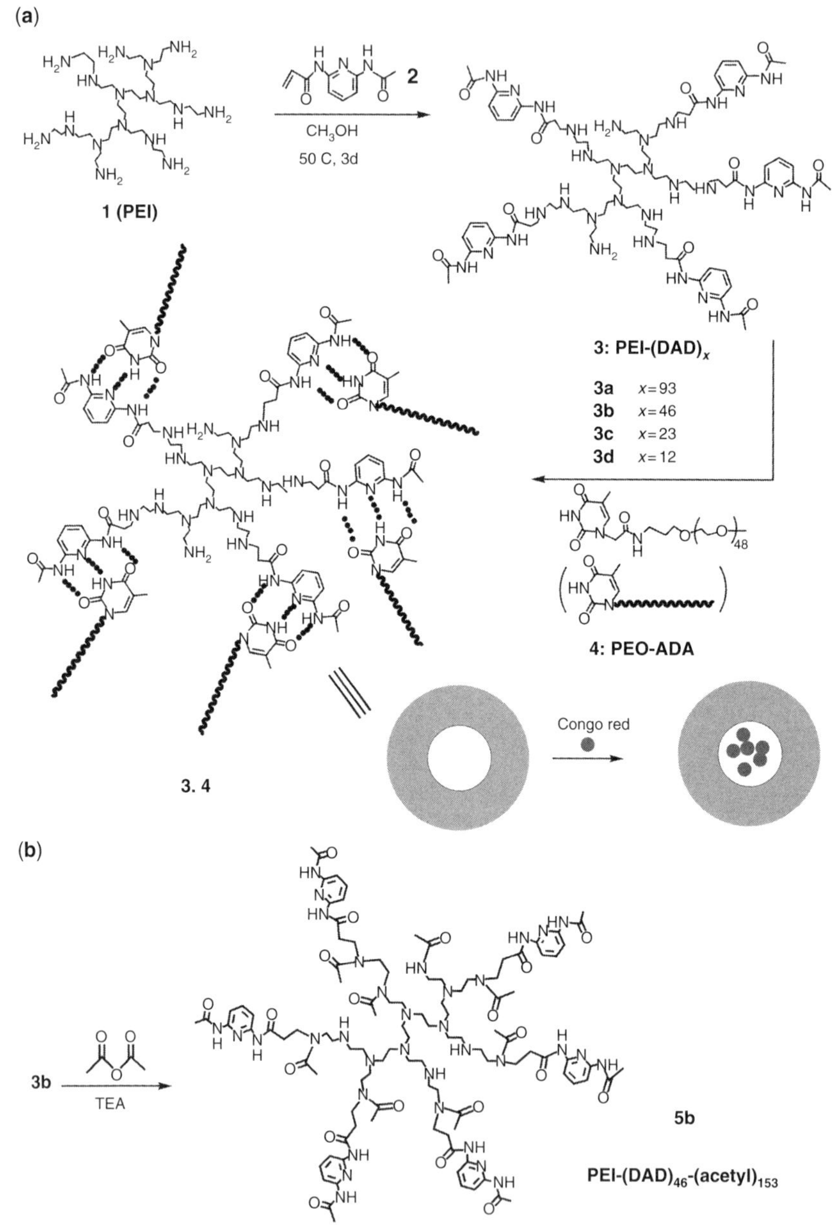

Figure 8.14 Physical micelles with "sheddable" shell. A) synthesis of physical micelles with multi triple-hydrogen-bonds; B) synthesis of a core with a lower basicity [67].

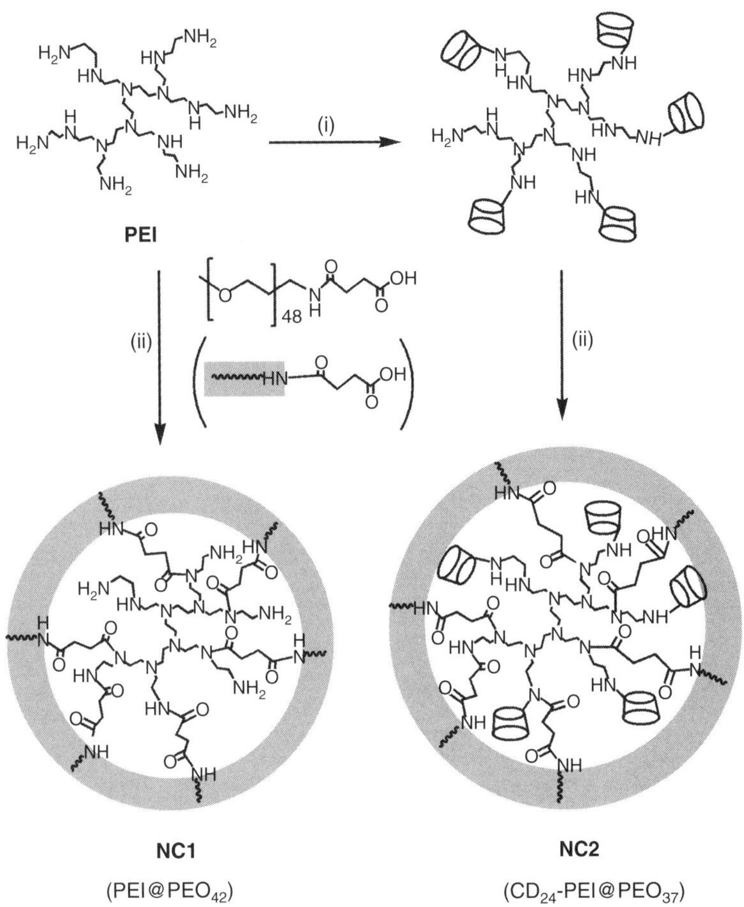

Figure 8.15 Outline of the synthesis of nanocapsule with (NC2) and without (NC1) CD moieties in the core. Nomenclature: e.g., CD24-PEI@PEO37 denotes PEI with 24 cyclodextrins as core and 37 PEO chains as shell [68].

naked pyrene. If the cyclodextrin was not attached to PEI, no triggered release was observed by either the pH or MO and RB. Guest release of a CAM could also be mediated by the structural design of the CAM. Wan *et al.* [11] studied the core structure–guest release behavior of several CAMs, and found that different cores led to different guest releasing rate of the guest MO. This experimental fact revealed that thermodynamic factors contribute to the guest release.

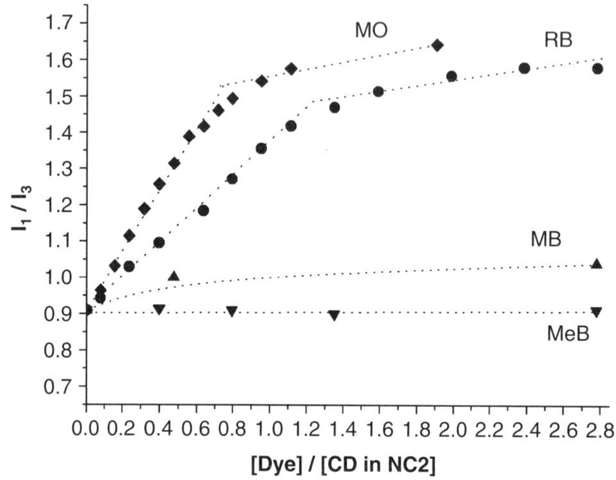

Figure 8.16 Dependence of the I1/I3 ratio of pyrene which was loaded in NC2 on the titration with aqueous RB, MO, MeB and MB. Conditions: NC2 (2.3×10^{-7} M) was saturated with PY; [dye] = 1×10^{-4} M; λex = 335 nm; pH 7.4 (PBS buffer) [68].

8.8 Concluding Remarks

A CAM with a hyperbranched polymer as the core is synthetically cost-effective and structurally widely available. The functional groups distributed throughout the entire hyperbranched polymer render the core of the CAM chemically designable. The electronic environment of the CAM is also relatively homogeneous due to the dense and random functional groups in the core, and this environment is conveniently adjustable. This feature is different from a dendrimer whose functional groups are arrayed regularly and exclusively on the periphery. Experiments have shown that tailoring the core of a CAM can lead to an enhanced unimolecularity, switchable guest affinity, designable guest selectivity and adjustable guest releasing rate.

PEI, a typical hyperbranched polymer, can be readily converted into an oil-soluble, reverse-micelle like CAM. The PEI-CAM can extract various hydrophilic solutes from water into organic media. The phase transfer extraction can be used for mixture separation, 100% charge selective separation can be widely available, and even separation of an anionic–anionic mixture and very similar components is possible. The separation is based on the nonlinearity of a complex system, namely, the nonlinear dependence of host–guest complementary strength on the electronic property of the host. Additionally, due to their multifunctionality, functional molecules, such as cyclodextrins, can be covalently introduced into the core, and this combination can result in new functions.

The multifunctionality has the potential to act as a platform for function integration. The dendritic framework is a useful component of catalytic material, optical materials and other functional materials but are not included in this chapter, thus readers are encouraged to read other chapters and comprehensive reviews elsewhere.

Acknowledgements

The authors are grateful for the financial support by the Natural Science Foundation of China (No. 21074094, 51273149) and the Japan Society for the Promotion of Science (JSPS) for this study.

References

1. C. Gao, D.Y. Yan. *Prog. Polym. Sci.* Vol. 29, p. 183, 2004.
2. D. Astruc, E. Boisselier, C. Ornelas. *Chem. Rev.* Vol. 110, p. 1857, 2010.
3. B.I. Voit, A. Lederer. *Chem. Rev.* Vol. 109, p. 5924, 2009.
4. S. Hecht, J.M.J. Frechet. *Angew.Chem. Int. Ed.* Vol. 40, p. 74, 2001.
5. J.F.G.A. Jansen, E.W. Meijer. *J. Am. Chem. Soc.* Vol. 117, p. 4417, 1995.
6. Y. Tomoyose, D.L. Jiang, R.H. Jin, T. Aida, T. Yamashita, K. Horie, E. Yashima, Y. Okamoto. *Macromolecules* Vol. 29, p. 5236, 1996.
7. U. Gupta, H.B. Agashe, A. Asthana, N.K. Jain. *Biomacromolecules* Vol. 7, p. 649, 2006.
8. D.C. Wan, H.T. Pu, M. Jin, G.W. Wang, J.L. Huang. *J. Polym. Sci., Part A: Polym. Chem.* Vol. 49, p. 2373, 2011.
9. D.C. Wan, Y. Lai, M. Jin, H.T. Pu. *Macromol. Chem. Phy.* Vol. 212, p. 1910, 2011.
10. D.C. Wan, H.T. Pu, M. Jin. *Macromolecules* Vol. 43, p. 3809, 2010.
11. D.C. Wan, M. Jin, H.T. Pu, H.Y. Pan, Z.H. Chang. *React. Funct. Polym.* Vol. 70, p. 916, 2010.
12. D.C. Wan, G.C. Wang, H.T. Pu, M. Jin. *Macromolecules* Vol. 42, p. 6448, 2009.
13. D.C. Wan, J.J. Yuan, H.T. Pu. *Macromolecules* Vol. 42, p. 1533, 2009.
14. D.C. Wan, H.T. Pu, X.Y. Cai. *Macromolecules* Vol. 41, p. 7787, 2008.
15. F. Vogtle. *Supramolecular chemistry: An introduction*. Chichester, John Wiley & Sons, 1991.
16. D. A. Tomalia, A. Naylor, W.A. Goddard III. *Angew. Chem., Int. Ed.* Vol. 29, p. 138, 1990.
17. G.R. Newkome, C.N. Moorefield, G.R. Baker, A.L. Johnson, R.K. Behera. *Angew. Chem., Int. Ed.* Vol. 30, p. 1176, 1991.

18. G.R. Newkome, C.N. Moorefield, G.R. Baker, M. J. Saunders, S.H. Grossman. *Angew. Chem., Int. Ed.* Vol. 30, p. 1178, 1991.
19. E. Burakowska, J.R. Quinn, S.C. Zimmerman, R. Haag. *J. Am. Chem. Soc.* Vol. 131, p. 10574, 2009.
20. K. Huang, J. Rzayev. *J. Am. Chem. Soc.* Vol. 133, p. 16726, 2011.
21. V. Balzani, P. Ceroni, S. Gestermann, M. Gorka, C. Kauffmann, F. Vogtle. *Tetrahedron* Vol. 58, p. 629, 2002.
22. L.A. Zadeh. *IEEE Trans Syst Man Cybernet* Vol. 3, p. 28, 1973.
23. M. Kramer, M. Kopaczynska, S. Krause, R. Haag. *J. Polym. Sci., Part A: Polym. Chem.* Vol. 45, p. 2287, 2007.
24. C. Aymonier, U. Schlotterbeck, L. Antonietti, P. Zacharias, R. Thomann, J.C. Tiller, S. Mecking. *Chem. Commun.* p. 3018, 2002.
25. M. Kramer, J.F. Stumbe, H. Turk, S. Krause, A. Komp, L. Delineau, S. Prokhorova, H. Kautz, R. Haag. *Angew. Chem., Int. Ed.* Vol. 41, p. 4252, 2002.
26. Y. Chen, Z. Shen, L. Pastor-Perez, H. Frey, S.E. Stiriba. *Macromolecules* Vol. 38, p. 227, 2005.
27. L. Antonietti, C. Aymonier, U. Schlotterbeck, V.M. Garamus, T. Maksimova, W. Richtering, S. Mecking. *Macromolecules* Vol. 38, p. 5914, 2005.
28. H.J. Liu, Y. Chen, D.D. Zhu, Z. Shen, S.E. Stiriba. *React. Funct. Polym.* Vol. 67, p. 383, 2007.
29. S.J. Xu, Y. Luo, R. Haag, *Macromol. Rapid Commun.*, Vol. 29, p. 171, 2008.
30. M. Adeli, R. Haag, *J. Polym. Sci. Part A: Polym. Chem.*, Vol. 44, p. 5740, 2006.
31. X.L. Cao, Z.Q. Li, X.W. Song, X.H. Cui, P.F. Cao, H.J. Liu, F. Cheng, Y. Chen. *Eur. Poly. J.* Vol. 44, p. 1060, 2008.
32. H.J. Liu, Z. Shen, S.E. Striba, Y. Chen, W.Q. Zhang, L.H. Wei. *J. Polym. Sci., Part A: Polym. Chem.* Vol. 44, p. 4165, 2006.
33. H.Y. Tian, X.S. Chen, H. Lin, C. Deng, P.B. Zhang, Y. Wei, X.B. Jing. *Chem. –Eur. J.* Vol. 12, p. 4305, 2006.
34. Y.R. Ren, X.S. Jiang, J. Yin. *J. Polym. Sci. Part A: Polym. Chem.* Vol. 47, p.1292, 2009.
35. R. Wang, B. Yu, X.S. Jiang, J. Yin. *Adv. Funct. Mater.* Vol. 22, p. 2606, 2012.
36. C.F. Di, X.S. Jiang, R. Wang, J. Yin. *J. Mater. Chem.* Vol. 21, p. 4416, 2011.
37. Y.Y. Mai, Y.F. Zhou, D.Y. Yan. *Macromolecules* Vol. 38, p. 8679, 2005.
38. Y.F. Zhou, W. Huang, J.Y. Liu, X.Y. Zhu, D.Y. Yan. *Adv. Mater.* Vol. 22, p. 4567, 2010.
39. Y.F. Zhou, D.Y. Yan. *Chem. Commun.* p. 1172, 2009.
40. C.J. Hawker, F.K. Chu. *Macromolecules* Vol. 29, p. 4370, 1996.
41. Y. Kitajyo, Y. Nawa, M. Tamaki, H. Tani, K. Takahashi, H. Kaga, T. Satoh, T. Kakuchi. *Polymer* Vol. 48, p. 4683, 2007.
42. Y. Kitajyo, T. Imai, Y. Sakai, M. Tamaki, H. Tani, K. Takahashi, A. Narumi, H. Kaga, N. Kaneko, T. Satoh, T. Kakuchi. *Polymer* Vol. 48, p. 1237, 2007.
43. T. Satoh, M. Tamaki, Y. Kitajyo, T. Maeda, H. Ishihara, T. Imai, H. Kaga, T. Kakuchi. *J. Polym. Sci., Part A: Polym. Chem.* Vol. 44, p. 406, 2006.
44. M.J. Maciejewski. *Macrom. Sci.-Chem.* Vol. 17A, p. 689, 1982.
45. A. Sunder, M. Kramer, R. Hanselmann, R. Mulhaupt, H. Frey. *Angew. Chem., Int. Ed.* Vol. 38, p. 3552, 1999.
46. S.E. Stiriba, H. Kautz, H. Frey. *J. Am. Chem. Soc.* Vol. 124, p. 9698, 2002.
47. T. Satoh. *Soft Matter* Vol. 5, p. 1972, 2009.
48. P.F. Cao, R.X Zhao, L. Li, W.W. Yang, F. Cheng, Y. Chen, C.H. Lu, S.C. Jiang. *J. Polym. Sci. Part A: Polym. Chem.* Vol. 50, p. 227, 2012.

49. P.F. Cao, R. Xiang, X.Y. Liu, C.X. Zhang, F. Cheng, Y. Chen. *J. Polym. Sci., Part A: Polym. Chem.* Vol. 47, p. 5184, 2009.
50. Y. Liu, Y. Fan, X.Y. Liu, S.Z. Jiang, Y. Yuan, Y. Chen, F. Cheng, S.C. Jiang. *Soft Matter* Vol. 8. P. 8361, 2012.
51. Z.L. Yu, F. Cheng, S.J. Zhao, J.W. Zhang, Z.C. Cai, Y. Chen. *Macromol. Res.* Vol. 19, p. 189, 2011.
52. D.C. Wan, Z.L. Yang, H.T. Pu, J.X. Zhao, G.J. Yang. *J. Appl. Polym. Sci.* Vol. 113, p. 3702, 2009.
53. F. Yuan, H. Pan, F. Cheng, Y. Chen, S.C. Jiang. *Polymer* Vol. 53, p. 2175, 2012.
54. G. Pistolis, A. Malliaris, D. Tsiourvas, C. M. Paleos. *Chem. –Eur. J.* Vol. 5, p. 1440, 1999.
55. M. Irfan, M. Seiler. *Ind. Eng. Chem. Res.* Vol. 49, p. 1169, 2010.
56. M.-C. Jones, J.-C. Leroux. *Soft Matter* Vol. 6, p. 5850, 2010.
57. T.M. Lodge, A. Rasdal, Z.B. Li, M.A. Hillmyer. *J. Am. Chem. Soc.* Vol. 127, p. 17608, 2005.
58. M.R. Radowski, A. Shukla, H. von Berlepsch, C. Bottcher, G. Pickaert, H. Rehage, R. Haag. *Angew. Chem., Int. Ed.* Vol. 46, p. 1265, 2007.
59. S. Sengupta, D. Eavarone, I. Capila, G.L. Zhao, N. Watson, T. Kiziltepe, R. Sasisekharan. *Nature* Vol. 436, p.568, 2005.
60. X.L. Lou, F. Cheng, P.F. Cao, Q. Tang, H.J. Liu, Y. Chen. *Chem. –Eur. J.* Vol. 15, p. 11566, 2009.
61. M.R. Radowski, A. Shukla, H. von Berlepsch, C. Bottcher, G. Pickaert, H. Rehage, R. Haag. *Angew. Chem. Int. Ed.* Vol.46, p. 1265, 2007.
62. Y. Liang, D.C. Wan, X.Y. Cai, M. Jin, H.T. Pu. *J. Polym. Sci., Part A: Polym. Chem.* Vol. 48, p. 681, 2010.
63. X.S. Fan, G.W. Wang, S. Zhang, J.L. Huang. *J. Polym. Sci., Part A: Polym. Chem.* Vol. 49, p. 4146, 2011.
64. D.C. Wan, M. Jin, H.T. Pu, G.W. Wang. *J. Polym. Sci., Part A: Polym. Chem.* Vol. 50, p. 1342, 2012.
65. K. Fukae, T. Terashima, M. Sawamoto. *Macromolecules* Vol. 45, p. 3377, 2012.
66. C.H. Liu, C. Gao, D.Y. Yan. *Macromolecules* Vol. 39, p. 8102, 2005.
67. D.C. Wan, F. Chen, T. Kakuchi, T. Satoh. *Polymer* Vol. 52, p. 3405, 2011.
68. D.C. Wan, S. Ohta, T. Kakuchi, T. Satoh. *Soft Matter* Vol. 7, p. 6422, 2011.

9

Polymer Layers by Initiated CVD for Thin Film Gas Barrier Encapsulation

D.A. Spee, J.K. Rath and R.E.I. Schropp

Debye Institute for Nanomaterials Science, Utrecht University, Utrecht, The Netherlands

Abstract

In this chapter a thorough description of the initiated chemical vapor deposition (iCVD) process will be given, concentrating on molecular weight and deposition rate of the deposited polymer, which are essential for large-scale application in hybrid gas barriers. Practical applications of coatings by iCVD are addressed, and it will be shown that iCVD single layers can be used individually as gas barriers. However, so far the intrinsic moisture barrier function of polymers is too low to meet the strict requirements that are needed for organic light emitting diodes (OLEDs) and organic solar cells. Ultra-high gas barriers, with a WVTR << 10^{-3} g/m^2/day, are an interesting area for the application of iCVD layers as well; thin polymer layers can be used as defect decoupling layers in multilayer hybrid organic/inorganic gas barriers. Although thin inorganic layers can be very impermeable, they inevitably contain defect or pinholes, through which moisture can permeate. Since these defects tend to propagate through the entire inorganic layer, an intermediate layer is necessary to decouple defects in consecutive inorganic layers. To be able to optimally fulfill their function in such a hybrid multilayer, there are certain required properties for the iCVD layers concerning their smoothness, stability, glass transition temperature and adhesion, which will be discussed. Actual multilayers containing polymer layers by iCVD developed in the groups of Prof. Gleason at MIT and Prof. Schropp at Utrecht University will be addressed, as well as scaling up of the iCVD process, and consequently commercialization.

Keywords: Initiated chemical vapor deposition, hot wire chemical vapor deposition, moisture barrier, hybrid organic/inorganic, flexible substrate, organic light emitting diode, solar cell, roll-to-roll, low temperature

Vikas Mittal (ed.) Encapsulation Nanotechnologies, (255–290) © 2013 Scrivener Publishing LLC

9.1 Introduction

Initiated chemical vapor deposition (iCVD) is a gas-phase technique to deposit polymer film, avoiding the use of high temperatures. Contrary to solution-based techniques or techniques that involve a plasma, it is very gentle and unlikely to damage the underlying substrate. It can be used to deposit on very fragile and soluable substrates.

iCVD belongs to the family of hot wire CVD (HWCVD) processes in which source gasses are decomposed at resistively heated wires. First reported in the 1980s [1] and further developed in the 1990s [2], HWCVD is a relatively new technique. Since it was almost simultaneously developed in different parts of the world, alternative names are used: "Cat-CVD" [3, 4], stressing that the wire material could have a catalytic effect on the reactions, or "hot filament CVD" [5, 6], pointing out the similarity between an incandescent light bulb and a hot wire reactor (the term "filament" was used in electronics for the tungsten wires in a light bulb). Although HWCVD is mainly used to deposit inorganic (semiconductor) materials, it can also produce organic layers. However, using high filament temperatures could result in unwanted side reactions during the deposition of chemically complex polymers and prevent the coating of delicate functional materials.

The use of an initiator, a second, thermally labile precursor which can be dissociated much easier than the actual monomer and starts the polymerization process was reported by Pryce Lewis *et al.* in 2001 [7]. This reduced the process temperatures drastically. Since then, the technique was further developed in the laboratory of Prof. Gleason at the Massachusetts Institute of Technology (MIT).

In iCVD, not only are processes at the substrate and at the hot wires separated, as they are in HWCVD, but also are processes involving monomer and initiator separated: while the initiator is dissociated, the monomer stays intact, creating a highly controllable process.

iCVD combines the great versatility of CVD with the many advantages of polymer materials [8], which is schematically depicted in Figure 9.1.

In the next section, first a thorough description of the iCVD process will be given, concentrating on aspects like molecular weight of the deposited polymer, which are important for stability and deposition rate. Both aspects, molecular weight and deposition rate, are essential for large-scale application in hybrid gas barriers.

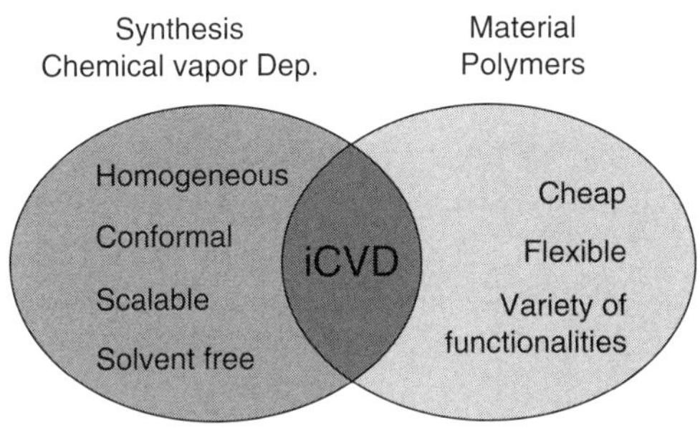

Figure 9.1 In initiated CVD the advantages of CVD deposition are combined with the possibility to maintain functional properties of polymer materials.

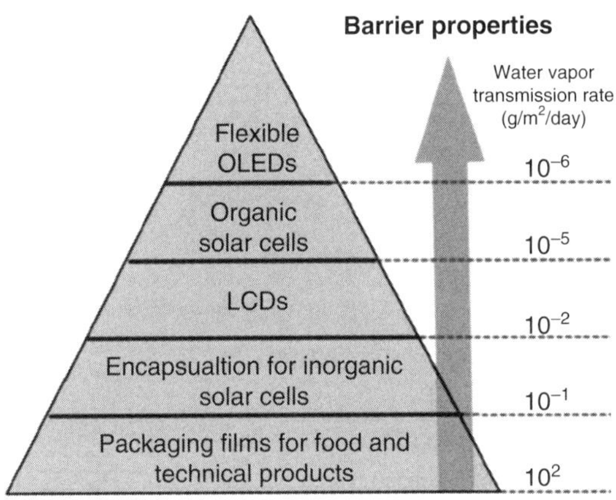

Figure 9.2 WVTR requirements of moisture barriers for various applications.

Afterwards, practical applications of coatings by iCVD are discussed in Section 9.3. In this section it will be shown that iCVD single layers can be used individually as gas barriers; a typical water vapor transmission rate (WVTR) of 10^{-3} g/m^2/day can be reached by a single polymer layer. However, so far the intrinsic moisture barrier function of polymers is too low to meet the strict requirements that are needed for organic light emitting diodes (OLEDs) and organic solar cells, which are shown in Figure 9.2.

Ultra-high gas barriers, with a WVTR << 10^{-3} g/m^2/day, are an interesting area for the application of iCVD layers as well; thin polymer layers can be used as defect decoupling layers in multilayer hybrid organic/inorganic gas barriers. In Figure 9.3, such a multilayer is shown schematically. Although thin layers of inorganic materials like silicon oxide (SiO_2), silicon nitride (Si_3N_4) or

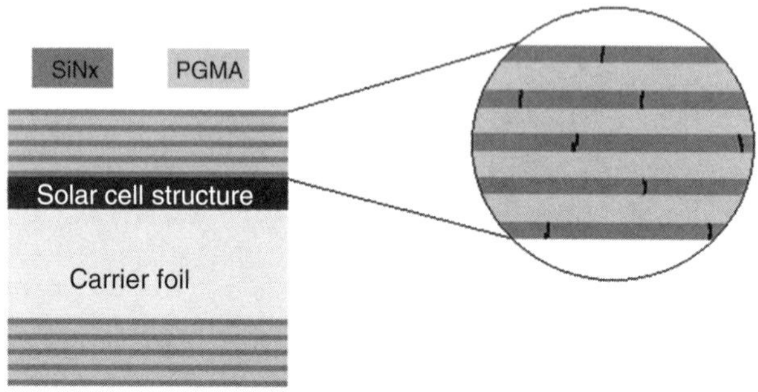

Figure 9.3 Schematic of the application of a hybrid organic/inorganic multilayer as moisture barrier on a flexible solar cell and the decoupling of pinholes or microcracks in consecutive inorganic layers, creating a tortuous path for diffusing moisture.

aluminum oxide (Al_2O_3) are transparent materials that are very impermeable, they inevitably contain defect or pinholes, through which moisture can permeate. This means their barrier function will not increase after a certain thickness [9]. Since these defects tend to propagate through the entire inorganic layer, an intermediate layer is necessary to decouple defects in consecutive inorganic layers.

From Section 9.4 on, layers by iCVD will be addressed in the context of multilayer gas barriers more specifically, starting with the advantages of the use of iCVD for multilayers.

To be able to optimally fulfill their function in such a hybrid multilayer, there are certain required properties for the iCVD layers concerning their smoothness, stability, glass transition temperature and adhesion, which will be addressed in Section 9.5.

Multilayers containing polymer layers by iCVD, developed in the groups of Prof. Gleason at MIT and Prof. Schropp at Utrecht University will be addressed in Section 9.6.

Eventually, scaling up of the iCVD process and consequently commercialization are included in the final section.

9.2 Initiated CVD Polymerization

The process of iCVD polymerization consists of different steps which are spatially separated. The radicals that are formed by thermal dissociation of initiators at hot filaments in the gas phase only start the second step of the process, the initiation, on the substrate. The polymerization that follows is determined by the amount of radicals reaching the substrate, the amount of monomers present at the substrate, and the substrate temperature. The polymerization process can be limited by: (i) the dissociation of the initiator at low filament temperatures, (ii) the propagation rate at the surface at low substrate temperatures, and (iii) monomer adsorption at the surface, when the partial pressure of the monomer is much lower than its saturation pressure (low p_M/p_{sat} ratio). The latter is again dependent on substrate temperature.

9.2.1 Reaction Mechanism

In Figure 9.4, a schematic of a typical iCVD reactor is shown. Radicals created by dissociation of initiator molecules at heated filaments start a polymerization reaction when they reach monomers adsorbed at the cooled substrate [10].

A complete reaction mechanism, which includes many steps and is given below in Table 9.1, was proposed by K.K.S. Lau and K.K. Gleason [11].

The main reaction which occurs in the gas phase is the decomposition of the initiator in the vicinity of the heated wires (formula 9.1). The radicals that are formed there diffuse to the substrate where they are adsorbed (9.2). Equilibrium conditions are expected for the adsorption of the monomer (9.3), since monomer gas is fed into

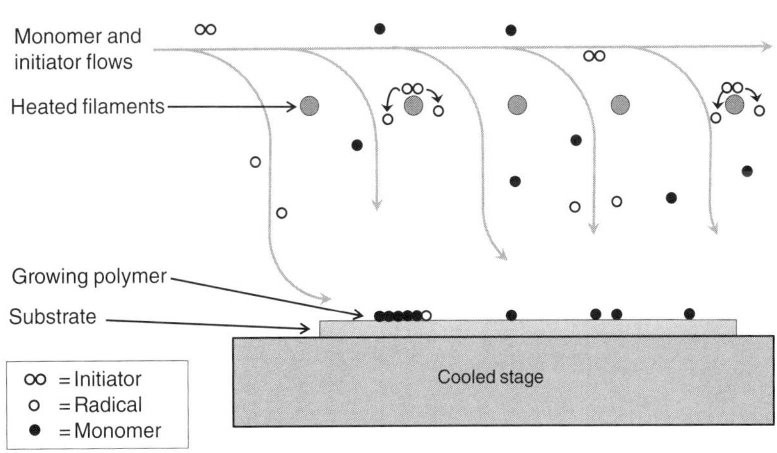

Figure 9.4 Schematic representation of the iCVD process.

Table 9.1 The reaction scheme in the iCVD process. If only surface reactions are considered, the kinetic equations from bulk phase radical polymerization can be applied directly to iCVD polymerization [11].

gas phase reactions:				
initiator decomposition	**I (g)**	→	**2 R· (g)**	(9.1)
gas-to-surface processes:				
primary radical adsorption	**R · (g)**	→	**R· (ad)**	(9.2)
monomer adsorption	**M (g)**	→	**M (ad)**	(9.3)
surface reactions:				
initiation	**R · (ad) + M (ad)**	→	$\mathbf{M_1}$**· (ad)**	(9.4)
propagation	$\mathbf{M_n}$ **· (ad) + M (ad)**	→	$\mathbf{M_{n+1}}$**· (ad)**	(9.5)
termination	$\mathbf{M_n}$ **· (ad) +** $\mathbf{M_m}$ **· (ad)**	→	$\mathbf{M_{n+m}}$ **(ad)** $\mathbf{M_n}$ **(ad) +** $\mathbf{M_m}$ **(ad)**	(9.6)
primary radical termination	$\mathbf{M_n}$ **· (ad) + R · (ad)**	→	$\mathbf{M_n}$ **(ad)**	(9.7)
primary radical recombination	**R · (ad) + R · (ad)**	→	$\mathbf{R_2}$ **(ad)**	(9.8)

the reactor in sufficient amount. Now that radicals and monomers are adsorbed at the surface, polymerization takes place through the pathways of initiation (9.4), propagation (9.5) and termination (9.6), similar to free radical polymerization in the liquid phase. In equation (9.6) termination can occur through coupling of two polymer radicals or, alternatively through disproportionation, the transfer of a hydrogen atom from one radical chain to another, eliminating both radical sites.

It was found that under certain conditions the concentration of radicals can be so high that radicals (the initiator) can terminate the polymerization (9.7) and recombine (9.8)[10].

If only surface reactions are considered, the kinetic equations of bulk phase polymerization, describing the polymerization rate, R_p, and the kinetic chain length, ν, in terms of R_p and the initiation rate R_i, can be applied [11]:

$$R_p = -\frac{d[M]}{dt} = k_p[M][M\cdot] \tag{9.9}$$

$$\nu = \frac{R_p}{R_i} = \frac{k_p[M][M\cdot]}{k_i[M][R\cdot]} \tag{9.10}$$

where $[M]$ is the monomer concentration, $[M\cdot]$ is the polymer radical concentration and $[R\cdot]$ is the primary radical concentration. More detailed information on the kinetic equations of (bulk phase) polymerization is given in ref. [12].

9.2.2 Radical Creation

A thermally labile initiator is fed into the reactor in the vapor phase and dissociated at hot filaments. Usually peroxides are used for this, for instance, tert-amyl peroxide [10], tert-butyl peroxide or tert-butyl peroxybenzoate [13], which are depicted in Figure 9.5, however non-peroxides like perfluorooctane sulfonyl fluoride [7] and triethylamine [14] have been utilized, all having different dissociation energies.

The most commonly used initiator, tert-butyl peroxide (TBPO), dissociates around 150°C. The filament temperature, however, needs to be higher, since one would like the initiator to dissociate not only at the filament, but also in the vicinity of it. Typically

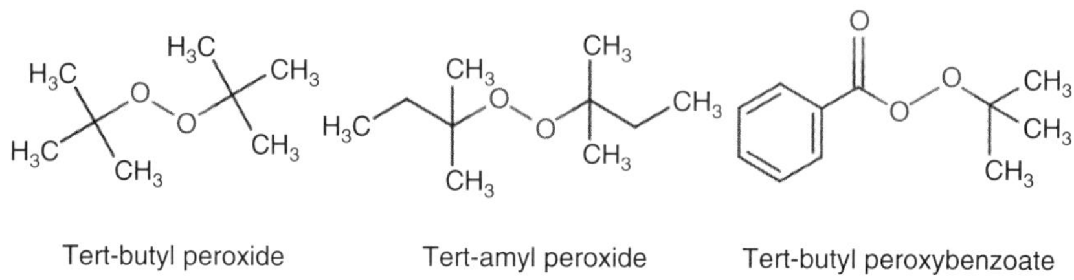

Figure 9.5 For an initiator usually peroxides are used, which are thermally unstable and can easily be dissociated into two radicals, by breaking the bond between the oxygen atoms.

filament temperatures between 200°C and 270°C are used. It was found by Xu and Gleason [13] that by using tert-butyl peroxybenzoate (TBPOB), compared to TBPO, the growth rate could be increased up to a factor 7 when using the same wire temperature and wire temperatures below 200°C can be applied.

Lowering the wire temperature can be important for several reasons. Firstly, in this way, radiative and conductive heating of the substrate [15] can be kept at a minimum. Since in a vacuum it is difficult to cool the substrate due to insufficient heat conduction, it is crucial to accurately control the substrate temperature. The importance of the substrate temperature as a process parameter will be addressed in Subsections 9.2.2 and 9.2.3. Secondly, avoiding high temperatures prevents the monomer molecules from dissociating and reduces unwanted gas phase reactions. These were found to occur above 220°C by Mao and Gleason [16].

The eventual amount of nucleation sites is influenced by both the amount of initiator fed into the reactor and the fraction of initiator molecules that is subsequently dissociated, as well as the amount of formed radicals eventually reaching the substrate. The latter is dependent on the total pressure in the reactor and flow rates. Although the increase in nucleation sites will increase the growth rate of the polymer layer, it can be easily seen from formula (9.10) that increasing the initiation rate R_i (i.e., the amount of nucleation sites) without increasing the polymerization rate R_p will result in smaller polymer chains.

Furthermore, it is important to understand that as soon as initiator gas is dissociated, the partial pressure of the (now) radical gas, relative to that of the monomer gas, becomes twice as high. Especially since in vacuum systems, only the total pressure in the reactor can be adjusted, meaning partial pressures of different gases can only be adjusted indirectly by adjusting the relative flows of these gases and the total pressure in the reactor.

9.2.3 Deposition Rate and Molecular Weight

The deposition rate of the polymer is dependent on both initiation rate, R_i, and propagation rate, R_p. In formula (9.10) it can be seen that by increasing R_i independently, although the deposition rate is increased, the average chain length of the polymer is decreased. Since some critical features of the polymer, such as stability and glass transition temperature T_g depend on this chain length, increasing *Ri* is usually not desirable. The other way to increase the deposition rate is by increasing R_p, which is, as can be seen in formula (9.9), dependent on both the monomer concentration, [M], and the polymer radical concentration at the surface, [M·]. The latter, however, is in turn dependent on R_i. To increase the deposition rate without decreasing the average chain length, one thus needs to increase the monomer surface concentration.

It was indeed found by Chan and Gleason that the polymer deposition rate increases linearly with monomer surface concentration, and moreover, also the average chain length (i.e., molecular weight) of the polymer [17]. This is shown in Figure 9.6.

Regimes exist in which this relation is of 2nd order, however, only when there are very few available monomers compared to the amount of radicals reaching the surface [10, 12].

The fact that deposition rate and molecular weight both increase with an increase of surface concentration of the monomer means that no trade-off between the two is needed. Since industry usually looks for high-throughput deposition methods, this is important for eventual commercial deposition of iCVD polymer layers.

Besides the polymer radical and monomer surface concentration, the propagation rate, and thus the deposition rate, is also dependent on the reaction rate constant k_p in formula (9.9). This constant is first of all dependent on the monomer used. Although in all commonly used monomers, of which some are shown in Figure 9.12, polymerization proceeds through the vinyl bonds of the monomer, the activation energy for this process is not equal for all of them. Another aspect is that when a monomer containing two or more vinyl bonds is used, which will result in a branched polymer, the alignment of monomers is thought to play a major role in propagation [18]: a steric hindrance can occur in the propagation, especially

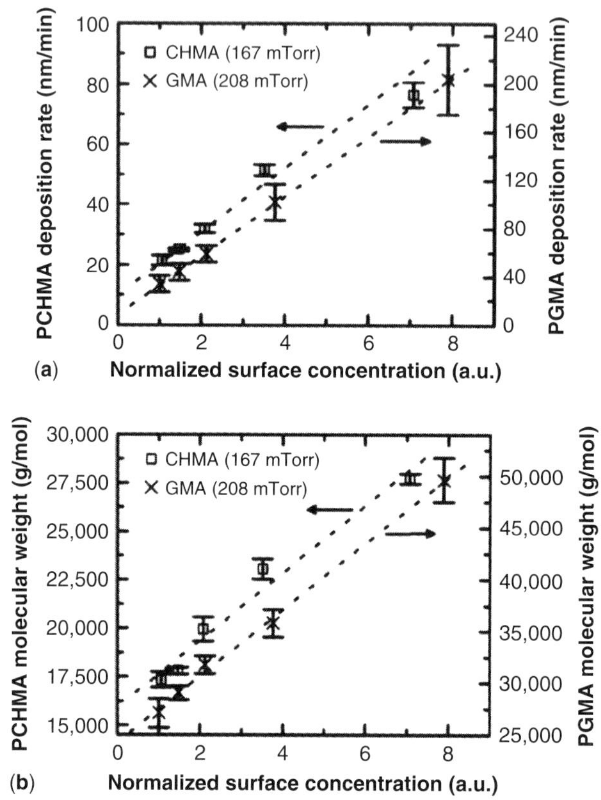

Figure 9.6 Keeping the partial pressures constant, the deposition rate (a) as well as the molecular weight (b) of poly(cyclohexyl methacrylate)(PCHMA) and poly(glycidyl methacrylate) (PGMA), is linearly increasing with monomer surface concentration. Surface concentrations were measured using a quartz-crystal microbalance [17]. Reprinted with permission from [17]. Copyright 2006 American Chemical Society.

when large monomers are used. Secondly, k_p is dependent on the surface temperature. The above mentioned steric hindrance in the propagation will have less effect at higher temperature, when the surface mobility of the monomers is higher. In general, iCVD kinetics will be enhanced by a higher surface temperature because rate coefficients of these events generally follow the usual Arrhenius dependence [10].

Summarizing, the deposition rate will increase with *decreasing* substrate temperature in an adsorption (surface monomer concentration) limited regime, and the deposition rate will increase with *increasing* substrate temperature in a regime that is limited by initiation or propagation processes. In the next section, however, it is shown that the monomer surface concentration is strongly negatively dependent on substrate temperature, meaning that the activated growth process is often only valid when large monomers with multiple vinyl groups are used.

9.2.4 Monomer Adsorption

The above section addressed the fact that the monomer adsorption (i.e., monomer surface concentration) is often one of the most important parameters, if not the most important, in the iCVD polymerization process. It was found experimentally by Chan and Gleason [17] that the monomer surface concentration is dependent on substrate temperature and partial pressure of the monomer (see in Figure 9.7).

The volume, V, of monomer that is adsorbed on the substrate can be related to the ratio of partial pressure of the monomer, p_M and the saturation pressure of the monomer, p_{sat} using the BET (Brunauer, Emmet and Teller) equation [19]:

$$\frac{p_M V_m c}{V(p_{sat} - p_M)} = \frac{p_M (c-1)}{p_{sat}} + 1 \tag{9.11}$$

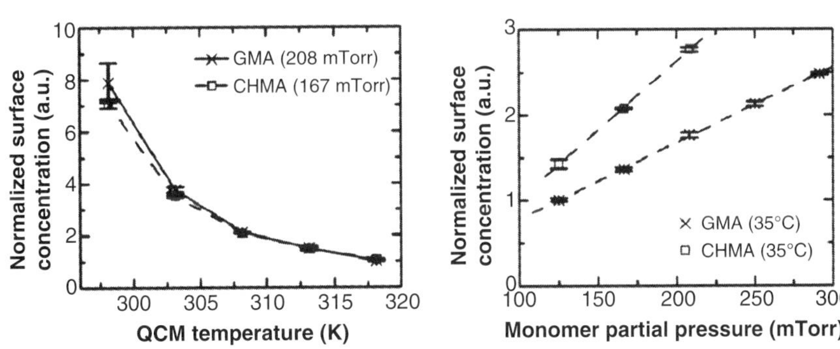

Figure 9.7 Temperature dependency at a constant partial pressure (left) and partial pressure dependency at a constant substrate temperature of the monomer surface concentration, for GMA and CHMA monomers, as found by Chan and Gleason [17]. Surface concentrations were measured using a quartz-crystal microbalance. Reprinted with permission from [17]. Copyright 2006 American Chemical Society.

in which V_m is the volume of a monolayer of monomer and c is given by:

$$c = \exp\left(\frac{\Delta H_{des} - \Delta H_{vap}}{RT}\right) \tag{9.12}$$

where T is the temperature, R is the gas constant, ΔH_{vap} is the enthalpy of vaporization of the monomer, and ΔH_{des} is the enthalpy of desorption of a monolayer of monomer from the substrate.

The enthalpy of vaporization, ΔH_{vap}, can be found experimentally using the Clausius-Clapeyron equation, which relates the boiling point and the vapor pressure at a fixed temperature of a gas-liquid system [20, 21]. Boiling points and vapor pressures for some monomers can be found in Afeefy *et al.* [22]. Intuitively one could predict that by using larger monomers, less of them will reside in the vapor phase under the same process pressure, compared to smaller monomers [10], i.e., ΔH_{vap} will be larger for larger monomers.

The enthalpy of desorption of a monolayer of monomer from the substrate is dependent not only on the monomer but also on the substrate [20]. It is, amongst others, dependent on the polarity or nonpolarity of the monomer combined with the non-hydrophobicity of the substrate. Desorption energies for some monomers used in iCVD are described by Alf *et al.* [23]. For example: when using GMA as a monomer and a clean crystalline silicon wafer, a value of 12 was calculated for c by Bakker [20].

It can be derived from formula (9.11) that at low p_M/p_{sat} ratios, the relation between p_M and monomer concentration becomes linear, following Henry's law [24, 25]. This is very useful, as it means that in this regime, the monomer surface concentration is directly proportional to p_M, as can be seen in the right side of Figure 9.7. Consequently, the deposition rate and molecular weight of the deposited polymer are directly proportional to p_M.

The BET equation can be rewritten in the more convenient form [20]:

$$\frac{V}{V_m} = \frac{cx}{(1-x)\cdot(1-x+cx)} \tag{9.13}$$

in which $x = p_M/p_{sat}$. Equation (9.13) is used to plot BET isotherms for different values of the BET constant c in Figure 9.8. The volume adsorbed, expressed in the number of monolayers, is plotted

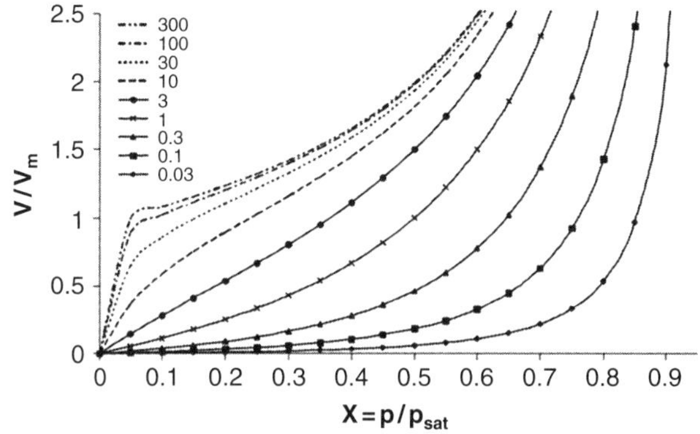

Figure 9.8 The number of monomer layers (V/V_m) plotted against x (p_M/p_{sat}). BET isotherms are shown for different values of the BET constant c [20]. Reprinted with permission from [20].

against x. Assuming that a volume of adsorbed monomers close to one monolayer is the ideal situation, since the amount of available monomers, i.e., $[M]$ in equations (9.9) and (9.10), is optimal and yet no liquid is formed on the surface, it can be seen in Figure 9.8 that a larger process window is available if the BET constant c is larger. Larger c values give a more flat isotherm around a V/V_m value of 1. In practice it is not necessary to avoid adsorption of more than one monolayer of monomer, however, the conformality of the deposition will, in this case, decrease [26].

It can be seen in Figure 9.8 that when p_M approaches p_{sat} ($x \rightarrow 1$), the monomer starts to condensate, meaning a liquid will form on the surface. This should be avoided for several reasons: Monomers that did not react can be trapped inside the growing polymer. When diffusing out afterwards they can cause a porous material, or even bubble-like cavities. Second, the conformality of the deposited polymer layer is highest when surface tension is absent in the process, meaning, when coating textured materials, one should avoid forming a liquid on the surface. This will be discussed in Section 9.3.2.

Summarizing, in general, when using iCVD it is beneficial to have adsorbed as many monomers on the substrate as possible, thereby increasing deposition rate as well as polymer chain length (the latter will improve material characteristics such as stability and glass transition temperature, addressed in Sections 9.5.2 and 9.5.3), as long as one avoids condensation of the monomer. There is one major exception: if extremely conformal coating is required, one should preferably have one monolayer of monomer or less adsorbed on the surface.

9.3 Coating by Initiated CVD

Using iCVD for the deposition of polymer layers, one does not need solvents like in solution-based polymerization, which leads to materials that are highly pure and stoichiometric. Many steps in the reaction mechanism take place separated in space, which means that they can be controlled independently, which gives a highly controllable processing. Also, since high energies are not required to activate the processes, all the functional groups of the monomers stay intact. In this way, many different functional coatings can be deposited very effectively on any kind of substrate, even on highly soluble plastics or soft tissue. By mixing different monomers the spectrum of possibilities even grows broader.

9.3.1 Thickness Control

An important aspect of iCVD is that the film thickness is highly controllable. Film thickness and deposition rate can be monitored *in situ* by laser reflection interferometry. By measuring the periodic interference of light waves reflected from the growing film surface and the film/substrate interface, and comparing the results with data collected using a second method, one can obtain a calibration that can be used to continuously monitor film growth. When using a transparent casing or viewports on the iCVD reactor, enabling real-time determination of film thickness, the deposition can be stopped once the desired thickness is deposited [27–29]. Typical iCVD growth rates are 10–100 nm/min and typical film thicknesses are between 100 and 1000 nm [8, 30].

9.3.2 Conformality

In applications where barrier coatings are needed, like electronics packaging or flat display or lighting panels, substrates are often textured (i.e., non-planar). In this case, protective coatings that are conformal to the geometry and features of the substrate are desirable [31, 32]. Since surface tension does not play a role in iCVD as it does in solution-based polymer processes, iCVD can be deposited extremely conformal. In Figure 9.9 high aspect ratio trenches coated by spin coating and iCVD can be seen, showing the high conformality of the iCVD deposited polymer layer compared to the spin coated layer.

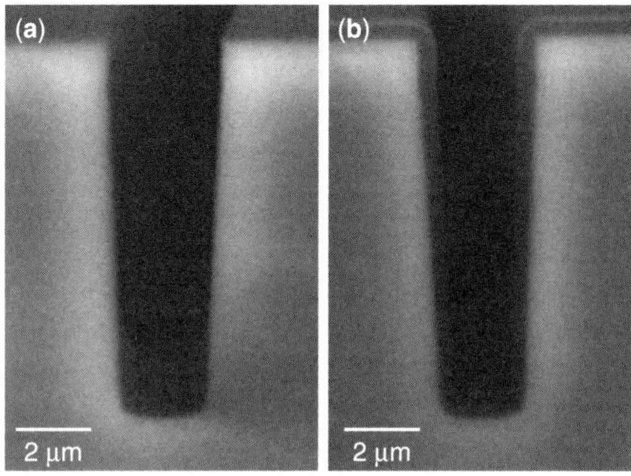

Figure 9.9 Trenches coated with polymeric films, by spin coating (a) and iCVD (b). Coating by iCVD yields more conformal films [33]. Reprinted with permission from [33]. Copyright 2008 Wiley-VCH Verlag GmbH & Co.

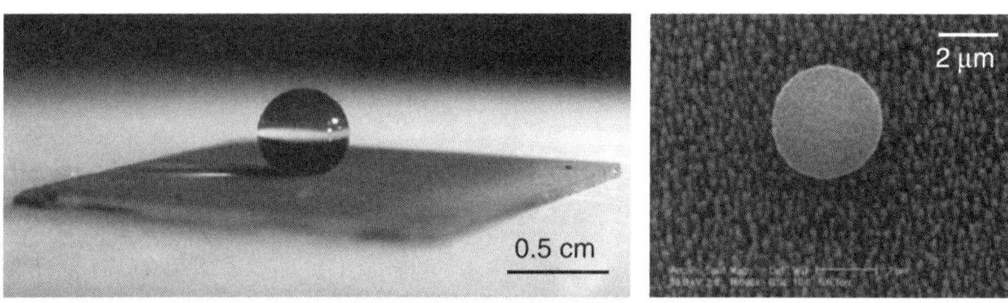

Figure 9.10 Superhydrophobic surface created by coating an array of multiwalled carbon nanotubes with a 40 nm thick coating of PTFE. Reprinted with permission from [35]. Copyright 2007 Elsevier.

It was shown by M. Gupta *et al.* that trenches with an aspect ratio of 80:1 (3 µm wide and 240 µm deep) can be conformally coated by iCVD [34]. The conformality is dependent on the sticking coefficient of the monomer to the surface, which in turn is dependent on the surface concentration of the monomer (the amount of adsorption): the higher the surface concentration of monomers, the higher are the chances are that a monomer sticks to the surface. This means that conformality is tunable by adjusting the fractional saturation p_M/p_{sat}. An excellent step coverage can be obtained at $p_M/p_{sat} = 0.1$ [26]. An example of extremely conformal coating is shown in Figure 9.10, where carbon nanotubes were coated with a 40 nm thick film of polytetrafluoroethylene (PTFE), resulting in a superhydrophobic material [35].

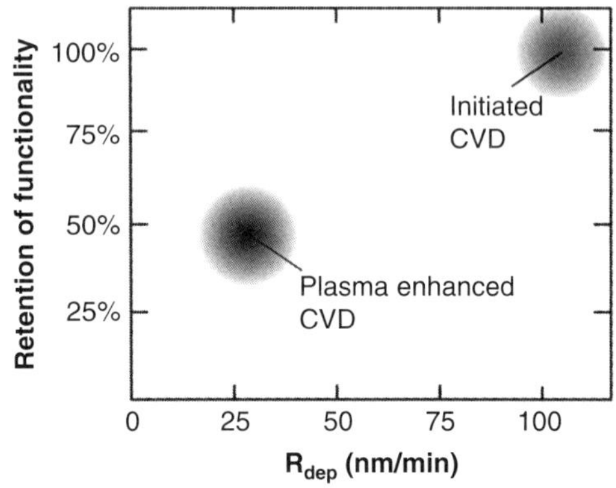

Figure 9.11 The functional group retention of polymers and possible deposition rates shown, for different polymer deposition techniques. Data from references [36] and [37] are used [8].

9.3.3 Retention of Functional Groups

No high temperatures are used in iCVD and since initiator dissociation is decoupled from the polymerization process, the molecular structure of the monomers is, except from the vinyl group, not changed in the polymerization process, even at high deposition rates. This makes iCVD, compared to other polymer deposition techniques like PECVD, an excellent method for depositing functionalized polymers, i.e., polymers containing functional groups. This is depicted in Figure 9.11.

For instance, the glycidyl methacrylate (GMA) monomer contains the reactive epoxide ring moiety (encircled in Figure 9.12), which will be retained during the iCVD deposition of poly(glycidyl methacrylate) (PGMA). Differently functional molecules can bind to the PGMA through a substitution ring opening reaction during post deposition chemistry. In this way particles were coated with fluorescent layers and, in another experiment, the refractive index of the coating could be adjusted from 1.5 up to 1.7 by adding thiophenol or 2-naphthalenethiol [8]. A refractive index adjustment can be very useful when iCVD layers are to be combined with inorganic materials in multilayers to reduce interference effects.

9.3.4 Tunable Properties by Combining Monomers

Deposition by iCVD has proven to be exceptionally versatile in growing different polymers. A few of them are shown in Figure 9.12, ordered after their function [38]. The main limiting factor in choosing

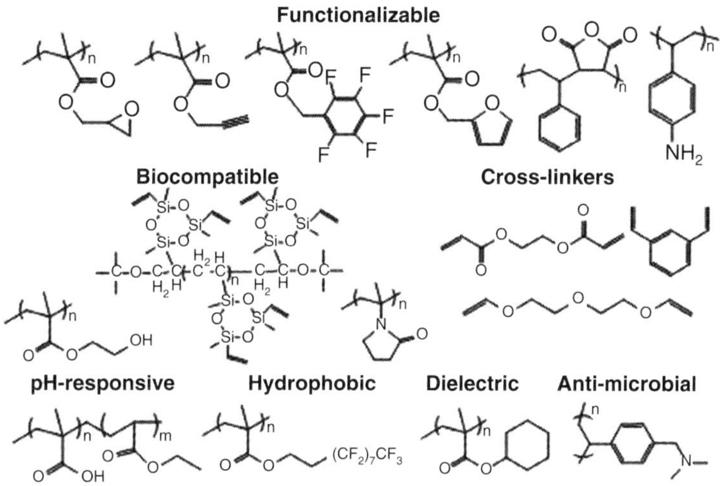

Figure 9.12 An overview of (a selection of) monomers that have so far been polymerized using iCVD. Encircled in the upper left corner is the reactive epoxide ring of PGMA. Reprinted with permission from [38]. Copyright 2010 Elsevier.

monomers is that they should have a high enough vapor pressure to be able to feed them into the reactor at a practical flow rate, generally excluding monomers with a very high molecular weight.

More than one monomer can be delivered into the reactor simultaneously, making the deposition of copolymers or terpolymers possible [39, 40]. For copolymerization, the control of surface concentration is required for two monomers simultaneously. This can practically be achieved when different monomers have a similar P_{sat} [23]. Recently, various combinations of monomers, for instance methacrylic acid and ethyl acrylate [41], have been shown to produce random copolymer layers [33]. Incorporating monomers with two or more vinyl groups in copolymerization presents the opportunity to deposit highly crosslinked films, increasing stability, i.e., structural integrity, and mechanical properties [42]. Varying the relative delivery rates of the monomers throughout the process makes it possible to deposit layers with gradient chemistries.

9.3.5 Barrier Coating by a Single Organic Layer

Thin polymer coatings are used in many industries as barrier layers to protect, for instance, metals from corrosion and electronics against moisture. Using iCVD, such barriers can be deposited extremely conformal and accurately. This was shown by Parker *et al.* [43], by coating 355 μm NaCl particles with metallic coatings with PGMA, thereby slowing down their dissolution rate in water by two orders of magnitude. However, the intrinsic barrier function of any polymer does not reach the level that is needed for coating, for instance, an OLED, as is shown in Figure 9.2.

By increasing the amount of crosslinking in polymer structure the mechanical properties like hardness and barrier function can be enhanced and brought closer to that of inorganic materials. J. Xu *et al.* [44] utilized the monomers 4-aminostyrene (4-AS) and maleic anhydride (Ma), depositing an alternating copolymer PASMa by iCVD. After annealing, an extremely high crosslinked polymer was obtained with high mechanical hardness and barrier properties, while retaining flexibility. Coating a 25 μm PDMS membrane with a 200 nm PASMa layer reduces the oxygen permeability by 7 orders of magnitude.

9.4 Advantages of iCVD in Hybrid Multilayer Gas Barriers

Given the high intrinsic permeability of common polymers, for ultra-high barriers one needs inorganic layers. Transparent materials, known to be good barrier materials, are metal (including silicon) oxides, nitrides, and oxynitrides (Al_2O_3, Si_3N_4, and SiO_2 are often used). Although the barrier performance of such materials increases with thickness initially, after a certain critical thickness there is no significant gain [45, 46], which is shown in Figure 9.13. This is due to substrate- and process-induced macro defects, such as pinholes or cracks, propagating through the entire layer [47].

To circumvent this problem a stack of alternating thin inorganic layers and organic interlayers is often used to create a structure, as shown in Figure 9.2. The organic layers in hybrid organic/inorganic multilayers are thought to have a positive effect on the multilayer barrier performance in three different ways: first of all, they decouple macro defects in consecutive organic layers and when they are thin enough, a tortuous path is created for the permeating species. Second, the polymer is thought to fill pores (defects of nanoscale size) in the inorganic layers, which reduced the permeation through these pores. Third, the organic layers smoothen the substrate, reducing defects in the inorganic layer that are induced by dust particles, or other features on the substrate.

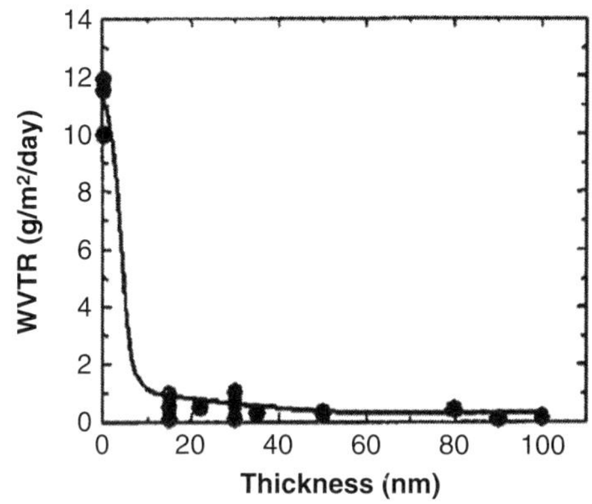

Figure 9.13 After a certain critical thickness, there is no significant gain in barrier performance of a single layer of inorganic material; here PECVD deposited silicon nitride [46]. Reprinted with permission from [46]. Copyright 2004 American Vacuum Society.

9.4.1 Using Thin Layers for Decoupling

Since the increase in barrier performance of a single layer of inorganic material saturates after a critical thickness, due to macro defects, defect decoupling interlayers are needed to create an ultra-high barrier material. The state-of-the-art solution is an alternated organic/inorganic layer stack [48]. This µm thick material known as Barix™, has shown moisture permeation rates as low as $<10^{-5}$ g/m^2/day. Graff *et al.* [49] concluded that the good performance of such a multilayer can be ascribed to the tortuous path that permeating molecules must follow through the organic layer from pinhole to pinhole in consecutive inorganic layers. The tortuous path is dependent on the organic interlayer thickness [50]. As soon as the interlayer thickness becomes less than the average lateral distance between defects in consecutive inorganic layers, one enters a regime in which the diffusion of permeating molecules becomes non-Fickian and is slowed down significantly [46]. This is shown in Figure 9.14.

Thus, since one should preferably use thin and conformal organic interlayers, iCVD is a very well-suited method to deposit these layers. It allows for the conformal deposition of films with nanoscale thicknesses with macroscale uniformity [46], and the thickness is highly controllable [29].

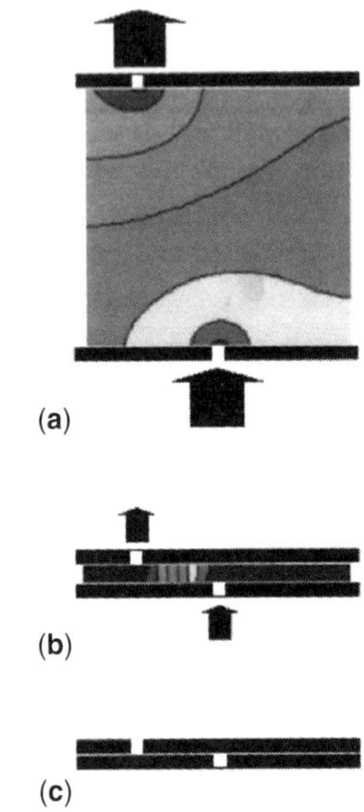

Figure 9.14 For permeation through a multilayer system the ratio of lateral distance between defects in consecutive layers and interlayer thickness is important. When the latter is smaller (b) the diffusion rate will be significantly lower. Ultimately, decoupling defects without an interlayer (c) results in a hermetically closed multilayer[46]. Reprinted with permission from [46]. Copyright 2004 American Vacuum Society.

9.4.2 Filling of Defects by Polymer

It was pointed out by Affinito and Hilliard [51] that in addition to permeation through macro defects, permeation through nanoscale defects comparable to the size of the permeating molecules in the inorganic material matrix plays an important role in permeation barriers. Permeation through such defects was confirmed by Roberts *et al.* [52] when modeling permeation through a single barrier layer on a polymer substrate. The organic interlayer is thought to enhance barrier performance of a multilayer by filling of such nanopores [51]. The ability of iCVD to conformally coat high aspect ratio pores makes the technique extremely useful for this purpose. This was shown by Aresta *et al.* [53], who deposited interlayers of trimethyl-trivinyl-cyclotrisiloxane (V_3D_3) by iCVD on top of PECVD deposited SiO_x-like inorganic barrier layers, which is depicted in Figure 9.15.

Their measurements point out the infiltration of monomer into the nano-defects and filling of them in the iCVD polymerization process.

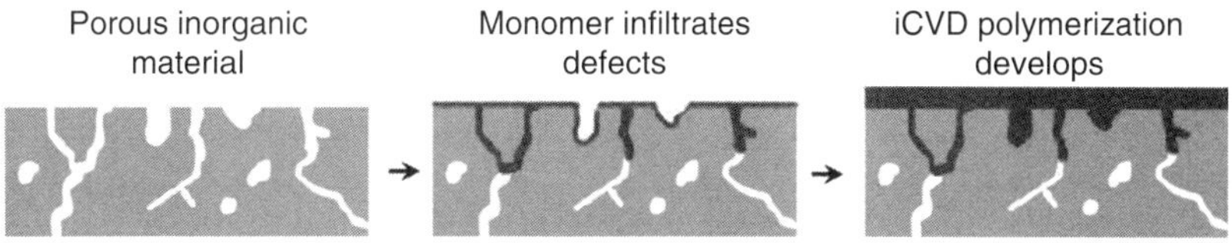

Figure 9.15 Schematic representation of the filling of nano pores in the inorganic material by polymer during the iCVD process.

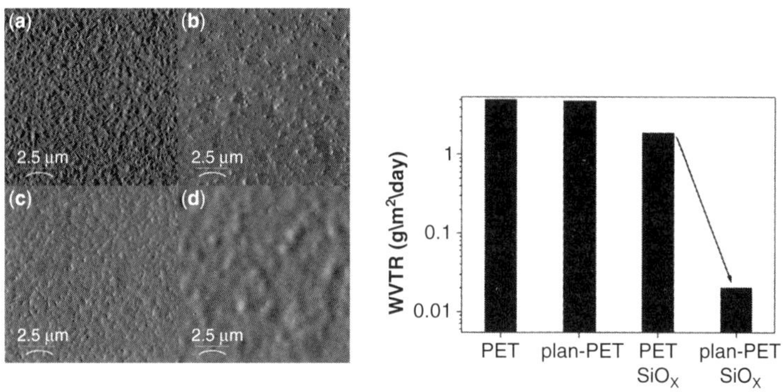

Figure 9.16 By applying a PGMA planarizing layer the surface rms roughness of a rough substrate can be decreased from 42.3 nm to 14.3 nm using a layer of only 335 nm thickness (left). Comparison of the WVTR of a bare PET substrate, a planarized PET substrate, a SiO_x coated PET substrate and a SiO_x coated planarized PET substrate (right) [55,56]. Reprinted with permission from [55]. Copyright 2012 American Institute of Physics. Reprinted with permission from [56]. Copyright 2007 Elsevier.

Additionally, in these studies the hypothesis of Affinito and Hilliard about the microstructure of the inorganic layer was confirmed.

9.4.3 Smoothening of the Substrate

The high surface roughness of commercially available plastic substrates induces many macroscale defects in deposited inorganic layers [54]. A third way in which organic layers are thought to enhance barrier performance in hybrid multilayer barrier is by smoothening of the layer or substrate underneath, avoiding a high amount of defects [46, 51]. That iCVD deposited layers are suitable for this was shown by Coclite and Gleason [55] by comparing a PET substrate with a 20-nm SiO_x layer, with and without applying a planarizing, 1-μm thick, iCVD deposited polymer layer first. The planarizing layer improves the barrier function by two orders of magnitude (Figure 9.16, right).

Bakker *et al.* [56] demonstrated that even thin iCVD layers of PGMA (of only 300 nm) are good planarizing layers by coating a textured Asahi U-type TCO substrate. Their results and those of Coclite and Gleason are shown in Figure 9.16. By applying a 335 nm PGMA layer, the *rms* surface rougness of the Asahi U-type TCO substrate was decreased from 42.3 nm to 14.3 nm [56].

9.5 Specific Requirements for the Use in Hybrid Multilayers

To be able to use iCVD polymer layers as inter-layers between typical inorganic layers like Si_3N_4, SiO_2 or Al_2O_3 they should exhibit certain properties. They should be very stable since the inorganic layers are usually deposited in PECVD, HWCD, or sputtering processes that involve (aggressive) highly reactive radicals, ion bombardment, and/or high temperatures. Furthermore, they should be planarizing to decouple the defects, and have a high glass transition temperature to facilitate controlled deposition of the high quality inorganic layers. The adhesion between inorganic and organic layers should be excellent to enable practical use in flexible devices.

9.5.1 Planarization

For use as a decoupling layer, the deposited layers should be, on the one hand, conformal to fill up pores in the underlying substrate and cover defect-inducing features tightly, while simultaneously being planarizing. This can conveniently be combined, since on the one hand planarization increases with the thickness of the layer, even at small thicknesses [56], and conformality is tunable by adjusting the fractional saturation p_M/p_{sat} of the monomer during the deposition [34]. Another aspect is the intrinsic smoothness of the polymer layers. In iCVD this is dependent on the amount of radicals available at the surface to start polymerization, i.e., the amount of nucleation sites [16]. This amount in turn is dependent on both filament temperature and monomer/initiator flow ratio. The effect of the filament temperature is shown in Figure 9.17. To avoid a coarse morphology and deposit smooth layers, a sufficient amount of radicals should be available [16].

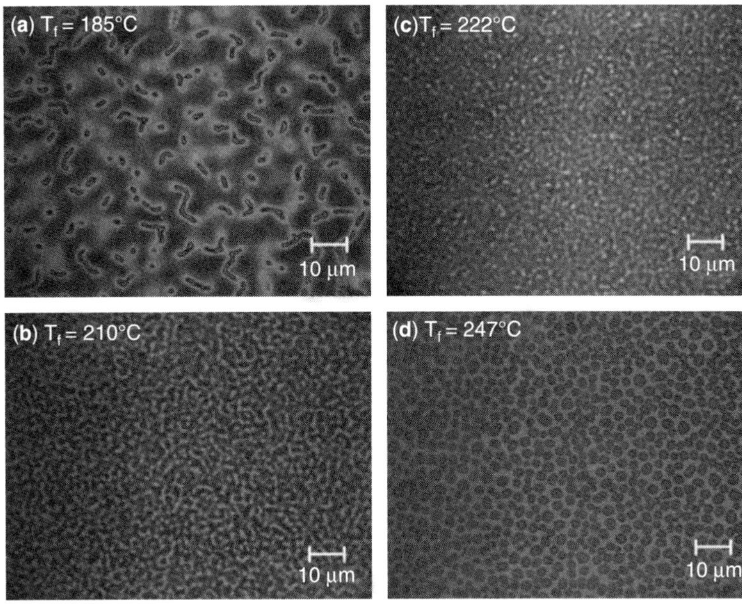

Figure 9.17 In a regime with relatively few radicals, the intrinsic smoothness of iCVD deposited layers is dependent on the amount of radicals available to start polymerization on the surface. This in turn is dependent on the filament temperature, T_f, when using low temperatures[16]. Smoothness increases from a to d with increasing filament temperature. Reprinted with permission from [16]. Copyright 2004 American Chemical Society.

9.5.2 Stability

During the deposition of inorganic layers by sputtering, PECVD, or HWCVD on top of polymers, generally elevated substrate temperatures are involved and highly reactive species like atomic hydrogen are present, which can easily degrade the polymer [57, 58]. Therefore, it is important to deposit polymer materials with a high (temperature) stability. A strong indication that the temperature stability of iCVD polymer layers depends on their molecular weight was found by Bakker *et al.* [56]. Their data, shown in Figure 9.18, reveals that degradation of polymer layers progresses in two steps. This is consistent with the data found earlier by Lee and Park [59].

The first step in material reduction is ascribed to depolymerization initiated by unsaturated chain ends [60, 61]. The second step, at higher temperatures, is ascribed to random chain scissions. If chains are, on average, larger, the amount of unsaturated chain

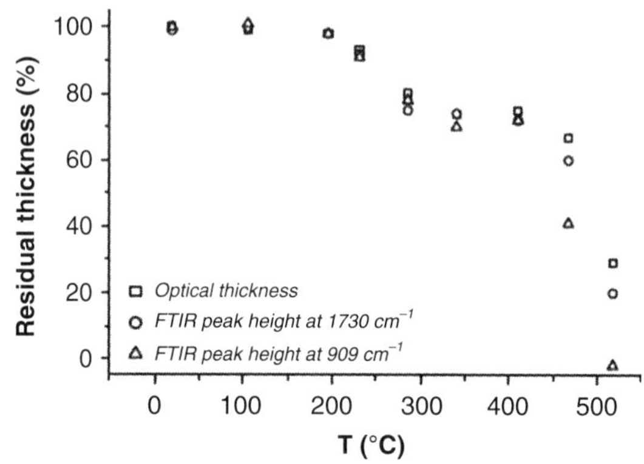

Figure 9.18 Relative optical thickness and FTIR absorption of PGMA layers after 4 hours of annealing in vacuum at different temperatures [56]. Reprinted with permission from [56].

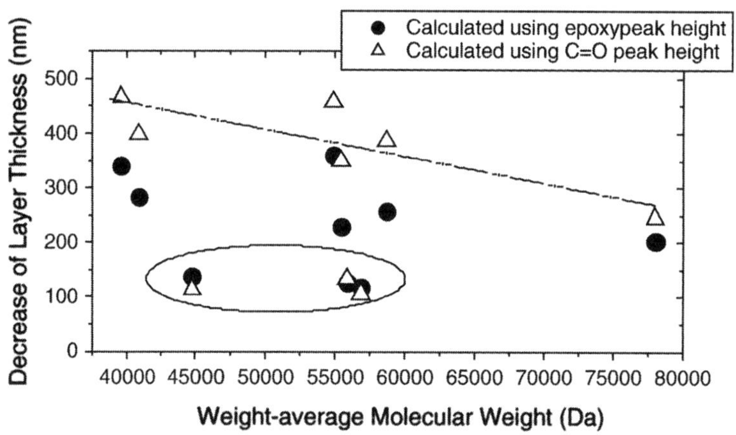

Figure 9.19 Thickness decrease after 550 s of H-treatment, calculated using the FTIR epoxy peak and C=O peak height, as a function of molecular weight, M_W. Samples made at a filament temperature of 220°C are encircled. Other samples were made at a filament temperature of 250°C [62]. Reprinted with permission from [62]. Copyright 2011 Elsevier.

ends will be relatively lower, making the material more stable. In an experiment in which PGMA layers were degraded in an atomic hydrogen environment, mimicking the deposition conditions of silicon nitride, it was found by Spee *et al.* [62] that, in addition to polymer chain length, the filament temperature used during the iCVD deposition is an important factor determining the stability of the polymer. Their data are shown in Figure 9.19. A reduced stability is found when filament temperatures above 220°C are used during deposition. This can be explained by gas phase reactions of the monomers occurring at high temperatures, causing defects in the polymer layer.

9.5.3 High Glass Transition Temperature

To be able to deposit smooth, defect free inorganic layers on the polymer, the glass transition temperature (T_g) of the polymer should not be exceeded. If it is exceeded, the material is easily deformed. A typical example of such deformation is shown in Figure 9.20.

For this reason, the T_g of the polymer should preferably be high. Although T_g in general is not a discrete value, as depicted in Figure 9.20, it is hard to ascribe an exact T_g to most polymers. Intuitively, it is easy to see that the transition from a crystalline into a glassy state is dependent on the ease of movement of the polymer chains relative to each other [63].

The glass transition temperature T_g increases with increasing polymer chain length. Also, the stiffness of the polymer backbones influences T_g. The third factor, the amount of crosslinking, is probably the most important factor determining T_g. In a branched polymer, an example of which is schematically shown in Figure 9.21, there is hardly any movement possible, making T_g high. Where T_g can be around 80°C for a material consisting of linear chains without crosslinking, such as PGMA, it can be above 120°C for a branched polymer such as V_3D_3.

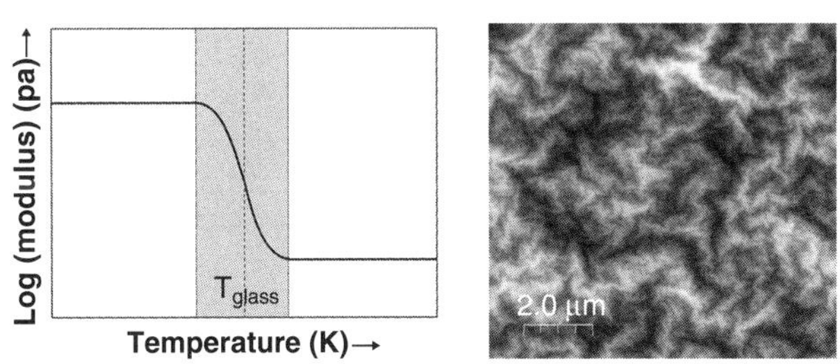

Figure 9.20 Although the glass transition temperature T_g is often given as a specific value, the stiffness of the material changes gradually. The modulus can decrease by a factor 10^3. On the right an atomic force micrograph of a 50 nm SiN_x layer on top of a 300 nm PGMA layer of which the T_g was slightly exceeded during the deposition is shown. The material will return to its initial state after the temperature drops again, but it is easily deformed during the process.

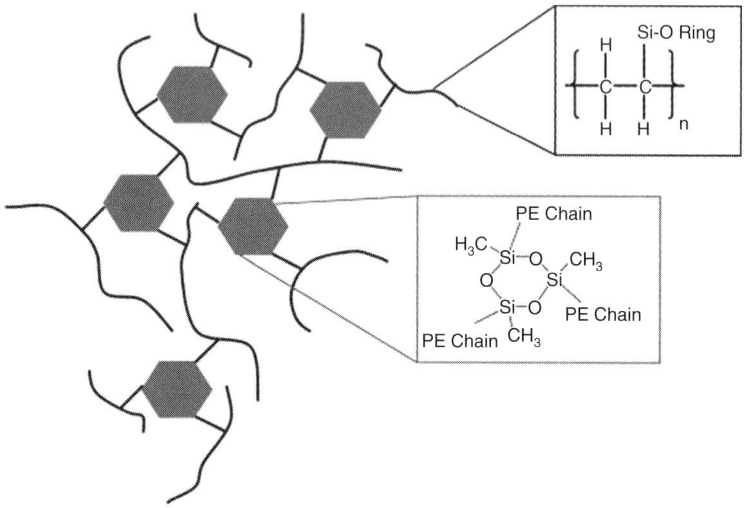

Figure 9.21 Schematic representation of the V_3D_3 polymer matrix. The intact siloxane rings act as cross linkers for multiple carbon backbones. The high degree af crosslinking increases the glass transition temperature [18]. Reprinted with permission from [18]. Copyright 2006 American Chemical Society.

When using thin layers, as is often the case using iCVD, the thickness of the layer and the underlying substrate also affect the T_g. If there is a high interfacial energy, a thin polymer layer will have a T_g higher than its bulk value. If, on the other hand, the interfacial energy is low, the T_g will decrease compared to the bulk material [64].

9.5.4 Adhesion

When the polymer layer is to be integrated into a device it is important to have high interfacial adhesion. Adhesion can be promoted by chemically activating the substrate. For organic substrates this can, for example, be done using a plasma glow discharge, and for inorganic substrates by using a piranha solution or an oxygen plasma treatment. The former method generates free radical species on the substrate, able to initiate polymerization with gas phase monomers [65]. The latter two methods create a high density of hydroxyl groups at the surface [66, 67].

However, since barrier layers are often applied on sensitive substrates or devices, methods like this cannot always be used. Another option is to use monomers with groups that can physically (or even chemically) attach to neighboring layers. The earlier

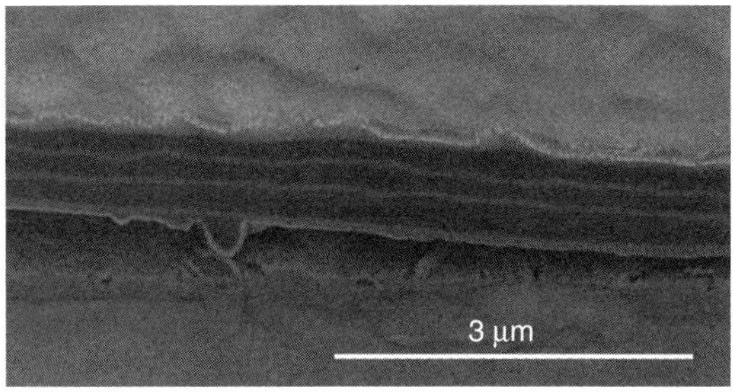

Figure 9.22 Cross sectional SEM picture of a PGMA/silicon nitride layer, which is detached from its substrate. It can be seen that the excellent adhesion between different interlayer causes the multilayer to retain its structural integrity even when it is free standing.

mentioned epoxide ring in the GMA monomer can be used for this. In Figure 9.22 a PGMA/silicon nitride multilayer being detached from its substrate is shown. The excellent adhesion between layers, due to the use of PGMA for the organic interlayers, makes the structural integrity of the free-standing multilayer very high.

Even another strategy is to entirely avoid a sharp organic/inorganic interface, thereby circumventing adhesion challenges. An example of this is shown in the next section.

9.6 Multilayer Gas Barriers Containing Polymers by iCVD

Although extensive research has been done on iCVD for use in hybrid organic/inorganic multilayers on subjects such as substrate planarization [56], nanopore filling [53] and stability [62], not many actual multilayer gas barriers containing iCVD interlayers have been made. In this section two kinds of multilayer barriers are addressed: one graded multilayer, combining PECVD with iCVD using only one precursor; and one multilayer, combining HWCVD SiN_x with iCVD.

9.6.1 Polymers by iCVD with PECVD Inorganics

The multilayer gas barrier described in this section was deposited by the MIT group of Prof. Gleason [68]. Since good barrier performances had been achieved before by graded organic/inorganic hybrid materials deposited by PECVD [69], this strategy was used to overcome the problem of poor adhesion between the organic and the inorganic material. A graded interface is naturally produced by PECVD deposition of the inorganic material, due to the ion bombardment and subsequent chemical reactions with the organic layer underneath. For both types of layers the same precursor was used: hexavinyldisiloxane (HVDSO). When depositing the polymer of HVDSO by iCVD, a smooth, and flexible polymer layer is deposited, which adheres to the underlying substrate, has a high degree of crosslinking and a high carbon content [70]. PECVD deposition using the same precursor results in a dense, C-depleted, SiO_x-like material. This is probably due to the ion bombardment and precursor fragmentation: since the vinyl groups of the monomer are labile they are easily cleaved off during the discharge. PECVD and iCVD were done in the same chamber, and since a single monomer was used for both materials there was no need to break the vacuum. This offers the possibility to produce high quality interfaces and good adhesion through the entire multilayer.

The formation of 60-70 nm thick graded interface was observed when depositing the plasma layers over the iCVD ones. A SEM cross section of a hexalayer, consisting of three organic/inorganic dyads is shown in Figure 9.23. WVTR of single as well as multilayer coatings was tested. Single 100-nm C-depleted (i.e., SiO_x-like) layers showed

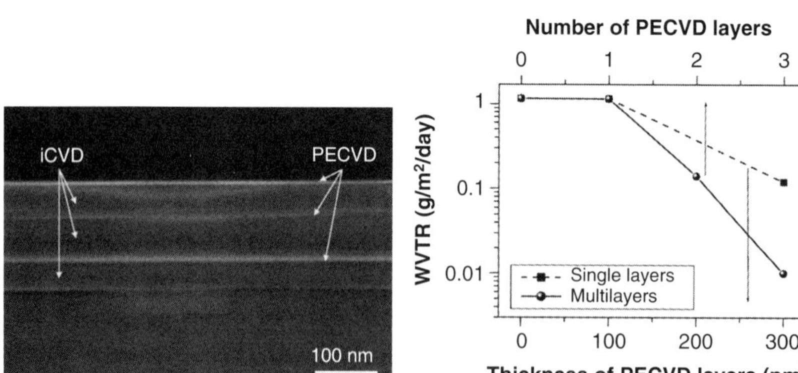

Figure 9.23 On the left a SEM cross sectional micrograph of a hexalayer, consisting of three SiO_x-like/$SiO_xC_yH_z$ dyads, made by PECVD and iCVD respectively of one precursor. On the right the WVTR of barrier films as a function of the number of C-depleted layers in the multilayer [68]. Reprinted with permission from [68]. Copyright 2010 Wiley-VCH Verlag GmbH & Co.

poor barrier properties, but when combined with iCVD deposited C-rich material, lower transmission rates were achieved. The WVTR as a function of number of PECVD layers is shown in Figure 9.23.

For a PET substrate coated with a hexalayer, the WVTR was found to be 10^{-2} g/m^2/day, an improvement in barrier function of two orders of magnitude over a single C-depleted layer. This good barrier performance of the multilayer is ascribed to the effective defect decoupling and smoothening properties of the C-rich layer.

9.6.2 iCVD Polymer and HWCVD SiN_x

Spee *et al.* [71] combined low temperature SiN_x layers deposited by HWCVD with iCVD deposited PGMA interlayers. One of the main reasons PGMA was chosen as interlayer material is the good adhesion, due to the reactive epoxide ring. For the deposition of the SiN_x layers, a dedicated low temperature HWCVD assembly was used, ensuring that temperatures never exceeded 100°C [72]. In Figure 9.24 there is a comparison of the WVTR results for 100 nm low temperature SiN_x, 100 nm state-of-the-art SiN_x and a multilayer consisting of two 100 nm low temperature SiN_x, sandwiching a PGMA layer. The use of iCVD allows for a PGMA interlayer of only 200 nm thick, which is very effective in decoupling defects in consecutive SiN_x layers. The WVTR rates were determined using a calcium degradation test [73]. It is clear that the barrier performance

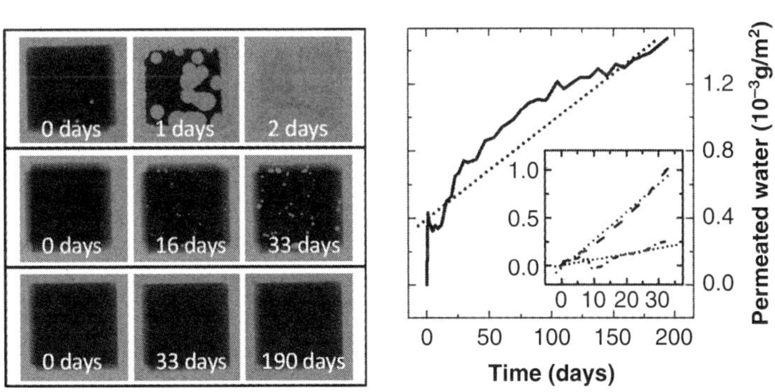

Figure 9.24 The development in time of Ca squares covered by 100 nm low T SiN_x (top), 100 nm state-of-the-art SiN_x (middle) and a low temperature multilayer on the left. On the right, the graph of permeating moisture through the three-layer structure. The inset shows permeation through the state-of-the-art SiN_x, including and without pinholes, for comparison [71]. Reprinted with permission form [71]. Copyright 2012 Wiley-VCH Verlag GmbH & Co.

of a single layer of low temperature SiN_x is poor, due to a high pinhole density. In combination with the iCVD interlayer, however, a simple three-layer structure was created, which has a WVTR rate as low as 5×10^{-6} $g/m^2/day$ and is pinhole free. Since the WVTR was determined using accelerated conditions of 60°C and a relative humidity of 90%, this value is low enough for any sensitive electronic device. Also shown in Figure 9.24 is the moisture permeation graph of this multilayer. The fact that permeation flattens over time indicates that the high barrier function is a consequence of a low equilibrium permeation rate rather than a high lag time of the water vapor [49].

The experiment shows that the structure is tolerant with respect to defects created in the process and originating from the substrate. It was difficult to avoid contamination with defect-inducing dust particles, since samples had to be moved in ambient between separated reactor chambers. Although in practical production this problem is circumvented, since transport will then take place in vacuum, an experiment was done using the same concept to examine the yield increase as a function of number of inorganic layers [74]. The total cumulative thickness of SiN_x layers was kept constant in the experiment: multilayers containing two 100 nm SiN_x layers, three 67 nm SiN_x layers and four 50 nm SiN_x layers, all separated by 200 nm PGMA layers, were examined. The results are shown, together with a SEM cross sectional micrograph of the multilayer containing four 50 nm SiN_x layers, in Figure 9.25. The yield of the samples, i.e., the fraction of undamaged samples, measured over 36 samples,

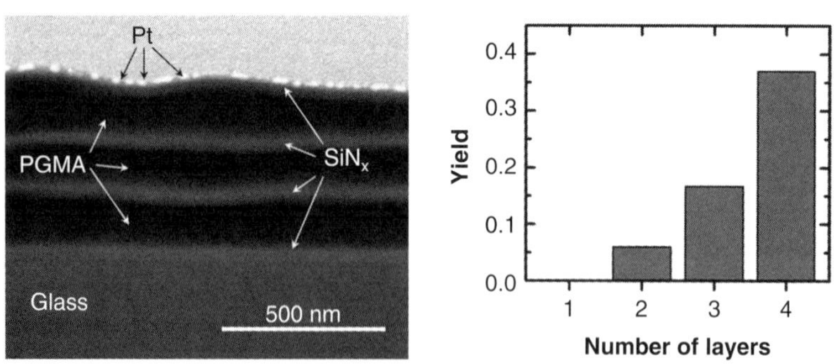

Figure 9.25 A SEM micrograph of a multilayer containing four 50 nm SiN_x layers (left) and the yield, which is affected by defect creating dust particles, as a function of number of SiN_x layers (right)[74]. Reprinted with permission from [74]. Copyright 2012 Cambridge University Press.

increases with the number of SiN_x layers, on the one hand because the tortuous path effect increases, on the other hand because the total PGMA thickness increases, better covering large dust particles.

9.7 Upscaling and Utilization

In the preceding sections the excellent gas barrier properties of multilayers utilizing polymer layers by iCVD were discussed. To make the iCVD deposition process and application of such devices commercially feasible upscaling is needed.

9.7.1 Roll-to-Roll and Inline Processing

Commercially it is generally desirable to enable automation, improving reproducibility, and increasing process throughput by scaling up reactors [76, 77]. Furthermore roll-to-roll production of thin films is desirable for further cost reduction. iCVD is a low temperature process, devoid of ion bombardment, and is compatible with almost any substrate, including cheap flexible materials like PET and PEN foils, which can be used in roll-to-roll processes. Moreover, iCVD is a vacuum technique, making it compatible with other vacuum processes like PECVD and HWCVD, as discussed in Section 9.6. Since the filaments provide a linear source of radicals, an iCVD deposition will be homogeneous in two dimensions when the substrate is moved perpendicular to the wires, allowing convenient implementation in roll-to-roll and inline processes [78]. A schematic representation of such a system is shown in Figure 9.26.

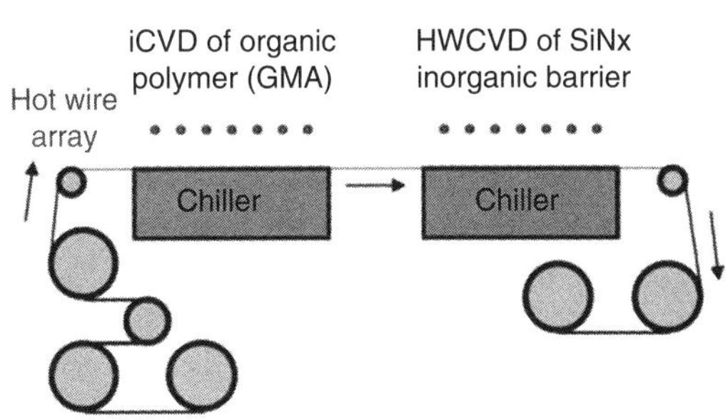

Figure 9.26 Schematic representation of an inline deposition system for multilayers. The number of deposition chambers can be increased without changing the concept.

The most critical issues affecting commercial reactors are film growth rate and the effective utilization of expensive precursors [23]. In reducing the average cost per coated area by increasing growth rate, even a tradeoff in barrier performance can sometimes be acceptable [76].

Appropriate dimensionless analysis of the convective and diffusive fluxes in both small and large reactor can ensure that process conditions can be translated between systems of different size scales [79, 80].

A roll-to-roll iCVD reactor was demonstrated by Gupta and Gleason [81]. The 30-cm wide substrate was moved through a 30 cm × 30 cm deposition zone, resulting in a coating with uniform thickness. Growth rates were observed to be the same as on a stationary substrate.

9.7.2 Commercial Availability

Although iCVD is a relatively new technique, iCVD deposited coatings are now becoming commercially available.

In 2001 GVD Corporation was established, a company specializing in iCVD coatings. It focused on commercial development of infusible, insoluble polymer coatings such as polytetrafluoroethylene (PTFE or Teflon®), and has scaled up production of its coatings from a 25-cm diameter R&D-scale reactor to a 100 cm × 50 cm commercial coating tool in 2006 [82]. In addition to this large size batch system, different standard reactors were developed, ranging form small R&D-sized systems to roll-to-roll coating systems. These are shown in Figure 9.27. Besides being used as separate

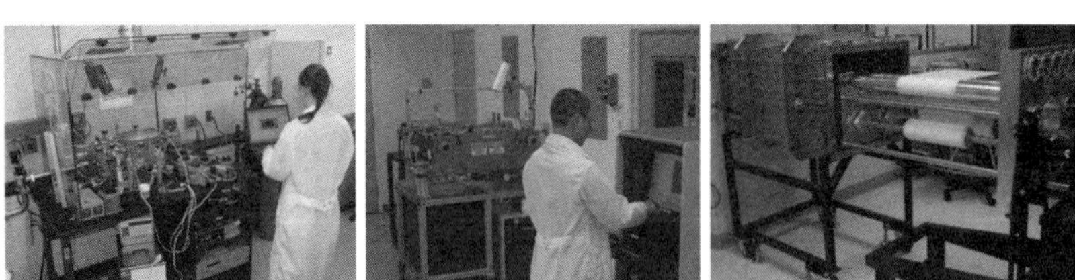

Figure 9.27 GVD Corporation (US) has developed a number of standard iCVD coating systems. From left to right: a small R&D coating system (with 15 cm coating area), a mid-sized production batch coater (50 × 75 cm coating area), and a roll-to-roll web coating system (75 cm in width) [81]. Reprinted with permission from [81]. Copyright 2009 Elsevier.

system, reactors like these can easily be implemented in larger or even existing production lines.

References

1. K. Shibuki, M. Yagi, K. Saijo, and S. Takatsu. *Surface & Coatings Technology* 36 (1988) p. 295.
2. R.E.I. Schropp, K.F. Feenstra, E.C. Molenbroek, H. Meiling, and J.K. Rath. *Phil. Mag. B* 76 (1997) p. 309.
3. H. Matsumura. *Japanese Journal of Applied Physics* 28 (1989) p. 2157.
4. H. Matsumura, Japanese Journal of Applied Physics 30 (1991) p. 1522.
5. N. Setaka, S. Matsumoto, and M. Kamo. *Journal of the Japan Society of Powder and Powder Metallurgy* 34 (1987) p. 395.
6. N. Kikuchi, T. Komatsu, and H. Yoshimura. *Materials Science and Engineering* 105–106 (1988) p. 525.
7. H.G. Pryce Lewis, J.A. Caulfield, K.K. Gleason. *Langmuir* 17 (2001) p. 7652.
8. S.H. Baxamusa, S.G. Im, and K.K. Gleason. *Phys. Chem. Chem. Phys.* 11 (2009) p. 5227.
9. M. Schaepkens, T.-W. Kim, A. Gün Erlat, M. Yan, K.W. Flanagan, C.M. Heller, and P.A. McConnelee. *J. Vac. Sci. Technol. A* 22.4 (2004) p. 1716.
10. K.K.S. Lau, and K.K. Gleason. *Macromolecules* 39 (2006) p. 3688.
11. K.K.S. Lau, and K.K. Gleason. *Macromolecules* 39 (2006) p. 3695.
12. G. Odian. *Principles of polymerization*. 4th ed. John Wiley and Sons, Hoboken NJ (2004).
13. J. Xu, K.K. Gleason. *Appl. Mater. Interfaces* 3 (2011) p. 2410.
14. K. Chan, K.K. Gleason. *Chem. Vap. Deposition* 11 (2005) p. 437.
15. R. Bakker, V. Verlaan, A.D. Verkerk, C.H.M. van der Werf, L. van Dijk, H. Rudolph, J.K. Rath, R.E.I. Schropp. *Thin Solid Films* 517 (2009) p. 3555.
16. Y. Mao, K.K. Gleason. *Langmuir* 20 (2004) p. 2484.
17. K. Chan, K.K. Gleason. *Macromolecules* 39 (2006) p. 3890.
18. W.S. O'Shaughnessy, M. Gao, and K.K. Gleason. *Langmuir* 22 (2006) p. 7021.
19. S. Brunauer, P.H. Emmett, and E. Teller. *Journal of the American Chemical Society* 60 (1938) p. 309.
20. R. Bakker. PhD thesis, Utrecht University (2010) p. 26.
21. D.A. McQuarrie, and J.D. Simon. *Physical chemistry – a molecular approach*. University Science Books, Sausalito CA (1997).
22. H.J. Afeefy, J.F. Liebman, S.E. Stein. Neutral thermochemical data. In *NIST Chemistry WebBook*. NIST Standard Reference Database Number 69, edited by P.J. Lindstrom and W. G. Mallard (National Institute of Standards and Technology) Gaithersburg, MD, (2005), http://webbook.nist.gov.
23. M.E. Alf, A. Asatekin, M.C. Barr, S.H. Baxamusa, H. Chelawat, G. Ozaydin-Ince, C.D. Petruczok, R. Sreenavasan, W.E. Tenhaeff, N.J. Trujillo, S. Vaddiraju, J. Xu and K.K. Gleason. *Adv. Mater.* 22 (2010) p. 1993.
24. W.F. Beach. *Macromolecules* 11 (1978) p. 72.
25. P.J. Flory. *Principles of polymer chemistry*. Cornell University Press, Ithaca NY (1953) p. 514.

26. S.H. Baxamusa, K.K. Gleason. *Chem. Vap. Deposition* 14 (2008) p. 313.
27. G.H. Chen, M. Gupta, K. Chan, K.K.Gleason. *Macromol. Rapid Commun.* 28 (2007) p. 1877.
28. X. Chen, M. Anthamatten, and D.R. Harding. *Polymer* 49 (2008) p. 1823.
29. G.H. Chen, K.K.S. Lau, and K.K. Gleason. *Thin Solid Films* 517 (2009) p. 3539.
30. T.P. Martin, K.K.S. Lau, K. Chan, Y. Mao, M. Gupta, W.S. O'Shaughnessy, and K.K. Gleason. *Surf. Coat. Technol.* 201 (2007) p. 9400.
31. N. Binh-Khiem, K. Matsumoto, and I. Shimoyama. *Appl. Phys. Lett.* 93 (2008) page?
32. D. Cheyns, K. Vasseur, C. Rollins, J. Genoe, J. Poortmans, and P.Heremans. *Nanotechnology* 19 (2008) page?
33. W.E. Tenhaeff, and K.K. Gleason. *Adv. Funct. Mater.* 18 (2008) p. 979.
34. M. Gupta, V. Kapur, N.M. Pinkerton, and K.K. Gleason. *Chem. Mater.* 20 (2008) p. 1646.
35. K.K.S. Lau, and K.K. Gleason. *Surface & Coatings Technology* 201 (2007) p. 9189.
36. K. Chan, and K.K. Gleason. *Langmuir* 21 (2005) p. 8930.
37. C. Tarducci, W.C.E. Schofield, J.P.S. Badyal, S.A. Brewer, and C. Willis. *Chem Mater.* 14 (2002) p. 2541.
38. A. Asatekin, M.C. Barr, S.H. Baxamusa, K.K.S Lau, W. Tenhaeff, J. Xu, and K.K. Gleason. *Materials Today* 13 (2010) p. 26.
39. Y. Mao, and K.K. Gleason. *Langmuir* 22 (2006) p. 1795.
40. W.E. Tenhaeff, and K.K. Gleason. *Chemistry of Materials* 21 (2009) p. 4323.
41. K.K.S. Lau, K.K. Gleason. *Macromol. Biosc.* 7 (2007) p. 429.
42. K. Chan, L.E. Kostun, W.E. Tenhaeff, K.K. Gleason. *Polymer* 47 (2006) p. 6914.
43. T.C. Parker, D. Baechle, and J.D. Demaree. *Surface & Coatings Technology* 206 (2011) p. 1680.
44. J. Xu, A. Asatekin, and K.K. Gleason. *Adv. Mater.* 24 (2012) p. 3692.
45. H. Chatman. *Surface & Coatings Technology* 78 (1996) p. 1.
46. M. Schaepkens, T.W. Kim, A.G. Erlat, M. Yan, K.W. Flanagan, C.M. Heller, and P.A. McConnelee. *J. Vac. Sci. Technol. A* 22 (2004) p. 1716.
47. A.S. da Silva Sobrinho, M. Latreche, G. Czeremuszkin, J.E. Klemberg-Sapieha, and M.R. Wertheimer. *J. Vac. Sci. Technol. A* 16 (1998) p. 3190.
48. P.E. Burrows, G.L. Graff, M.E. Gross, P.M. Martin, M.K. Shi, M. Hall, E. Mast, C. Bonham, W. Bennet, and M.B. Sullivan. *Displays* 22 (2001) p. 65
49. G.L. Graff, R.E. Williford, and P.E. Burrows. *Journal of Applied Physics* 96 (2004) p. 1840.
50. J. Greener, K.C. Ng, K.M. Vaeth, and T.M. Smith. *Journal of Applied Polymer Science* 106 (2007) p. 3534.
51. J. Affinito, and D. Hilliard. *47th S.V.C. Annual Tech. Conf. Proc.* (2004) p. 563.
52. A.P. Roberts, B.M. Henry, A.P. Sutton, C.M.R. Grovenor, G.A.D. Briggs, T. Miyamoto, M. Kano, Y. Tsukahara, and M. Yanaka. *J. Membr. Sci.* 208 (2002) p. 75.
53. G. Aresta, J. Palmans, M.C.M. van de Sande, and M. Creatore. *Micropor. Mesopor. Metar.* 151 (2011) p. 434.
54. M.S. Weaver, L.A. Michalsky, K. Rajan, M.A. Rothman, J.A. Silvernail, J. Brown, P.E. Burrows, G.L. Graff, M.E. Gross, P.M. Martin, M. Hall, E. Mast, C. Bonham, W. Bennet, and M. Zumhoff. *Applied Physics Letters* 81 (2002) p. 2929.
55. A.M. Coclite, and K.K. Gleason. *Journal of Applied Physics* 111 (2012) p. 073516.

56. R. Bakker, V. Verlaan, C.H.M. van der Werf, J.K. Rath, K.K. Gleason, and R.E.I. Schropp. *Surface & Coatings Technology* 201 (2007) p. 9422.
57. S. Klein, F. Finger, R. Carius, and M. Stutzmann. *Journal of Applied Physics* 98 (2005) p. 1.
58. A. Gordijn, J.K. Rath, and R.E.I. Schropp. *Progress in Photovoltaics: Research and Applications* 14 (2006) p. 305.
59. M.S. Lee, and W.H. Park. *J. Polym. Sci. A* 40 (2001) p. 351.
60. S. Zulfiqar, M. Zulfiqar, M. Nawaz, I.C. McNeill, and J.G. Gorman. *Polymer Degradation and Stability* 30 (1990) p. 195.
61. I.C. McNeill. *European Polymer Journal* 4 (1968) p. 21.
62. D.A. Spee, R. Bakker, C.H.M. van der Werf, M.J. van Steenbergen, J.K. Rath, and R.E.I. Schropp. *Thin Solid Films* 519 (2011) p. 4479.
63. H. Sillescu. *Relaxation and thermodynamics in polymers-glass transition*, by E. Donth. Akademie Verlag, Berlin (1992) p. 355.
64. D.S. Fryer, R.D. Peters, E. Jun Kim, J.E. Tomaszewski, J.J. de Pablo, P.F. Nealey, C.C. White, and W. Wu. *Macromolecules* 34 (2001) p. 5627.
65. P.K. Chu, J.Y. Chen, L.P. Wang, and N. Huang. *Metr. Sci. Eng. R* 36 (2002) p. 143.
66. R.R. Rye, G.C. Nelson, and M.T. Dugger. *Langmuir* 13 (1997) p. 2965.
67. S.W. Choi, W.B. Choi, Y.H. Lee, B.K. Ju, M.Y. Sung, and B.H. Kim. *J. Electrochem. Soc.* 149 (2002) p. G8.
68. A.M. Coclite, G. Ozaydin-Ince, F. Palumbo, A. Milella, and K.K. Gleason. *Plasma Process. Polym.* 7 (2010) p. 561.
69. T.W. Kim, M. Yan, A.G. Erlat, P.A. McConnelee, M. Pellow, and M. Schaepkens. *J. Vac. Sci. Technol. A* 23 (2005) p. 791.
70. A.M. Coclite, G. Ozaydin-Ince, R. d'Agostino, and K.K. Gleason. *Macromolecules* 42 (2009) p. 8138.
71. D.A. Spee, C.H.M. van der Werf, J.K. Rath, and R.E.I. Schropp. *Phys Status Solidi RRL* 6 (2012) p. 151.
72. D.A. Spee, C.H.M. van der Werf, J.K. Rath, and R.E.I. Schropp. *J. Nanosci. Nanotechnol.* 11 (2011) p. 8202.
73. G. Nisato, P.C.P. Bouten, P.J. Slikkerveer, W.D. Bennet, G.L. Graff, N. Rutherford, and L. Wiese. *Proc. Asia Display* (2001) p. 1435.
74. D.A. Spee, M.R. Schipper, C.H.M. van der Werf, J.K. Rath, and R.E.I.Schropp. *MRS Proceedings* (2012) p. 1447.
75. T.W.F. Russel, V. Dalal, R. Gay, and S. Guha. *Prog. Photovoltaics* 5 (1997) p. 353.
76. V. Hopfe, and D.W. Sheel. *Plasma Processes Polym.* 4 (2007) p. 253.
77. R.E.I. Schropp, C.O. van Bommel, C.H.M. van der Werf, M. Brinza, G.A. van Swaaij, J.K. Rath, H.B.T. Li, and J.W.A. Schuttauf. *Proc. 24th European Photovoltaic Solar Energy Conference* (2009) p. 2328.
78. C.R. Kleijn. *Thin Solid Films* 365 (2000) p. 294.
79. Y.K. Chae, Y. Egashira, Y. Shimogaki, K. Sugiwara, and H. Komiyama. *J. Electrochem. Soc.* 146 (1999) p. 1780.
80. M. Gupta, and K.K. Gleason. *Thin Solid Films* 519 (2006) p. 1579.
81. H.G. Pryce Lewis, N.P. Bansal, A.J. White, and E.S. Handy. *Thin Solid Films* 517 (2009) p. 3551.

10

Polymeric Hollow Particles for Encapsulation of Chemical Molecules

Jong Myung Park

Pohang University of Science and Technology (POSTECH), Gyeongbuk, Korea

Abstract

This review describes recent progress in the fabrication and application of polymeric hollow particles (capsules) for encapsulation of chemical molecules. The development of reliable synthetic routes to nanoengineered polymer capsules with tailored structures and functions is integral to advances in diverse fields including advanced materials science and biotechnology. Several synthetic methods have been developed to prepare a range of polymer capsules, which include the colloidosome approach, internal phase separation, self-assembly, layer-by-layer deposition, unimolecular micelles approach, and heterophase polymerization. Herein, the advantages and limits of each approach are discussed. For instance, layer-by-layer deposition is one of the most widely employed methods in the biomedicine area due to its capability of precise control over size, shape, composition and wall thickness. This approach, however, has several intrinsic disadvantages, ranging from the inherent difficulty of achieving high product yields to the lack of structural robustness of polymer walls upon core removal and incorporation of active chemical molecules. On the other hand, the heterophase polymerization approach can allow an easy preparation of a large variety of polymeric capsules with simultaneous encapsulation of various active chemicals during preparation of the polymer capsules. However, this method has a critical disadvantage of the lack of precise control on the shell properties in a nanometer precision.

In addition, key design features for applications of hollow polymer particles such as morphology, release behavior and functionalization of the capsules are also discussed in this review.

Keywords: Polymer, hollow particles, encapsulation, synthesis, morphology, release behavior, functionalization

---

Vikas Mittal (ed.) Encapsulation Nanotechnologies, (291–346) © 2013 Scrivener Publishing LLC

10.1 Introduction

Technology for the encapsulation and release of various materials (e.g., drugs, oils, or perfumes) has received considerable scientific interest in recent years due to the many advantages afforded by the encapsulated systems. For example, encapsulation may allow the safe handling of toxic materials; masking of odor or taste; protection of unstable, sensitive materials from their environments before use; and controlled, sustained, or timed release. Therefore, this area of research has quickly become one of the most rapidly developing areas of research in modern materials science, biotechnology, cosmetics, and medicine. Among the various types of nano- or microcapsules, polymer capsules, which are also known as hollow polymer particles, offer considerable versatility for encapsulation and triggered release applications because of the availability of a variety of natural and synthetic polymers as shell materials, and the rather easy manipulation of the surface functionality and permeability of the polymer shell.

Several approaches have been developed for synthesizing polymeric hollow micro/nanoparticles. These methods have their own unique characteristics that will be outlined in this article.

As shown in Table 10.1, the preparation method can be divided into 3 primary categories, including chemical, physico-chemical and physico-mechanical approaches. Although several comprehensive review articles on this subject are available, the present discussion will focus on the chemical and physico-chemical methods that are more relevant to the advanced coating technology and biotechnology. Among these methods, the colloidosome approach and the phase separation; layer-by-layer deposition; self-assembly of block copolymers, dendrimers or hyper-branched polymers; and heterophase polymerization (emulsion polymerization and interfacial polymerization) methods are the most widely employed and will be described in detail in this article.

A discussion of the function and applications of polymer capsules will be addressed in the following section. The unique core/shell nanostructures of polymer capsules offer many new opportunities for a large variety of application. On the one hand, properties such as the dielectric constant, refractive index [1], density, and thermal conductivity could be significantly tuned by the void of the hollow polymer particles, which leads to many emerging functional materials such as anti-reflective coatings [2], opaque polymers [3] and

Table 10.1 Overview of different encapsulation methods.

	Advantages	**Limits**
Chemical processes		
Suspension polymerization	-Process Simplicity	-The size of hollow particles is normally greater than a micrometer and is not uniform
(Mini)emulsion polymerization	-Simple, convenient, economical and environmentally friendly -Thick and high strength shell walls -Large scale synthesis -Narrow size distribution can be obtained	-Surfactant and polymerization specific -Difficult to encapsulate aqueous cores -Can be loaded once -Often large size distributions
Interfacial polymerization	-Suitable for both oil cores and aqueous cores -Simple fabrication procedures	-Shell formation is diffusion controlled and consequently slow
Dendrimer / Hyperbranched	-Controllable geometry; several nanometers in diameter -Well-defined and predictable cavity	-The dendrimer synthesis procedure is costly and tedious
Physico-chemical processes		
Phase separation	-High strength shell walls -Carbon-rich polymers can be used -Ideally suited for thermal triggers -More suitable for oil core encapsulation -Microcapsules with relatively thick shells obtained -Narrow size distribution	-Limited triggered capabilities -Hydrophobic cores are required -Limited core/shell polymer combinations -Can be loaded once -Often large size distributions -Use of organic solvents required -Less than 100% release of active ingredients

(Continued)

Table 10.1 (cont.)

	Advantages	**Limits**
Colloidosome	-Suitable for biological encapsulation due to no contact with harsh solvents -Good degree of control on shell permeability -Possibility of dual levels of encapsulation with gelled core	-Further shell stabilization stage required to ensure robust structure - Risk of incomplete shell formation leading to leakages and/or core contamination
Self-assembly	-Environmental friendly -Capsules with size in the range of several to hundreds of nanometers	-Dependent on the relative block length, composition of the block copolymers, ionic content, solvent composition, solution concentration
Layer-by-layer deposition	-Compatible with aqueous or organic cores -Easy trigger incorporation -Post-fabrication core loading -More common with aqueous cores due to electrostatic attraction as driving force -Controllable shell thickness by number of times process is repeated -Possible biological encapsulation due to non-use of harsh solvents	-Laborious fabrication -Often poor structural integrity -Dry isolation difficult -Some cores require strong acid in preparation -Long term stability dependent on surrounding conditions -High tendency for flocculation -Only possible with low particle concentration
Physico-mechanical processes		
Spray drying Fluid-bed coating Centrifugal techniques	-Large scale production	-Not suitable for liquid core encapsulation -Only large capsules feasible

super thermal insulation materials [4]. On the other hand, hollow nanoparticles could be used as nano-containers and nanoreactors, which catalyze many new applications. The applications for hollow nanoparticles in lithium batteries [5], catalysts [6] and sensors [7]; functional coatings; phase change materials [8] and biomedical applications [9, 10] are emerging. The precise control over permeability of the shell and triggered responsiveness are the most critical features for possible applications in self-healing coatings and drug delivery [11–13].

The purpose of this chapter is to provide an overview of the current status of polymer capsule technology, with a specific focus on the preparation methods and their areas of application. This article consists of two primary subsections: the preparation of polymer capsules and their general features for applications.

10.2 Colloidosome Approach

Colloidosomes are microcapsules whose shells consist of coagulated or fused colloid particles at the interface of emulsion droplets, which provides a highly promising approach for efficiently encapsulating active ingredients and their controlled release based on size exclusion. Colloidosomes are fabricated from the self-assembly of colloidal articles onto the emulsion droplets (Figure 10.1). An aqueous suspension of colloidal polymer particles is introduced into an organic phase to form a water-in-oil emulsion, in which the polymer particles self-assemble at the oil/water interface and stabilize the water-in-oil emulsion droplets by minimizing the total interfacial energy of the system. Subsequently, the colloidal shell

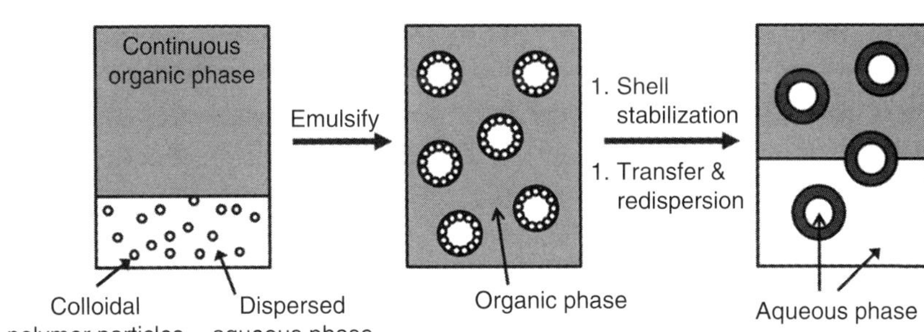

Figure 10.1 General overview on the fabrication of colloidosomes.

structures of the water-in-oil droplets are transferred to an aqueous phase either by centrifugation or repeated washing. Therefore, the effective self-assembly at the interface and immobilization of the self-assembled colloidal particle layers are critical for the successful preparation of stable colloidosomes. Surface modifications of colloid particles have been employed to increase their suitability for interfacial self-assembly. For example, in the pioneering work of Velev *et al.*, electrostatic interactions were used to effectively self-assemble micron-sized polystyrene particles on the surface of an octanol droplet [14]. In addition, the formed colloidosomes must be mechanically stabilized by permanently locking the particle layer together by either chemical or physical means, such as thermal annealing, chemical crosslinking or physical bridging through the adsorption of high molecular weight polymers (e.g., polyelectrolytes). For example, Dinsmore *et al.* stabilized droplets of vegetable oil and toluene in water using polystyrene latex particles. These particles were then immobilized at the interface either by heating to fuse the particles or by use of a polyelectrolyte to bridge-flocculate them [15]. Armes *et al.* utilized the thermal transition and the reactive amine groups of the polymer chains adsorbed on polystyrene latex particles for thermal annealing and chemical crosslinking to lock the latex particle monolayers at the interface [16–18]. The colloidosomes can be transferred into an aqueous continuous phase that is equivalent to the encapsulated environment.

The encapsulation and release behaviors of such colloidosomes are likely to occur on the basis of size exclusion because the pores of the shell originate from the interstices within the shell layer. Therefore, a considerable degree of control over the permeability (diffusion) of the entrapped species can be achieved by varying the size and/or degree of fusing of the colloid particles. For example, Hsu *et al.* tailored the permeability of the polymer shell by controlling the sintering of the particles and with polystyrene particles; a sintering temperature of approximately 100°C was required [19]. By using different polymers with lower glass transition temperatures, sintering can occur at considerably lower temperatures. Laib *et al.* used polystyrene-co-butylacrylate latex, which has low glass-transition temperatures in the range of 30–42°C, in a water-in-oil system [20]. The particles were suspended in an aqueous phase and then dispersed in an oil medium that contained a surfactant or electrolyte (e.g., Span 80) to stabilize the aqueous droplets. Colloidosomes were prepared through thermal annealing at the glass-transition temperatures of the bulk particles. In this approach, three interfacial tensions between the three involved materials (oil, water and particle) should be set to thermodynamically favor the full engulfing configuration. Another method of immobilizing colloidal particles at the interface was introduced by Cayre *et al.*, who applied a gel trapping technique [21]. Instead of a liquid-core, the aqueous gel-core leads to the formation of robust and water-dispersible colloidosomes. The functions of the gel cores are to support the particle shells and to provide the microcapsules with sufficient stiffness and structural integrity to "survive" their separation from the diluted oil phase and the transfer into water. This method offers the advantage of an additional level of encapsulation provided by the gel network of the core.

As previously mentioned, the drawbacks of the conventional colloidosome fabrication method, which involves the adsorption of particles onto the surface of droplets in single emulsions, include the need for exchanging the continuous liquid phase after the colloidosome forms and the low encapsulation efficiency. In contrast, the fabrication of colloidosomes in microfluidic devices using double emulsions as templates provide various advantages, such as high flexibility and efficient loading and capsule formation in a one-step process. Lee and Weitz used this approach to create monodisperse semipermeable nanoparticle colloidosomes with a precisely tuned structure and composition because this technique provides the ability to independently control the thickness of the shell and to prepare multicomponent or composite colloidosomes [22] (Figure 10.2).

Diffusion through the interstitial pores between colloidal particles is the primary mode for the release of materials from colloidosomes. Diffusion by itself is an inadequate mechanism for applications that require the bulk release of materials in a short time. Such applications require an additional material-release mechanism to be engineered within the colloidosomes. The incorporation of a mechanism that can be preferably triggered by an external stimulus would further enhance the properties of colloidosomes and expand their application portfolio. To date, only a few colloidosome systems have demonstrated the possibility of using responsive materials within the microcapsule membrane to control the release of encapsulated species. For example, some systems have been designed using the responsive properties of microgels to enable such control [23, 24]. The properties of the microgel

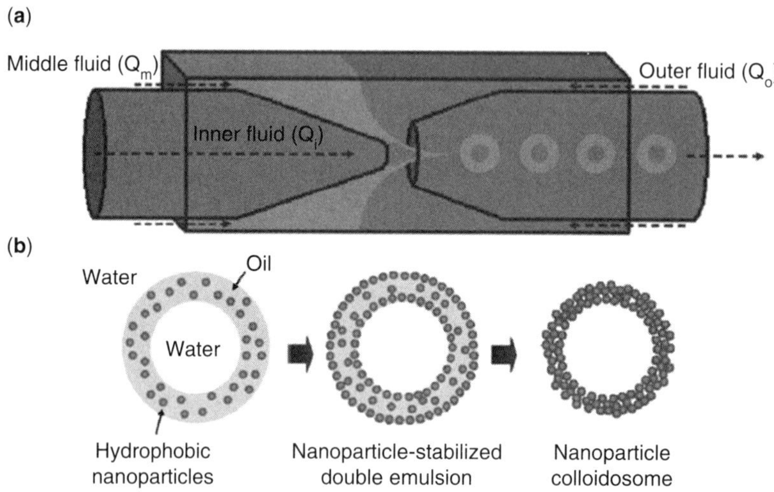

Figure 10.2 Schematic illustration of the formation of monodisperse colloidosomes by the combination of (a) the double emulsion generation process in a double microcapillary device and (b) the subsequent removal of solvent in the middle fluid phase (adapted from [22]).

particles are used here to prepare capsule membranes that swell in response to temperature. In one of these examples, the authors infiltrated the microcapsules with fluorescently-labeled dextran and demonstrated varying release rates of the 70 kDa sugar as a function of temperature. In another recent article, San Miguel *et al.* used a solvent extraction method to prepare polymer particles that can be completely dissolved as the pH of the suspension is increased [25]. The authors used these particles to prepare double emulsions where the middle oil phase could be extracted into the aqueous phase to create a particle bilayer around the inner aqueous droplets, thus forming colloidosome microcapsules. The authors demonstrated the pH-triggered dissolution of the microcapsules and revealed that the encapsulated labeled Dextran molecules of 500 kDa could be retained within the inner droplets. Such types of colloidosome microcapsules hold significant potential for initiating a rapid delivery in response to external stimuli; however, their use might be limited by issues such as active compatibility with the solvent used as the middle phase of the double emulsions and the accessible range of active ingredient molecular weights that can be retained within the microcapsules.

Another distinct advantage of the colloidosome approach is that the colloidal particles that serve as modular building blocks allow the properties of the particle to be incorporated into the functional capabilities of the capsules. For example, the particles can serve as appropriate antennae to induce a response to external triggers (e.g., magnetic fields or laser) for the controlled release of the encapsulated materials. For example, magnetic nanoparticles were used as the stabilizers for the initial emulsions, and the microcapsules obtained from these emulsions could be manipulated using an external magnetic field, which is an important characteristic for a targeted drug delivery application [26]. The laser-initiated release of fluorescently labeled polymers from polyelectrolyte-multilayer microcapsules has been demonstrated inside living cancer cells. A polymer was incorporated in capsules that had metal nanoparticles in their walls, which serve as light-absorbing centers. The capsules were internalized by cancer cells, and near-infrared light ruptured the walls of the capsules, which released the contents of the capsules into the cells [27].

10.3 Internal Phase Separation/Precipitation Approach

There are two primary approaches for the formation of hollow microcapsules through phase separation or the precipitation of a shell-forming polymer: (i) polymerization-induced phase separation, and (ii) solvent extraction and evaporation.

Both approaches consist of two production steps: first, an emulsification step in which stable emulsion droplets, e.g., oil (s)-in-water (w), form and second, a solidification step either by subsequent polymerization of the monomers in the droplet or by the phase separation and precipitation of the polymer (p) induced by solvent evaporation or displacement (Figures 10.3 and 10.4). If the balance of the interfacial tensions (i.e., γ_{op}, γ_{ow}, and γ_{pw}) is correct, the liquid content of the dispersed phase is entrapped inside the polymer after solidification is finished. The size and shape of the final capsules are expected to be equal to that of the original emulsion droplets, which serve as liquid templates for the capsules. Normally, an oil-in-water type emulsion is used.

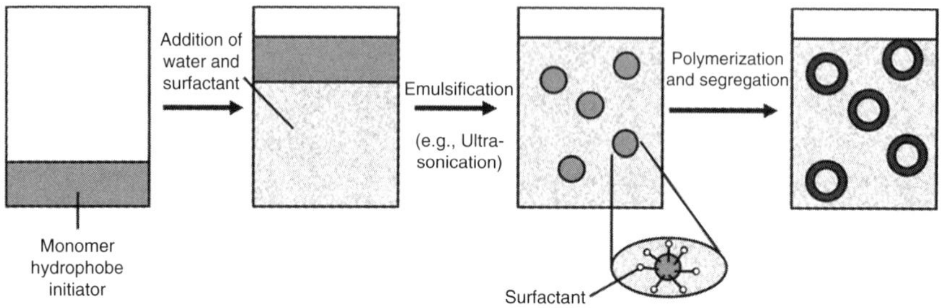

Figure 10.3 Polymerization-induced phase separation fabrication (adapted from [28]).

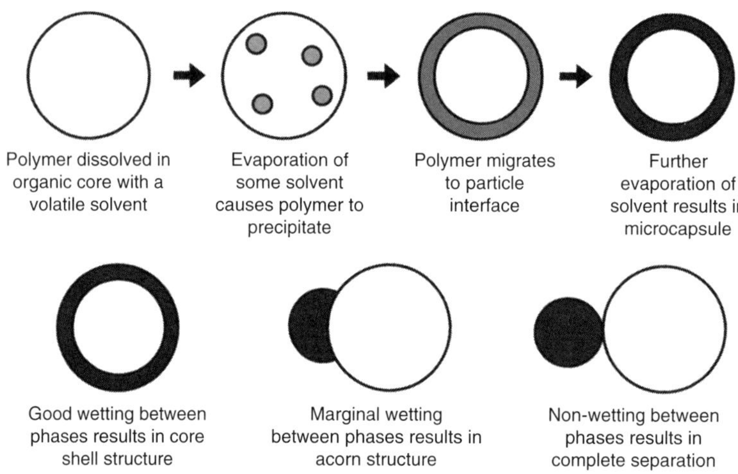

Figure 10.4 Solvent extraction and evaporation fabrication and possible equilibrium configurations corresponding to three different wetting conditions.

10.3.1 Polymerization-Induced Phase Separation

The polymerization-induced phase separation method uses an emulsion droplet that contains active target liquid materials (e.g., hydrocarbons) dissolved in the monomer [28]. This method is similar to the miniemulsion polymerization process, which will be described in the following section. In the polymerization-induced phase separation approach, as the polymerization process proceeds, the growing polymer chains become immiscible with the dispersed phase. The polymer phase subsequently separates, which leads to deposition at the interface and shell formation when the appropriate wetting conditions for the complete engulfing of the original droplet are established. In this system, two important factors should be seriously considered to obtain desirable particle morphologies, such as the core-shell morphology. First, the formation of a stable emulsion droplet is essential, especially when submicron-sized capsules are to be prepared. Because of Ostwald ripening, the destabilization or growth of the emulsion droplet likely occurs with the dissolution of smaller droplets. Therefore, there is often a limitation on the selection of core materials. On the one hand, the liquid content to be encapsulated should possess high hydrophobicity and very low water-solubility to depress the Ostwald ripening. On the other hand, because a polymeric solid shell around the liquid droplet is formed due to phase separation of the polymer, the composition of the core is usually chosen to ensure the phase separation, which means that the resulting polymer should be soluble neither in the core material nor in the continuous phase. The insolubility should be established in advance; otherwise, one cannot ensure the formation of the capsules.

Second, thermodynamic and kinetic influences should be carefully controlled to obtain a complete engulfing configuration, which leads to the core-shell particle morphology. The required conditions for the formation of the microcapsule can be determined by considering the various interfacial tensions between the (shell) polymer (p), the oil phase (o), and the continuous water phase (w), i.e., γ_{op}, γ_{ow}, and γ_{pw}. However, kinetics are also involved in the phase-separation process because the development of the final morphology of the polymer particles involves the mobility or diffusion of at least two molecular species influenced by some driving force to attain the phase-separated structure, which is determined by the phase viscosity and dynamic behavior of surface-active agents in the system. The most common method is to use conventional oil-in-water emulsions, although inverse water-in-oil and oil-in-oil emulsions have also been used for this polymerization-induced phase separation approach.

10.3.2 Phase Separation by Solvent Evaporation or Displacement

The second method, solvent evaporation and displacement, also predominantly uses oil-in-water emulsions, but the phase separation relies purely on physical changes such as the insolubilization of the polymer. The shell-forming polymer is dissolved in a solvent mixture that is composed of a good volatile solvent and a non-volatile non-solvent. A sufficient amount of the good solvent is present to ensure that the polymer is completely dissolved. As the good solvent is removed by evaporation, the polymer phase separates as small droplets of polymer-rich liquid within the emulsion droplets (a coacervate phase). Provided the appropriate wetting conditions for the complete engulfing are achieved, these droplets will migrate to the interface and coalesce to form a polymer shell around the original droplet. Further solvent removal encourages more polymer precipitation into the shell and stabilizes the core-shell morphology.

10.3.2.1 Single Emulsion Method

This method is based on the combination of mini-emulsification and solvent evaporation techniques. The first systematic study on the preparation of microcapsules using the phase-separation-based method was performed by Loxley and Vincent [29], where poly(methylmethacrylate) precipitated from within the droplets of the dispersed phase, a mixture of methylene chloride and octane, upon selective evaporation of the good, low-boiling cosolvent, methylene chloride. Different from the coacervation method that is based on the controlled precipitation of a polymer from the continuous phase of an emulsion around the droplets of the dispersed phase, the titled method uses internal phase separation-induced nano-precipitation at the interface of oil-in-water single emulsion droplets. A driving force other than the change of solvent composition in the droplets to induce the phase separation was reported by Shulkin and Stöver [30], who utilized the photo-stimulated precipitation of azobenzene-functionalized polymers, which occurs because the solubility of the photo-responsive polymer in the core oil is altered upon UV irradiation, to form a stable shell. The phase separation techniques outlined above are primarily suitable for encapsulating hydrophobic cores. This method has been extended by Atkin *et al.* for the preparation of microcapsules with aqueous cores from a water-in-oil emulsion [31]. The advantage of this method is that microcapsules with aqueous cores, dispersed in an aqueous medium, can be produced.

These methods can produce robust microcapsules while providing good control over the thickness of the shell. However, the need to remove large quantities of a co-solvent is a significant drawback for industrial applications. In addition, the polymer/co-solvent system has to be chosen such that the wall-forming polymer is driven by interfacial tension to precipitate at the interface rather than throughout the oil droplet. Therefore, more facile and eco-friendlier methods for the preparation of aqueous core microcapsules have been intensively investigated. One of these methods is based on the double emulsion templating concept, which is explained in the following section.

10.3.2.2 Double Emulsion Method

Another appealing method for the preparation of microcapsules is the double emulsion method, in which microcapsules are obtained via the removal of organic solvent from the preformed double emulsion (water-in-oil-in-water). Double emulsions are typically produced in a two-step process, in which the aqueous droplets are first emulsified in the middle fluid (polymer dissolved in solvent) and then the organic phase is emulsified in a large volume of water. The volatile solvent is removed as it diffuses into the external aqueous medium and then evaporates. The removal of the solvent precipitates the polymer, which consequently encapsulates the inner aqueous phase. This method was used to encapsulate hydrophilic chemicals (drugs, dyes), as reported by Zydowicz *et al.* [32] and Lorenceau *et al.* [33]

Each emulsification step during the double emulsion method, however, causes a highly disperse distribution of droplets, which results in the final double emulsions being polydisperse. Therefore, the resulting microcapsules are poorly controlled in terms of their overall size, wall thickness, and structures. With the aid of the microfluidics technique, monodisperse double emulsion droplets and the corresponding microcapsules could be formed [34]. In addition, by combining the flexibility of a block copolymer during the self-assembly process, the control over the properties of the polymer capsules could be increased; the characteristics of each block of the diblocks can be tuned to fit the desired application. For example, the release behavior could be manipulated by varying the degree of polymerization of the individual diblock molecules, the glass transition temperature of the hydrophobic block and the nature of the individual polymer blocks [35].

Similarly, these techniques suffer from the multiple processing steps required for double emulsions and the corresponding formation of the microcapsules. Therefore, the preparation of biodegradable polymer microcapsules with a tunable capsular size and internal structure in a reproducible single-step process still remains a challenge. Recently, a facile preparation method for biodegradable polymer microcapsules was proposed by Yu *et al.*, which was based on a modified self-emulsification process within the emulsion droplets by simply adding sodium dioctyl sulfosuccinate (Aerosol OT or AOT) as a cosurfactant to the initial polymer solution followed by the formation of a double emulsion due to the coalescence of the internal water droplets [36]. Microcapsules with tunable sizes (ranging from hundreds of nanometers to tens of micrometers) and morphologies were obtained using this technique. The capsules can encapsulate hydrophobic or hydrophilic dyes and hydrophobic nanoparticles, such as oleic-acid coated Fe_3O_4 nanoparticles and quantum dots.

10.3.3 Controlled Precipitation Method

In addition to the solvent evaporation and solvent diffusion based approaches, there is another method for forming polymer capsules based on the phase separation of a preformed polymer from the continuous phase liquid and its migration to the droplet interface. This method is the polymer precipitation method, also called the coacervation method, that has been widely used in various applications, including protection, oxidation prevention, perfume trapping and controlled release. The controlled precipitation technique is based on the interfacial deposition of a polymer (dissolved in a continuous phase) following the displacement of a good solvent in the continuous phase. The solvent displacement can be achieved by heating the system to remove the good solvent from the continuous phase. Polymeric nanocapsules that contained an aqueous antiseptic agent (chlorhexidine digluconate) were obtained through this controlled nanoprecipitation onto inverse (water-in-oil) miniemulsion droplets [37]. The advantages of this fabrication technique are the reasonably narrow size distributions (due to the mini-emulsification technique involved), controllable shell thickness and the economical characteristics compared to the previously mentioned solvent evaporation method. However, the drawbacks of this technique include less than 100% release of the active ingredient and lack the generality of the fabrication method due to the difficulty of selecting the necessary ternary system.

10.3.4 Other Methods

Hollow polymer capsules can be prepared using the phase-inversion method. The phase inversion technique is commonly employed to disperse hydrophobic polymer solutions into a water-based system to produce low volatile organic compound (VOC) coatings. Interestingly, this process could directly produce hollow polymer microspheres without any further treatment when the neutralized solution of hydrophobic chlorinated polypropylene modified with carboxylic or amino groups was diluted with deionized water [38]. This approach provides a simple and facile method for preparing polymer capsules. However, this technique also suffers in the generality of the fabrication method with regard to the choice of the shell-forming polymers.

A simple route for generating hollow polymer nanospheres from the precursor polymer particles, which involves swelling-evaporation processes, was proposed by Han *et al.* [39]. When the ethanol-swollen poly(o-toluidine) (POT) dispersion in water was heated, the solvent inside the POT nanoparticles along with the POT chains moved outside, which created a void at the center of each POT nanoparticle. It was reported that the size and the thickness of the shell can be tuned by varying the type of swelling solvents and the evaporation conditions. The fact that there have been no additional reports on this strategy for preparing hollow polymer particles implies the lack of generality of this method for preparing hollow polymer particles.

10.4 Self-Assembly of Amphiphilic Copolymers (Copolymer Vesicles)

Amphiphilic block copolymers composed of at least two parts with different solubilities are able to self-assemble to form a thin molecular membrane, which can enclose an inner core via two different routes [40] (Figure 10.5). It is quite reasonable that the internal cavity of these aggregates, which are the so-called polymer vesicles or polymersomes, should render them suitable as precursors for the preparation of stable nanocapsules. The flexibility afforded by the use of various block copolymers significantly increases the control over the properties of polymersomes because the physical properties of their polymer shells can be controlled to a large extent by

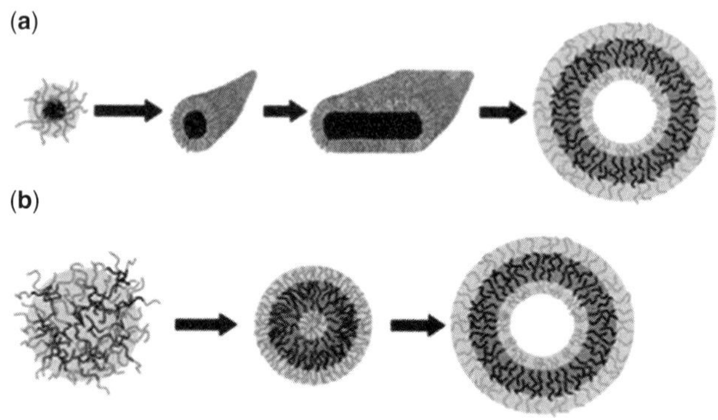

Figure 10.5 Schematic representation of the two mechanisms for the formation of polymersomes in block copolymer systems. (a) Mechanism 1: small micelles, to worms, to bilayers, to polymersomes. (b) Mechanism 2: phase separation grows to large micelles that rearrange to yield vesicles [40].

the block lengths, the ratio of each block of the copolymers or the chemical nature (hydrophobicity, the glass transition temperature) of the shell-forming polymer molecules.

10.4.1 From Amphiphilic Copolymers

The two most common methods for the preparation of polymersomes are the "solvent-switch" method and the film rehydration method. The solvent-switch method is most commonly used for preparing polymersomes, where the diblock copolymer is initially dissolved in an organic solvent that is a good solvent for both blocks. Then, the organic solvent is diluted with or injected into water, which is not a solvent for the hydrophobic block, and the hydrophobic blocks tend to associate to form a polymersome membrane and hydrophilic segments are solvated to form the corona, which colloidally stabilizes the aggregates. The subsequent removal of the residual organic solvents by dialysis or evaporation is often necessary. The use of organic solvents is not favorable for applications where bioactive compounds have to be encapsulated. To a certain extent, the film rehydration method can avoid the direct contact of biomolecules with the solvent. There are two rehydration methods: bulk rehydration and electroformation. In the former case, an organic solvent that dissolves the amphiphilic diblock copolymers is first thoroughly dried to form a thin film, and then an aqueous buffer solution is added to rehydrate the film for the formation of polymersomes. Rehydration causes the lamellar copolymer to buckle, which consequently forms the vesicles. In the latter case, an alternating electric field is applied to effectively generate the vesicles from the polymer film-coated electrodes. The assembly was originally submerged in a sucrose solution, and the formed vesicles were then dissociated by lowering the field frequency. This method is a type of organic-solvent-free preparation method; however, the resulting polymersomes are highly polydisperse.

Alternatively, polymersomes can be spontaneously formed by precipitating the block copolymers by adding a poor solvent for one of the diblocks or by direct dissolution in water [41]. In this approach, the copolymer was initially dissolved in an organic solvent, which was then added drop-wise into a stirred aqueous phase to form the vesicles. Despite the simple synthesis methods, the formed microcapsules are typically polydisperse and coexist with other ordered structures. Therefore, Utada and coworkers improved on the polymersome formation by using a double emulsion solvent evaporation technique coupled with microfluidics [42]. The key to this technique lies in the use of a microcapillary device to generate the water/oil/water double emulsion, in which the inner and outer fluids were always kept separate. The copolymers were initially dissolved in the organic phase. As the emulsion droplets formed, the copolymers migrated to the concentric interfaces and self-assembled. The microcapillary device enables the formation of uniform vesicles with high encapsulation efficiencies and ease of control over the particle size and architecture, including multi-inner-compartment structures. The primary disadvantage of this technique is the lack of scale-up capability because the number of formed vesicles is limited by the droplet formation frequency of the device.

Another solvent-free preparation method based on the electrostatic interaction-induced assembly was proposed by Du *et al.* [43] The poly(2-(methacryloyloxy)ethyl phosphorylcholine-block-poly(2-(diisopropylamino)ethyl methacrylate) vesicles were directly prepared in a pure aqueous solution without any solvents. These vesicles exhibited pH-responsive association-dissociation, which suggested the possibility for the intracellular delivery of water soluble drugs.

10.4.2 Crosslinked Polymer Vesicles

Similar to conventional lipids, polymer vesicles are held together solely by noncovalent interactions. Hence, these vesicles can disintegrate under certain conditions (e.g., after dilution or in the presence of surfactants) into individual block copolymer molecules.

Fixing the morphology of block copolymer aggregates by crosslinking (within either the membrane bilayer or the hydrophilic corona) is, therefore, necessary to explore vesicle applications and has been achieved using reactive block copolymers. For example, the block copolymers that bear photodimerization active segments (e.g., cinnamoyl groups) have been applied to fix the vesicles generated in organic solvent [44]. If the hydrophobic block is polybutadiene, the fixation of the vesicles can be achieved through photo-polymerization by using carbon-carbon double bonds of the polybutadiene [45]. Similarly, terminal methacrylate groups can be used for fixing the vesicles, as reported by Meier *et al.* The methacrylate end groups of a poly(2-methyloxazoline)-*block*-poly(dimethylsiloxane)-*block*-poly(2-methyloxazoline) (PMOXA-PDMS-PMOXA) triblock copolymer can be polymerized in the vesicular aggregates using a UV-induced free radical polymerization process [46].

Epoxy-amine reaction chemistry can be used to achieve covalent crosslinking within the membranes of poly(ethylene oxide)-block-poly(glycidyl methacrylate) diblock copolymer vesicles using akyldiamines [47]. Du *et al.* reported that poly(ethylene oxide)-*block*-poly[3-(trimethoxysilyl)-propyl methacrylate] (PEO-*b*-PTMSPMA) prepared by controlled radical polymerization self-assembled into vesicles and underwent silicification crosslinking when a small amount of triethylamine was added [48].

10.4.3 Vesicular Templating Approach

A similar concept simply uses the geometry of the vesicular aggregates as a template for the formation of the polymersome. In this case, it is not the amphiphilic molecules themselves that are polymerized to freeze in the whole superstructure of the supramolecular aggregate, they simply provide a geometrically restricted environment for dissolving and polymerizing conventional monomers. The synthesis of polymersomes via vesicle-templating has been explored using two main strategies: (i) membrane-restricted reaction within the bilayers (Figure 10.6; I), and (ii) surface-reactive templating and synthesis at the vesicle outer surface (Figure10.6; II). The first strategy utilizes the interior of the vesicle bilayer membrane as a spatially restricted microreactor. Typically, hydrophobic monomers are solubilized in the hydrophobic part of the bilayers, and the polymerization reactions of the organic monomers can be restricted to the bilayer interior. In this process, a

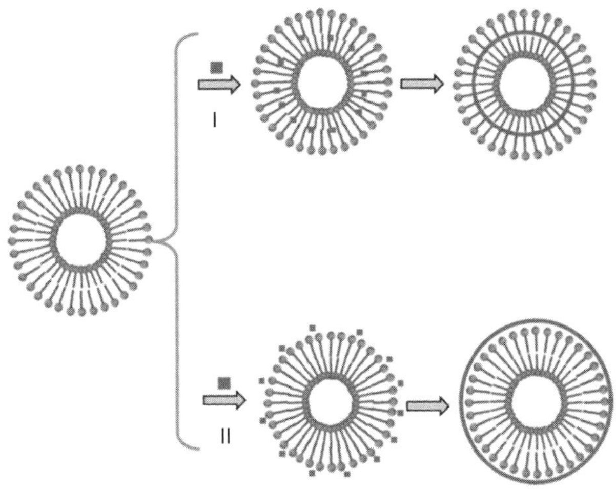

Figure 10.6 Schematic routes of the two practical uses of vesicles in the synthesis of polymersomes: (I) membrane-restricted microreactor and (II) surface-reactive templating and synthesis.

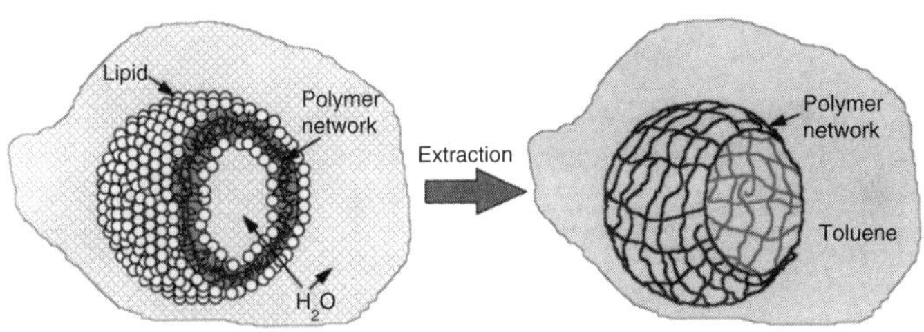

Figure 10.7 Isolation of hydrophobic polymer hollow spheres formed by polymerization within monomer swollen lipid bilayers of vesicles [49].

homogeneous distribution of monomers favors the formation of polymer chain networks that can retain the shape of the template to form hollow polymer capsules. For example, Meier and coworkers reported that the crosslinking polymerization of hydrophobic methacrylate monomers in the interior of the surfactant bilayer of dimethyldioctadecyl ammonium chloride (DODAC) vesicles and subsequent extraction of the surfactant matrix resulted in hollow polymer particles with dimensions ranging from several nanometers up to several hundred micrometers [49] (Figure 10.7).

In the second route, the outer surface of the vesicles is considered to be a specific reaction site for forming polymer shells, which can lead to a direct, transcriptive templating process (Figure 10.6; II).

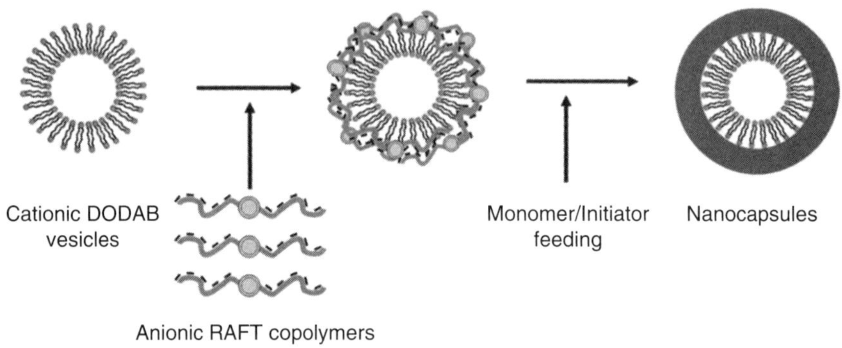

Figure 10.8 Schematic representation of the synthesis of vesicle-templated nanocapsules by aqueous starved feed emulsion polymerization using RAFT copolymers as stabilizers [51].

A key factor in this approach is to use charged vesicle bilayers such that the precursors can initially adsorb at the interface between the vesicle and the solution via electrostatic interactions. For example, hollow structures on the submicrometer scale were obtained with the LbL deposition of the biocompatible polyelectrolyte complex composed of alginate and chitosan on a vesicular template composed of didodecyldimethylammonium bromide (DDAB) [50]. Intriguingly, Ali *et al.* synthesized polymer nanocapsules by encapsulating a dimethyldioctadecyl ammonium bromide (DODAB) vesicle using a reversible addition-fragmentation chain transfer (RAFT)-based encapsulation approach [51] (Figure 10.8). The anionic polymers that contained acrylic acid and butyl acrylate units were first synthesized, subsequently adsorbed onto the surface of cationic DODAB vesicles, and then chain extended to form a polymeric shell by starved feed emulsion polymerization. Taking the concept a step further, they prepared pH-responsive crosslinked polymer nanocapsules [52].

10.5 Layer-by-Layer (L-b-L) Deposition

Another method for generating polymer hollow spheres is to form a polymer shell around a preformed template particle that can subsequently be removed, thus leaving an empty polymeric shell. There are several methods for realizing such a template synthesis of hollow polymer particles. Among the various available methods, the layer-by-layer deposition method has been the most widely explored because this approach provides precise tuning of the properties of the resulting polymer capsules by controlling the materials used (templates and polymers deposited), the deposition conditions, and subsequent processing conditions for stabilization and functionalization. There are three types of deposition in terms of intermolecular interactions for self-assembly, including electrostatic, hydrogen bonding and covalent bonding.

10.5.1 Electrostatic Deposition

The basic principle behind the electrostatic deposition technique is the sequential and repeated electrostatic adsorption of positively and negatively charged polymers onto a charged particle from a dilute solution. A charged particle (e.g., a negative surface charge) is initially placed into a dilute solution of a polyelectrolyte with the opposite charge (i.e., a polycation). The electrostatic driving force causes the polymer to coat the particle, thus changing its apparent charge. After cleaning any excess polyelectrolyte with cycles of centrifugation and washing, the deposition is repeated with a polyelectrolyte solution of opposite charge (i.e., a polyanion), and the process is repeated as many times as desired. Finally, the core is dissolved to obtain a hollow microcapsule. Such sequential deposition produces ordered polyelectrolyte multilayers, and the thickness of these layers can be exactly controlled by the number of deposition steps. Poly(styrene sulfonate) is typically used as the polyanion and poly(allylamine hydrochloride) as the polycation [53, 54].

Various solid templates have been employed, including organic materials such as latex and melamine formaldehyde particles and inorganic or metallic particles. For example, weakly crosslinked melamine–formaldehyde particles have been used [55]. Exposure of the coated particles to an acidic solution ($pH < 1.6$) dissolves the melamine–formaldehyde core without affecting the layered polyelectrolyte shells. Functionalized polystyrene latex particles that carry surface charges are also suitable substrates for the polyelectrolyte self-assembly technique.

The electrostatic nature of interaction allows for the extension of this concept to the preparation of hybrid composite layer systems that incorporate other charged materials than the simple polyelectrolytes. Examples of other charged species used to create hybrid materials include charged dye molecules, inorganic nanoparticles and biological macromolecules [56]. For example, SiO_2/ poly(diallyldimethylammonium chloride)(PDADMAC) composite capsules could be obtained via repeated depositions of nanometer-sized SiO_2 particles with a negative surface charge and cationic (PDADMAC) polyelectrolytes and the subsequent removal of the polystyrene core, which provided enhanced mechanical stability and exceptional permeability behavior compared to those with only the polyelectrolyte [57].

Recent interest has been devoted to developing deposition methods based on other interactions because of the following problems associated with electrostatic interaction-based deposition: (1) a polyelectrolyte-induced particle flocculation occurs at rather high particle concentrations, (2) excess polyelectrolyte not adsorbed to the surface must be carefully removed after each step, (3) difficulty in designing materials that are responsive within biologically relevant conditions (e.g., pH 4–8 or at 37°C), and (4) electrostatically assembled layers being typically highly charged, which leads to issues with fouling in biological systems.

10.5.2 Hydrogen Bonded L-b-L Deposition

Alternative production methods utilize *in situ* coupling reactions rather than electrostatic attractions to encourage polyelectrolyte deposition, which include hydrogen bonding, covalent bonding, base-pair interactions, guest–host interactions and van der Waals interactions. Among these methods, the most notable is hydrogen-bonding-based deposition, whose process is almost identical to that of electrostatic assembly. Hydrogen-bonding multilayer film assembly is based on the alternate deposition of polymers that contain a hydrogen bond acceptor and a hydrogen bond donor [58, 59]. Commonly used acceptors include poly(ethylene glycol), where the oxygen atoms on the polymer backbone act as hydrogen bond acceptors, and poly(N-vinylpyrrolidone) (PVPON), where the carbonyl group acts as the acceptor. The most commonly used donors include polyacids, such as poly-(methacrylic acid) and poly(acrylic acid), which contain carboxylic acid groups. When protonated, the carboxylic acid groups act as hydrogen bond donors.

The advantage of this method is to extend layer-by-layer assembly from aqueous (which is the basis for electrostatic assembly) to non-aqueous systems. Thus, these developments are invaluable because they allow a diverse range of materials to be assembled into the capsule walls and additional control over the structures and properties of obtained capsules. However, further stabilization is required for biomedical applications because the majority of these multilayers will be disassembled under physiological conditions. Crosslinking is an effective way to enhance the stability and tune the properties of multilayer capsules. Even for the multilayer capsules assembled through electrostatic interactions, crosslinking is still necessary in some cases for the capsules to survive in harsh conditions, such as high ionic strength, extreme pH and strong polar organic solvents. Furthermore, crosslinking can effectively manipulate the permeability and mechanical strength of the capsules. The first crosslinking method is carbodiimide chemistry. Click chemistry, which has the features of high efficiency and selectivity under mild conditions, is another powerful tool for crosslinking of the hydrogen-bonded multilayers and microcapsules [60]. In a general strategy, one component is first modified with alkyne moieties and then alternately assembled with another component on silica particles via hydrogen bonding. The films are crosslinked with a bisazide linker, followed by removal of the template and uncrosslinked component at physiological pH through the disruption of hydrogen bonds, which yields single-component hydrogel capsules. By selecting different alkyne-modified polymers, bisazide linkers and the multilayer assembly sequence, the properties of the capsules can be well manipulated. For example, the assembly of alkyne-modified PVPON and poly(ethylene glycol) results in low-fouling capsules, whereas the combination of pH sensitive alkyne-modified polymers and reduction-sensitive bisazide linkers yields dual-responsive capsules.

One of the significant advances in the hydrogen bonded L-b-L deposition technique is the reversible stabilization of hydrogen-bonded L-b-L capsules via disulfide bonds. In this strategy, the key step is to modify at least one of the components, for example, poly(methacrylic acid) with thiols, which can be further crosslinked under oxidative conditions to stabilize the capsule wall. The uncrosslinked component, poly(vinylpyrrolidone), can be selectively removed, which yields stable single component hydrogel capsules. Under reductive conditions, such as inside cells, the disulfide linkages can be cleaved by glutathione, which results in the disassembly of the capsules (Figure 10.9).

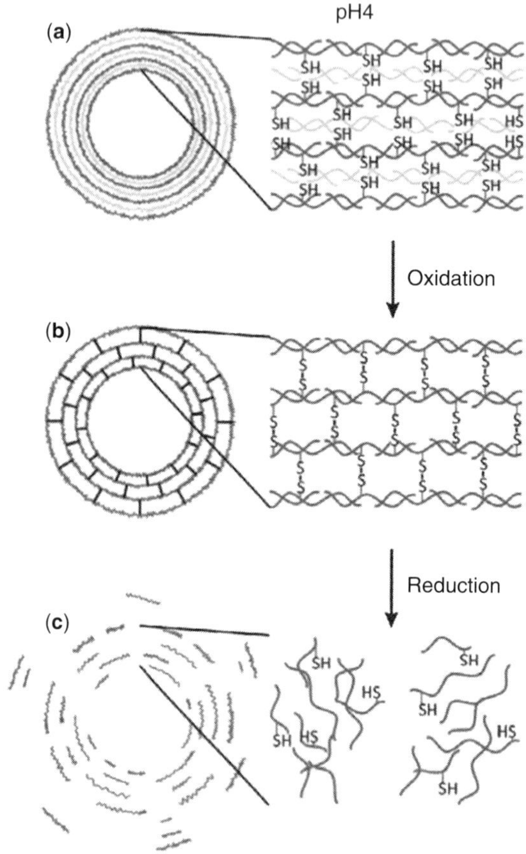

Figure 10.9 Reversible stabilization of hydrogen-bonded L-b-L capsules via disulfide bonds.

10.5.3 L-b-L Deposition on a Liquid Core

Using the L-b-L technique, the multilayer capsules with well-controlled sizes and shapes, finely tuned capsule wall thickness and compositions, and tailored functionalities can be successfully fabricated. Despite all of these attractive advantages, the primary drawbacks of the L-b-L technique with the solid templating technique are the tedious and time-consuming fabrication process and the waste of materials. Furthermore, the substance to be encapsulated should first permeate through the container shell; i.e., the latter has to be switched to the open state. After loading, the opposite change of the surrounding conditions is again necessary to close the shell.

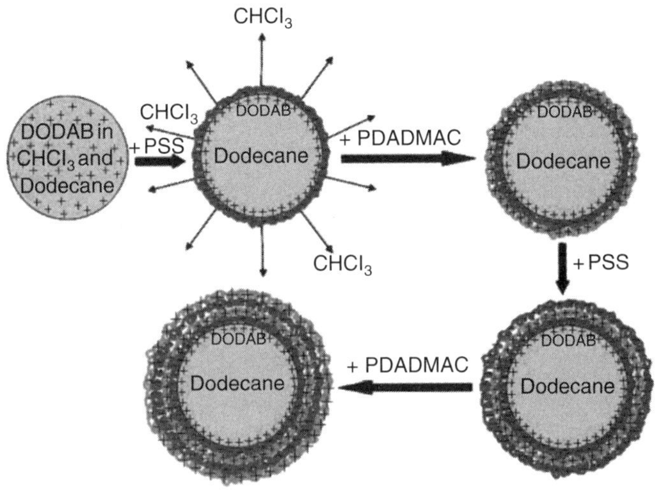

Figure 10.10 Schematic representation of several steps during L-b-L polyelectrolyte emulsion encapsulation. (Didodecyldimethylammonium bromide (DODAB), poly(sodium 4-styrenesulfonate)(PSS), poly(diallyldimethylammonium chloride) (PDADMAC)) [61].

However, different one-step pathways allowing the preparation of mechanically robust and already loaded microcontainers do not leave any possibilities to control and finely manipulate the properties of the shell.

Therefore, the combination of methods that combine the advantages of the one-step container preparation techniques with the accuracy provided by L-b-L deposition is of high practical importance. One example of a successful approach for the preparation of loaded micro- and nanocontainers was based on the oil-in-water emulsion encapsulation by L-b-L deposition directly on the droplets of the dispersed phase [61] (Figure 10.10). In this work, the liquid colloidal particles simultaneously played the role of the template and of the container load. This approach was, however, restricted to the preparation of oil-filled capsules in oil/water/polyelectrolyte systems.

10.6 Unimolecular Micelles Approach

Core-shell type globular structures that can induce the formation of polymer capsules can be produced via the direct polymerization of specially structured monomers. A variety of amphiphilic dendrimers, hyper-branched polymers and multiarm star polymers can form unimolecular micelles that can accommodate the guest molecules in their cores, which provides the possibility for molecular encapsulation and subsequent catalytic properties within these tailored confines. Similar to the block copolymer micelles, these unimolecular micelles are intrinsically stable upon dilution.

10.6.1 Dendrimer Approach

Dendrimers are highly branched macromolecules that grow from a central core through a step-wise repetitive reaction. If divergent branching reactions are controlled to have a small initiator core with a low density and multiple branching units, then the density of the dendrimer molecule increases with increasing separation from the core, which eventually leads to a rather densely packed shell. By reacting peripheral multi-functional groups in the shell with capping agents, the so-called dendritic box is constructed, in which guest molecules can be trapped inside. For example, these dendritic boxes were constructed from a flexible poly(propylene imine) dendrimer with 64 amine end groups and an L-phenylalanine derivative. Because the dendrimer shell is close-packed due to the bulky H-bonded surface groups, it can act as a monomolecular container that is capable of retaining Rose Bengal [62]. In addition to these dendritic boxes, a variety of amphiphilic dendrimers, hyper-branched polymers [63], and multiarm star polymers [64] have been demonstrated to have the characteristics of unimolecular micelles (in the form of hydrophilic core and hydrophobic shell) that can accommodate the hydrophilic guest molecules in their cores. Due to their amphiphilic nature, these systems are also able to selectively solubilize guest molecules within their core domain and sometimes within the shell layer.

Dendrimers are, however, generally not real hollow polymer particle systems because the core is covalently linked to the "dendritic wedges" of the molecule. It is possible to produce real hollow particles by removing the internal core from the dendrimer, whose peripheral groups are extensively crosslinked. For example, as shown in Figure 10.11, the dendrimers with three ester bonds at the core and homoallyl ether groups on their periphery are synthesized by the ring opening metathesis reaction. The selective crosslinking of homoallyl ether groups at their periphery by ring-closing metathesis and subsequent degradation of the core region by alkali hydrolysis resulted in the hollow polymer capsules [65].

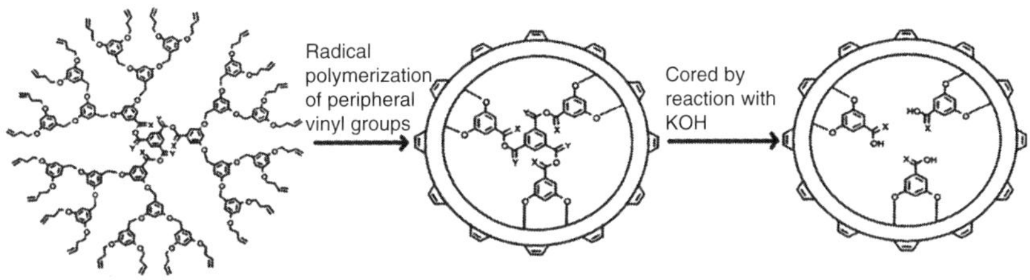

Figure 10.11 Preparation of a cored dendrimer (adapted from [65]).

Crosslinked hollow PS nanoparticles were prepared using a hyper-branched polymer (poly(ethyl methacrylate) (PEMA) with DC groups on the outside of molecule) as the core for the core-shell polymer particle [66]. The inactive dithiocarbamate (DC) radicals and the initiating methacryloyl ethyl radicals were produced from 2-(N,N-diethyldithiocarbamy)ethyl methacrylate (DTCM) under UV irradiation. Polymerization of DTCM produced the hyper-branched polymer. Subsequent polymerization of the EMA and styrene under UV irradiation yielded core–shell particles with a crosslinked PS shell and a hyper-branched PEMA core. Crosslinked hollow PS particles were obtained upon removal of the PEMA core by hydrolysis or electron beam irradiation. Although this synthetic protocol has generality, complicated multi-step reactions have limited their widespread applications.

Interestingly, by combining dendrimer and self-assembly approaches, the one-step preparation of a vesicular structure is possible. Similar to the self-assembly of block copolymers to create polymer vesicles, Cao *et al.* prepared the novel, large covalently stabilized vesicle (CSV) via the self-assembly and subsequent crosslinking of amphiphilic multiarm star polymers (with a hyper-branched polyethylenimide core and a poly(ε-caprolactone) shell) that have the characteristics of unimolecular micelles [67]. These CSVs have a diameter of more than 100 nm, which is a preferable size range for *in vivo* drug delivery, and can host hydrophobic and hydrophilic guests in the bilayer and in the void core, respectively. Furthermore, the guest-encapsulation capacity of these CSVs was superior to that of the corresponding multishell star-like polymer as a unimolecular micelle.

Similarly, Tao *et al.* [68] prepared supramolecular linear-hyper-branched block molecules through noncovalent host-guest coupling between the β-cyclodextrin (CD)-functionalized hyper-branched polyglycerols (HPG) and the adamantine (AD)-functionalized long alkyl chains (Figure 10.12) The obtained supramolecular

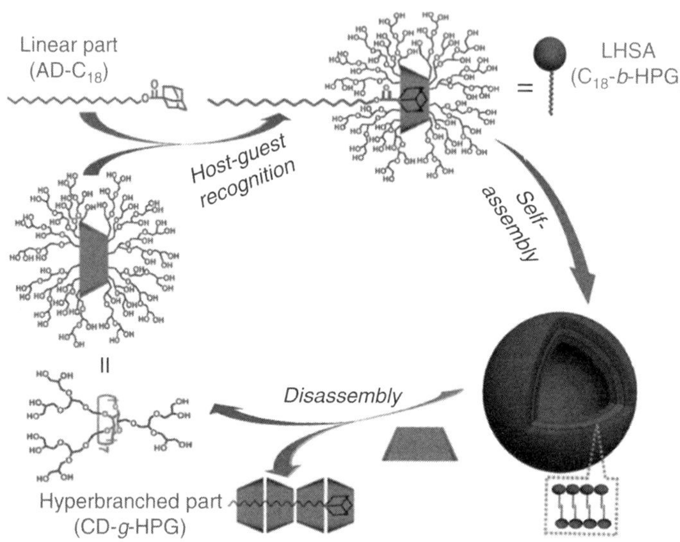

Figure 10.12 Preparation, self-assembly and disassembly processes of supramolecular amphiphiles through non-covalent coupling of β-cyclodextrin-functionalized hyper-branched polyglycerols and adamantane-functionalized long alkyl chains [68].

amphiphiles further self-assembled into vesicles in water, which can be readily disassembled under a competitive host of β-cyclodextrin. The vesicles were very stable and flexible, and they exhibited great ductility under an external force.

10.6.2 Polymerization of Cucurbituril

Thiol-ene photo-polymerization of a rigid, disk-shaped host molecule with a cavity and multiple polymerizable groups at the periphery ((allyloxy)12cucurbit[6]uril) led to the direct synthesis of polymer nanocapsules, as reported by Kim *et al.* [69] (Figure 10.13). This method, which appears to be applicable to any monomer with a flat core and multiple polymerizable groups at the periphery, directly produces polymer nanocapsules with a highly stable structure and relatively narrow size distribution without the need for any preorganized structure, emulsifier, or template. Another feature of this method is that the polymer shell, which comprises a host molecule, allows facile tailoring of its surface properties in a noncovalent and modular manner by virtue of the unique recognition properties of the accessible molecular cavities exposed on the surface.

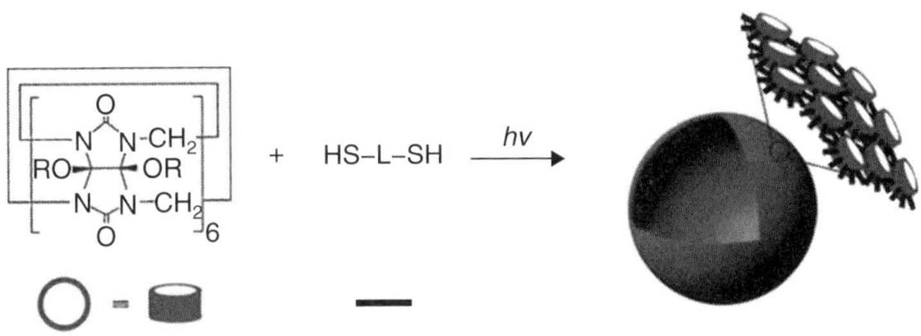

1, R = $CH_2CH{=}CH_2$ **2a**, L = $CH_2CH_2(OCH_2CH_2)_2$ **3a**
2b, L = $CH_2CH_2(OCH_2CH_2)_4$ **3b**
2c, L = CH_2CH_2 **3c**

Figure 10.13 Synthesis of the polymer nanocapsule (3) by the thiol-ene photopolymerization of (allyloxy)12cucurbit[6]uril (1), a rigid disk-shaped molecule with a cavity and 12 polymerizable allyl groups at the periphery, and dithiol (2) [69].

10.7 Heterophase Polymerization

10.7.1 Emulsion Polymerization

10.7.1.1 Double Emulsification Polymerization

Water-in-oil-in-water (W/O/W) multiple emulsions are polydisperse vesicular systems in which the dispersed oil drops contain even smaller dispersed droplets, which generally consist of a liquid that is identical to the continuous phase. Because of the presence of a reservoir phase inside droplets of another phase that can be used to prolong the release of active ingredients, multiple emulsions find many applications in industries such as pharmaceuticals and cosmetics. The most common method for the preparation of multiple emulsions is the two-step emulsification method using a homogenizer or high-speed mixer. Combining this approach with subsequent polymerization, liquid globules in the W/O/W emulsion could be transformed into solid polymer capsules that are usually in the micron size range. An important feature of this method is that oil-soluble or water-soluble active chemicals can be directly incorporated in the separate phases of W/O/W droplet during the double emulsification step. Single void or multi-void particles can be produced depending on the type of emulsifier and the viscosity of middle phase, which is the oil phase in the W/O/W emulsion, after the displacement of the inner water molecules. The first attempt to prepare hollow polymer particles using this approach was approximately half a century ago to improve the scattering efficiency of paint films [70]. Currently, due to the biocompatible compartments and controllable release behaviors, a variety of applications have shown great interest in such multiple systems. Generally, when preparing a double emulsion, the primary emulsification should be more intense than the secondary one, which results in each oil globule containing a significant number of water droplets. Thus, the freshly obtained globules were usually endowed with a multiple-core morphology. However, multi-cell microcapsules templated by multicore globules would be short in volume of each compartment and would slow mass transportation across the shells.

Microcapsules with single hollow cavities could be prepared during the two-step emulsification process by controlling the coalescence of internal water droplets and the stabilization of the two interfaces, and thus preferably forming single-core water-in-oil (W/O) globules from their multicore precursors (Figure 10.14). These single-core globules were further utilized as templates for solid microcapsules by the subsequent polymerization process. Due to this facile fabrication of single-core microcapsules without relying on microfluidic devices, it is expected that these capsules can be further exploited as microreactors with functional cores to be loaded and would be especially suitable to encage bioactive materials.

In general, the W/O/W emulsion polymerization method is a convenient and economical route for the preparation of hollow polymeric micro/nanospheres. The selection of emulsifiers is critical to the process. However, this process is less suitable

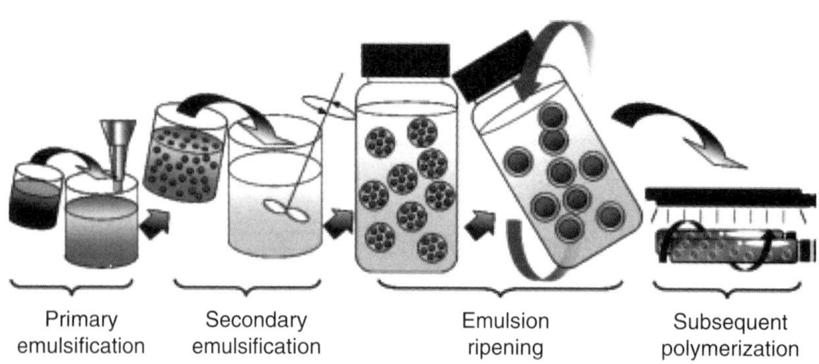

Figure 10.14 Flowchart for the preparation of double emulsion template microcapsules.

for preparing monodisperse particles that have particle sizes less than 1000 nm.

10.7.1.2 *Phase Separation During Miniemulsion Polymerization*

Another method for fabricating hollow polymer particles via heterophase polymerization, which is termed miniemulsion polymerization, uses the difference of interfacial tension and the phase separation process during polymerization. During miniemulsion polymerization, both the particle nucleation and the subsequent propagation reactions primarily occur in submicrometer monomer droplets. Each of those droplets can thus be regarded as an individual nanophase reactor. Under very strict experimental conditions, the miniemulsion can be polymerized without a change of particle identity, which is the characteristic feature of miniemulsion polymerization as an advantageous encapsulation method. The process initially involves polymerizing a monomer in a dispersed hydrocarbon-monomer mixture, which phase-separates during the polymerization. As the polymerization proceeds, phase separation occurs between the polymer and the solvent. When conditions of the three involved interfacial tensions are satisfied to obtain a full engulfment configuration, core-shell polymer particles (solvent as the core) will be formed. For example, in the case of poly(methylmethacrylate) and hexadecane as a model oil to be encapsulated, the pronounced differences in hydrophilicity are suitable for the direct formation of a nanocapsule. PMMA is regarded as rather polar, whereas hexadecane is very hydrophobic; therefore, the spreading coefficients are of the right order to stabilize a structure in which a hexadecane droplet core is encapsulated in a PMMA shell surrounded by water. However, in the case of the polystyrene and hexadecane system, the cohesion energy density (solubility parameter) of the polymer phase is closer to that of the oil, and consequently, a variety of different morphologies can be obtained. A powerful approach to improve the quality of the capsules is the addition of a comonomer to the oil phase. Depending on the polarity of the monomer, it will enter one of the two interfaces, polymer-water or polymer-oil, and reduce the corresponding interfacial tensions and spreading coefficients. The addition of a small amount of hydrophilic monomer such as acrylic acid was observed to dramatically improve the quality of polystyrene nanocapsules [28].

Miniemulsion polymerization is a promising method for direct encapsulation because of its high efficiency and ease of scaling up. However, the encapsulation is very sensitive to the recipe and other system parameters because of the strict thermodynamic and kinetic requirements, and thus obtaining a well-defined core-shell structure is difficult. Therefore, confining the loci of polymerization at the oil-water interface during the miniemulsion process may be the most preferable approach for obtaining well-defined polymer capsules in the nano- to micrometer range.

10.7.1.3 *Interfacially Confined Miniemulsion Polymerization*

There are five different approaches for confining the polymerization loci at the droplet interface: (a) isolating the initiating radical (e.g., water droplet) and monomer (supplied from oil phase), (b) alternating radical polymerization of hydrophilic and hydrophobic monomers, (c) using a redox interfacial initiation polymerization system, (d) growing oligomer radicals from aqueous continuous phase and oil-soluble monomers in the dispersed droplet, and (e) using a surface active initiator system. A representative example of each case is given as follows;

a. An interfacial radical polymerization method for synthesizing polymer capsules with a hydrophobic poly(*tert*-butyl acrylate) shell and a hydrophilic poly(allylamine) interior was proposed by Sarkar *et al.* [71]. This approach is based on the generation of the initiating polyradical on a water-soluble amine polymer in the aqueous phase (of the inverse emulsion) by hydrogen peroxide and subsequent grafting of a hydrophobic vinyl monomer to the polyradical from the water/oil interface. The macroradicals generated *in situ* act as emulsifier molecules and remain at the water/oil interface of the inverse emulsion, which is further stabilized by a water-in-oil emulsifier such as Span 80. The acrylate monomers are grafted to the macroradicals from the radical sites at the interface of the inverse emulsion and propagate in the oil phase. In the presence of a difunctional crosslinker in the oil phase, narrowly dispersed polymer nanocapsules can be produced.

b. A one-step approach for preparing polymer capsules with cores of liquid oil through the alternating free-radical polymerization of hydrophilic vinyl ethers and hydrophobic maleates at the oil-water interface was also reported by Scot *et al.* [72]. The low solubilities of the hydrophobic maleate in water and the hydrophilic monomer in oil, coupled with the nature of the alternating copolymerization and reluctance of either monomer to radically homopolymerize constrain the polymerization to the interface. Conceptually, this approach is similar to the interfacial condensation polymerization of hydrophilic diamines and hydrophobic diacid chlorides to form nylon. However, unlike interfacial condensation polymerizations, which proceed uncontrollably upon contact of the monomers, this free-radical-based interfacial polymerization allows for thorough emulsification before initiation by heat or UV irradiation.
c. Redox interfacial initiation miniemulsion polymerization was suggested to be an efficient method for controlling the site of free radical production and monomer polymerization [73]. A redox interfacial initiation system usually consists of a hydrophobic oxidant and a hydrophilic reductant, such as benzoyl peroxide/sodium formaldehyde sulfoxylate (BPO/SFS); the hydrophobic BPO will meet the hydrophilic SFS at the droplets and water interface where free radicals will be produced, and the primary BPO radicals initiate the polymerization of monomers near the interface to limit the escape of the encapsulant (e.g., hydrocarbon) from within droplets. The polymer chains will gradually grow, which leads to the formation of polymer nanocapsules.
d. Cao and Shan proposed that a water-soluble comonomer, N-isopropylacrylamide (NIPAM), and an oil-soluble crosslinker, divinylbenzene (DVB), have been combined in a system for the synthesis of nanocapsules with crosslinked shells through interfacial miniemulsion polymerization by encapsulating a liquid non-solvating hydrocarbon [74]. Oligomers of poly(N-isopropylacrylamide) (PNIPAM) were

dehydrated and separated from the aqueous phase and were adsorbed by the nanodroplets or latex particles and then anchored at their interfaces through a crosslinking reaction. Nanocapsules were then formed through encapsulation of the hydrocarbon by the newly produced polymers at the interfaces of the droplets. The crosslinked structure gradually grew to stabilize the shell morphology (Figure 10.15).

e. An amphiphilic RAFT oligomer of styrene and maleic anhydride has been used to confine the polymerization to the outer shell of the minidroplets. Amphiphilic RAFT agents could self-assemble on the interface of oil droplet/water, and therefore the radicals transferring among the RAFT agent were anchored onto the interface to confine the polymerization reaction. The polymer chains separated out on the interface, which led to the formation of a polymer shell. The particle size distribution was quite broad, and the shell thickness was heterogeneous. When a poly(acrylic acid)-block-polystyrene RAFT agent was used instead of the poly(styrene/maleic anhydride) RAFT agent, the nanocapsules with uniform structures, including particle size, shell thickness, and shape symmetry, were achieved [75].

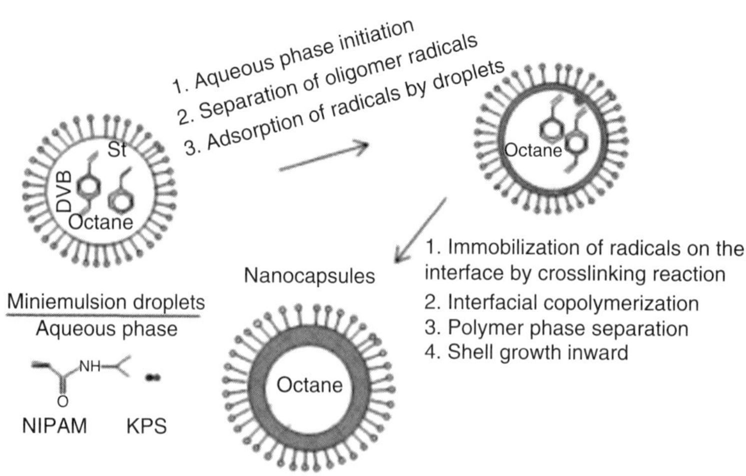

Figure 10.15 Schematic representation of the formation of nanocapsules via the adsorption of growing oligomer radicals at the interfaces [74].

10.7.1.4 *Osmotic Swelling/Solvent Swelling Method*

Various chemicals can be encapsulated in the hollow polymeric microspheres. A prominent approach for the preparation of hollow microspheres is based on the osmotic swelling of a structured latex particle that contains an ionizable core [76]. A typical example of the structured latex particle consists of a carboxylic acid-containing core with a thermoplastic polystyrene or acrylic shell. The composite particles are primarily fabricated by the multi-stage emulsion polymerization method. Then, the particles with an acid-containing core become swollen when the core is neutralized by bases. The bases permeate the shell polymer layer and form a polyelectrolyte salt that builds up osmotic pressure, which in turn causes water to be imbibed into the particle. A void is formed during the drying process at ambient temperature, in which water is dried out from the hollow microspheres. Park *et al.* encapsulated chemical materials in the hollow microspheres prepared using the osmotic swelling method [77]. A process similar to the above-mentioned synthetic approach was used. Phosphoric acid partial esters (PAPEs) were employed as the target materials for encapsulation. Polymer capsules loaded with PAPEs were prepared through multi-stage polymerization, in which PAPEs were contacted with the hydrophilic core polymer before the subsequent shell forming stage (Figure 10.16). The composite particles loaded with PAPE were neutralized with

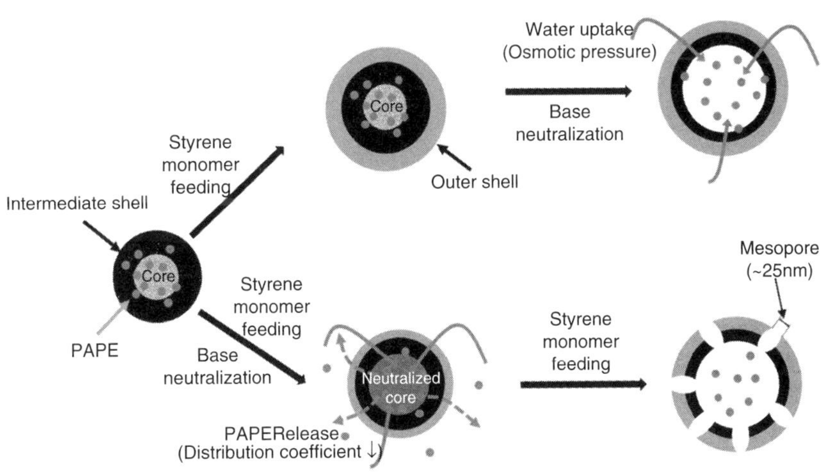

Figure 10.16 Schematic illustration of the formation of hollow particles with mesopores in their surfaces [77].

base to form a void in the polymer particle. The amount of PAPE within the capsule when it was neutralized by ammonia after the styrene shell forming stage was 5 wt %.

Alternatives to the osmotic swelling method have been developed to prepare hollow polymer particles. Okubo *et al.* reported a stepwise acid/alkali method for the fabrication of multi-hollow polymer particles [78–80]. Multi-hollow particles were fabricated by the stepwise acid/alkali treatments of acid-swellable composite particles produced with emulsion terpolymerization using dimethylaminoethyl methacrylate as an alkaline monomer. The multi-hollow particle can also be employed as a polymer reservoir for guest materials.

The particle size of the hollow microsphere prepared using the osmotic swelling method, however, was primarily less than 1 μm. In some cases, a larger hollow polymer particle can be beneficial because of its large storage capacity of guest materials. To produce monodisperse particles that have a diameter of several microns, the dynamic swelling method (DSM) was introduced [81, 82]. Dynamic swelling of seed polymer particles proceeded with a considerable amount of monomer. Micron-sized monodisperse PS seed particles were swollen with DVB and toluene. Subsequently, seeded polymerizations for the dispersions of (solvent/DVB)-swollen PS particles were performed at 70°C. When the solvent was evaporated at the decreased temperature, a void in the particle was formed due to the absorption of PS to the inner surface of the PDVB/PS shell. Im *et al.* reported the preparation of a hollow polymer microspheres with controllable holes in their surfaces [83]. PS hollow particles with holes in their surfaces were formed in three major stages. First, a PS solid particle in water suspension was swollen by the addition of toluene. Second, after the addition of toluene, the internal void was created by the cooling with liquid nitrogen due to the volume shrinkage of toluene. Finally, upon increasing the temperature to greater than 0°C, a hole was formed in the surface of the PS hollow particles because of the evaporation of toluene. The guest functional materials could be loaded via the created hole, and after the loading of the materials, the holes could be closed by annealing the polymer shell.

10.7.1.5 *Templated Heterophase Polymerization*

Hollow polymeric nanocapsules can be fabricated via the sacrificial core-template approach. This templating method can provide extra advantages, such as ease of fabrication and tunable sizes of the hollow void. The sacrificial core-template approach typically involves the covalent or noncovalent attachment of polymer shells onto the surface of inorganic or organic core templates, which is followed by the subsequent core etching step. Core templates can be coated with polymer shells using the layer-by-layer (L-b-L) adsorption or heterophase surface polymerization techniques. Heterogeneous polymerization in the presence of magnetic nanoparticles is by far the most frequently used technique in relevant industrial applications. This technique involves polymerization in a continuous (often aqueous) phase in the presence of inorganic particles by suspension, dispersion, emulsion, miniemulsion, microemulsion, surface-initiated polymerization methods, etc.

There are many literature reports on this subject. In this section, miniemulsion polymerization in the presence of core templates is described, where the core-shell morphology is the optimal structure as a precursor for the hollow polymer capsules. However, accurate control over the shell thickness of the hollow nanostructures is difficult because the free radical polymerization process cannot be solely restricted at the surface of the core templates.

The basic concept behind the successful design of obtaining a high degree of encapsulation is controlling the dispersion stability of the template particles in the continuous phase before polymerization and exclusively polymerizing the monomer onto the surface of the nanoparticles, which leads to sufficient encapsulation efficiency without generation of a new crop of secondary polymer particles. Therefore, the success in polymer encapsulation depends on the nature of template particle surface. For example, successful incorporation of hydrophilic particles into hydrophobic polymer particles relies on the surface modification to make them compatible with the template/polymer by hydrophobization with functionalization through a surface chemical reaction (e.g., with silane coupling agents [84]) or simple adsorption methods (e.g., with oleic acid [85], surface-active monomer [86]) in the case of direct miniemulsion polymerization. Thus, inverse miniemulsion polymerization methods are more preferable for the encapsulation of hydrophilic inorganic particles such as silica in hydrophilic polymer shells without relying on additional surface modifications.

Alternatively, nanoparticles with surface polymerizable or initiating groups are used as sacrificial templates to obtain polymer shells that are selectively grown on the template during the surface-initiated polymerization approach. Reactive groups can be incorporated onto the surfaces of the particles using macromonomers, monomeric surfactants or vinyl/methacrylic silanes. For example, Espiard and coworkers described the use of a polymerizable silane coupling agent, 3-trimethoxysilyl propyl methacrylate, to covalently attach the polymer shell onto the surface of the silica seed [87, 88]. The silane molecule allowed the grafting of a significant amount of polymer during the early stages of polymerization. The grafted polymer chains formed tight loops on the silica surface into which the free polymer chains were entangled. However, in these approaches, the surface modification and polymerization processes are always accompanied by aggregation, and the surface modification and polymerization processes are time consuming and difficult to control. Furthermore, the reagents used for removing the inorganic templates (e.g., HF for silica) are toxic. To circumvent such problems, the "self-templating" approach was proposed for fabricating the crosslinked polymeric nanocapsules [89]. The self-templating approach consists of the following four steps: (i) preparation of the PVAc latexes by the emulsion polymerization of VAc; (ii) surface hydrolysis of the PVAc latexes; (iii) crosslinking the PVA segments on the surface of the surface-hydrolyzed PVAc latexes, and (iv) removal of the PVAc core of the core–shell structures through dissolution in methanol. The surface segments of the poly(vinyl acetate) (PVAc) latexes were hydrolyzed into poly(vinyl alcohol) (PVA) segments. Then, the surface PVA segments were crosslinked with glutaraldehyde. The crosslinked polymeric nanocapsules were obtained after the PVAc molecules encapsulated in the crosslinked polymer shells were removed by dissolution in methanol.

10.7.2 Interfacial Polycondensation

Similar to the interfacially confined miniemulsion polymerization method explained in the previous section, the basic principle of interfacial polycondensation is that the polymerizations are made to occur at interfaces or to produce polymers that concentrate at the interface, thereby producing polymer capsules. Thus, the formation of a microcapsule can be performed in oil-in-water, water-in-oil, or oil-in-oil emulsion systems.

There are three basic types of interfacial polycondensation in terms of the location and supplying direction of the reactants for the polymerization; (a) the system where reactants are presented separately in each phase, (b) the system where reactants are transported from the continuous phase, and (c) the system where

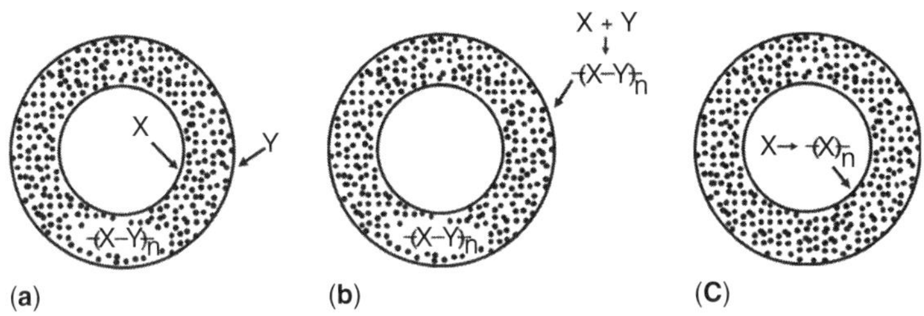

Figure 10.17 Schematic diagrams that illustrate the different types of interfacial polymerization reactions used to form microcapsules. Reactants: X, Y; polymerization product: $(X\text{-}Y)_n$ or $(X\text{-})_n$. See text for descriptions of cases (a)–(c) (adapted from [90]).

reactants exist in the dispersed phase and the shell is formed via internal phase separation induced by the polymerization reaction [90] (Figure 10.17). The typical example of the first approach (Figure 10.17a) is the formation of polyurethane microcapsules in which a water-miscible diol is in the aqueous phase and a polyisocyanate is in the dispersed oil phase. A polyurethane shell is formed at the emulsion droplet interface due to the reactants in each phase diffusing and rapidly reacting there to produce a polymeric shell. The dispersed phase normally contains the target materials to be encapsulated. Extending this concept, polyurea capsules can be prepared when a polyisocyanate-containing oil phase is dispersed in a water phase. The aqueous phase reacts with some of the isocyanate groups to produce primary amine functionalities. These amine groups react with the unreacted isocyanate in the droplets to produce a polyurea capsule shell. The second approach (Figure 10.17b) involves the formation of a capsule through the deposition of, for example, urea-formaldehyde type condensates from the aqueous phase. Due to the formation of the dense and polar wall, this approach is suitable for creating microcapsules that can retain hydrophilic chemicals for long periods of time and thus can be successfully employed as external additives for self-repairing coatings. The third approach (Figure 10.17c) represents interfacial polymerization processes in which a solution of water-immiscible (but solvent soluble) reactants dispersed in an aqueous phase is polymerized and the formed polymer is phase separated and precipitated or deposited at the droplet interface. This system is similar to the internal phase separation method described in the previous section, except that the phase separation is induced by the progression of the polymerization reaction.

The first two approaches have most widely been used to prepare microcapsules that contain target chemicals inside the capsule. For example, urea-formaldehyde- or polyurethane-based capsules have been employed for self-healing materials in which crack healing is typically accomplished by dispersing capsules that contain a healing agent and a solid catalyst within the polymer matrix [91]. However, there are some limitations in these systems. For example, the handling of low molecular weight isocyanate requires considerable care because of its considerable toxicity, and the reactants can react with some of the target chemicals, e.g., nucleophilic agents such as alcohols, which impacts the release behavior. To circumvent these problems, the simple polyaddition reaction-based capsule preparation method was proposed. The capsule membranes were formed by polyaddition at the interface between styrene-maleic acid copolymers dissolved in a dispersed relatively hydrophilic oil phase and a polyamine dissolved in the continuous aqueous phase. Dodecyl acetate and dodecanol, as model compounds for insect sex pheromones, were successfully encapsulated in the microcapsules by varying the solubility of the copolymer. The fact that the anhydride groups in the shell polymer can be used for further surface functionalization is another benefit of this system [92]. Double-walled polyurethane/urea-formaldehyde microcapsules were proposed to be used in self-healing materials. By combing two chemistries to form more robust capsule shell walls in a single process, more potential towards commercial implementation of this technology was revealed [93].

Microcapsules are traditionally templated by either water-in-oil or oil-in-water emulsions. The composition of the emulsion dictates both the type of material that may be encapsulated and the properties of the capsule wall. Because most emulsions consist of water and a nonpolar organic solvent, the material to be entrapped must be soluble either in water or in a nonpolar solvent. This strict solubility profile limits the types and/or amounts of materials that can be encapsulated. An alternative protocol that enables the encapsulation of materials that are soluble in polar organics was reported by Kobaslijia and McQuade [94], in which polyurea capsules were obtained via interfacial polymerization at the interface of methanol-in-cyclohexane and formaldehyde-in-cyclohexane (oil-in-oil) emulsions. Coumarin dye, as a model compound, was efficiently encapsulated using this method.

Note that the sizes of polymer capsules prepared using the conventional interfacial polymerization methods range from 1–1000 μm with a broad size distribution due to the inherent nature of mechanical atomizations involved. Therefore, considerable research efforts have been devoted to developing a novel preparation method for monodisperse submicron-sized polymer capsules. The utilization of electrocapillary emulsification [95] and the use of an ultrahydrophobe together with sonication [96] were proposed, but the challenge of developing economical and scalable fabrication methods still remains. One interesting approach recently reported by Cui *et al.* was based on the sol-gel-based monodisperse particle formation strategy [97]. Monodisperse polydopamine capsules were prepared by the interfacial polymerization of dopamine onto dimethyldiethoxysilane emulsion droplets and the removal of the templates with ethanol (Figure 10.18). Low polydispersity in the

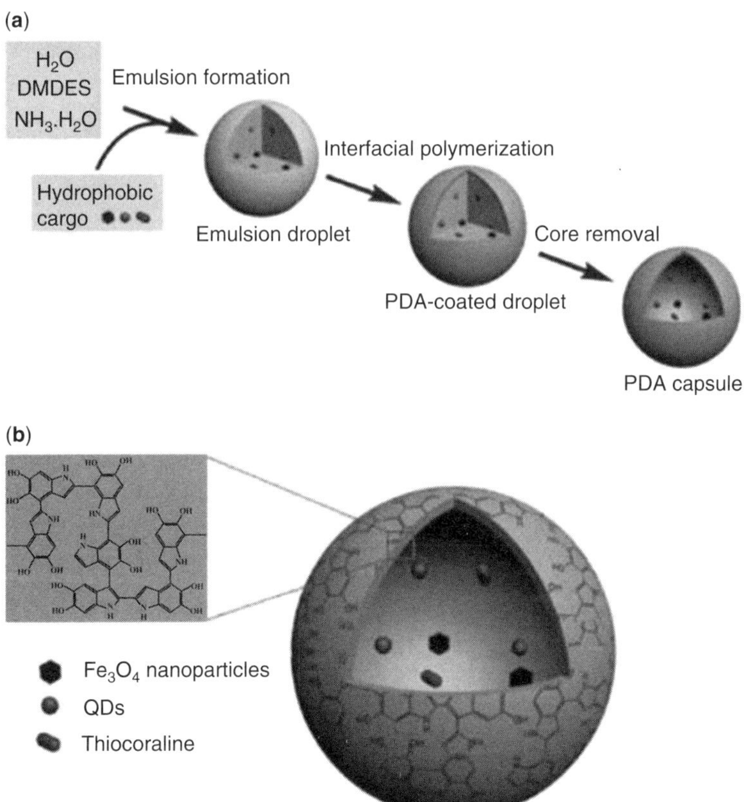

Figure 10.18 a) Schematic representation of the encapsulation of hydrophobic species in PDA capsules, which were obtained using DMDES emulsion templates. b) An enlarged schematic of a loaded PDA capsule [97].

diameters of the capsules is attributed to the inherent nature of the sol-gel chemistry of hydrolysis and the partial condensation of dimethyldiethoxysilane.

10.8 Key Design Features for Applications of Hollow Polymer Particles

There are some important features of polymer capsules to be considered when preparing them for specific applications, which include morphological attributes such as size, size distribution, structure and shape of the capsule, composition and thickness of the polymer capsule wall, stability and compatibility, and versatility and suitability of the synthesis methods. For instance, if monodisperse polymer capsules in the nanometer range are to be used as bio-carriers, harsh chemicals and processing conditions should be avoided, and the release behavior should be optimized by carefully manipulating the capsule morphologies. If the polymer capsules are to be used in self-healing coating applications, good compatibility with the matrix components and control of the permeability responsiveness on external stimuli are more important than other attributes.

10.8.1 Morphology

1. *Structure/Shape*
   In microencapsulation applications, a specific morphology is almost always required to use the encapsulation system for a specific application. For example, sustained-release applications prefer matrix-structured assays to deliver an active substance over a certain period of time [98]. Similarly, burst-release applications such as crack-healing composites prefer microparticles within a core-shell morphology for the instantaneous delivery of an active substance at a specific site [99]. The particle morphology is dependent not only on the employed encapsulation technology but also on the materials (templates and polymers) and processing conditions. Shape plays a critical role in biological functions. For instance, in drug delivery,

the particle shapes affect cellular uptakes and vascular dynamics. There was an interesting report on the preparation of hollow hydrogel particles with a pH-triggered shape switch for the potential application as smart carriers for controlled drug delivery [100].

2. *Size and size distribution*
   When polymer capsules are used as bioreactors or carriers for drug delivery applications, they are required to have sizes in the submicron range (< 1 μm). The carrier with a submicron-sized diameter avoids capillary blockage or filtration, which leads to an efficient uptake by the cells. Therefore, L-b-L deposition on the selected nanoparticle templates and miniemulsion polymerization-related techniques may be the most appropriate ones. Monodispersity in the particle sizes is also important, especially for biological applications such as magnetically targeted delivery and hyperthermia because of the reliable and precise dosage of drugs. For preparing such submicron-sized capsules, the L-b-L technique together with the microfluidic-assisted emulsification is recommended.
3. *Porosity*
   Pore size is one of the most important factors that determine the permeability of polymer capsules. Generally, a mesoporous wall is good for the controlled release applications and the pore-sealed wall for the phase change materials application. Although it is challenging to create small hollow nanocapsules with a mesoporous shell, some efforts have been made towards this goal. The successful preparation of polycaprolactone (PCL) nanocapsules with a hollow core and a mesoporous shell was recently reported [101], in which PCL polymer chains and a surfactant were co-deposited onto the sacrificial silica nanoparticles followed by the removal of the template silica nanoparticles and the surfactant to form PCL nanocapsules with a hollow core and a mesoporous shell.

Furthermore, the leakage of active materials from the capsules is often undesirable, especially in the case of phase change materials that contain polymer capsules. This undesired leakage is exacerbated when there is a gradient in the concentration of the active ingredients across the shell and the repeated solid-liquid phase transitions. Therefore, effective strategies for avoiding such leakage are essential if these structures are to find practical applications. One representative approach was reported by the Weitz group [102], in which two components that can form solid precipitates upon mixing were added, one each to the microcapsule core and to the continuous phase. The components diffuse through the shell in the same manner as the active materials, but upon meeting, they precipitate to form solid particles within the shell; this significantly reduces leakage through the shell of the microcapsules.

4. *Stability*

   Hollow polymer particles with crosslinked shells exhibit good resistances to organic solvents and also to dilution or phase inversion during the subsequent applications. The addition of crosslinkable groups during the fabrication of hollow polymer capsules is the most common method for preparing crosslinked hollow polymer particles. Vinyl, trialkoxysilyl or epoxy groups on the shell polymers can undergo crosslinking reactions via radical initiated polymerization, sol-gel reaction, Michael addition reaction or the photo-irradiation reaction. A new crosslinking strategy based on "click" chemistry, such as thiol-ene and azide-alkyne, has also been used to prepare crosslinked polymer capsules [103].

5. *Shell composition*

   When polymer capsules are designed for biomedical needs to function in water environments, the capsules that feature hydrophilic outer surfaces are preferable. However, for many other important applications, such as in catalysis, cosmetics, agrochemistry, or for smart coatings, polymer capsules that have hydrophobic outer surfaces (to provide dispersibility in organic solvents) and a hydrophilic interior for the encapsulation of polar compounds are strongly desired. Biotoxicity or biodegradation should be considered for biological applications.

Conductive polymers have been employed as capsule shell materials to improve their functions as supporting materials for catalysts, biosensors and electronic devices because of their advantageous properties such as low effective density and high specific surface areas [104]. One interesting example was recently reported in which polyaniline hollow spheres were obtained using MnO_2 or Cu_2O particles as a self-sacrificing template during the oxidation polymerization reactions [105]. As mentioned previously, solid particles of PANI derivatives can be transformed into hollow structures through a swelling-evaporation strategy.

6. *Yolk-shell type polymer capsules and hybrid capsules*

Polymeric yolk-shell spheres, which possess a hollow shell and an encapsulated spherical core, have generated considerable interest because of their unique morphological features and possible applications in the catalysis and biomedical fields. One representative process for preparing polymer yolk-shell microspheres was based on the seeded emulsion polymerization of monomer-swollen seed particles and the subsequent removal of the seed polymers after the phase separation in the resulting particles [106]. Following this proposal, yolk-shell microspheres, which contain an ~200 nm hollow shell of crosslinked poly(styrene-co-acrylamide) and a spherical core of crosslinked polystyrene with a coordinative segment (β-diketone), were fabricated. Inorganic/organic polymers and metal/polymer hybrid particles have also attracted considerable attention because of their synergistic and hybrid properties derived from the two components. Because of the unique properties of magnetic particles (e.g., site-specific delivery, easy separation in biochemical assays, and better imaging contrast property), polymer/iron oxide hollow nanospheres [107, 108] have been widely investigated (Figure 10.19).

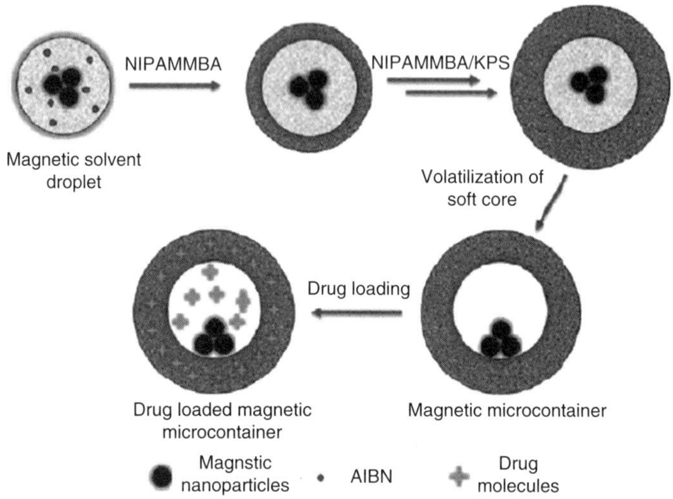

Figure 10.19 Illustration of the synthesis of magnetic/polymer hollow spheres for biomedical applications [108].

10.8.2 Release Behavior

1. *Permeability – release control*

   The release profile of the active ingredient primarily determines the utility of the polymer capsules for any given application. For a given core liquid and release medium, the release profile is determined by the physical size of the microcapsule, the solubility of the active ingredient in the polymer shell, and the release medium and the properties of the microcapsule wall, primarily its thickness and permeability. In principle, diffusional release from microcapsules should vary inversely with the thickness of the capsule wall. In addition to the shell thickness, there are other factors that influence the permeability of the polymer capsules, including the porosity, capsule size, crosslinking density and hydrophilicity of the shell polymer, and the chemical interaction between the core liquid and the capsule wall. Among these factors, shell thickness and pore size are perhaps the most influential factors. For polyamide microcapsules formed by interfacial polymerization, Mathiowitz and Cohen [109] have shown that the rate of azobenzene release decreases with increasing shell thickness and also with the addition of a crosslinking molecule. Shulkin and Stöver [110] have shown that, for capsules formed by the interfacial reaction between styrene-maleic anhydride copolymers and water-soluble polyamines, the microcapsules that have thick, porous walls release their content slowly relative to those that have a thin, dense wall. The observed slow release at room temperature from the microcapsules that possess porous and thick walls was attributed to the hydrophilic nature of the copolymer. Several methods for reducing the rate of release after the capsule has been formed have also been proposed, including the effects of post-crosslinking the shell to reduce its porosity and of heating the microcapsules above the T_g of the polymer shell.

2. *Stimuli-responsiveness*

   Stimuli-responsive polymer capsules are finding a variety of existing and potential applications, such as drug carriers, confined reaction vessels, gene therapy and protective shells for cells, enzymes, dyes and catalysts. The responsiveness is, in general, dependent on the interaction between the material of the shell and the environment surrounding the capsules. The shell of the capsules should be sensitive to an external impact or changes in the local environment; furthermore, the shell should selectively react to only one or two triggers that change its permeability, whereas the others should keep the shell intact. For the controlled release (opening/closing) of the capsule shell, the following triggers are utilized: local pH changes, temperature changes, electromagnetic irradiation (magnetic waves, UV, visible and near infrared), mechanical stress (crack propagation), humidity, electric and electrochemical potential (electric field and reduction environment), and biological triggers (enzymes). Because different parts of the human body can have different pH and temperature levels, specifically in the case of diseases, and different redox conditions, responsive polymers based on these three triggers are widely explored for biomedical applications. The simplest trigger is the pH shift in the local environment (i.e., biologically relevant pH condition is 4-8 and the cathodic area under the organic coating becomes an alkaline pH value after the onset of local corrosion reaction). Polymer capsules composed of various polyelectrolytes, such as polyacrylic acid, polyacrylamide and polystyrene sulfonate, revealed pH responsiveness due to the reversible and/or irreversible changes of the shell permeability over a wide range of pH values (e.g., at low pH <4 or high pH >9) [111]. Polymer capsules fabricated using the L-b-L assembly of multilayers through hydrogen bonding also exhibited reversible pH-responsive swelling and shrinking. Hydrophobic units in the polyelectrolyte can be used to tune the responsiveness. The primary feature of the pH-responsive polymers is that their volume and conformation or permeability can be altered (reversibly) by a change in the pH. Temperature changes can cause the burst release of core materials via the melting of a microcapsule wall or evaporation of core liquid, or it can result in a phase transition (e.g., lower critical solution temperature behavior of poly(N-isopropylacrylamide)), such as transforming a swollen state to a shrunken state. L-b-L capsules stabilized via disulfide bonds can undergo reductive cleavage by glutathione, which results in the disassembly of the capsules [112].

The other important triggers include external light irradiation and mechanical impact. For opening by light irradiation, the capsule shell should be modified with light-sensitive components, such as metal (gold) nanoparticles for IR light [113], dyes (e.g., azo dye Congo red) for visible light [114] and photosensitive moieties incorporated into the self-immolative polymers for UV light [115]. Near infrared laser light is interesting for drug delivery applications because most tissues exhibit negligible absorption in this wavelength range and it is safe. For responding to direct mechanical impact, polymer capsules should be larger than 100 nm, and their walls should have a certain level of rigidity or brittleness to rupture [116].

10.8.3 Functionalization

In addition to modulating the morphology, permeability and trigger-responsiveness, the functionalization of polymer capsules is required to improve their performance for practical applications. For instance, for the self-healing application, the surface functionalization of polymer capsules is necessary for the capsules to be homogenously dispersed in the matrix, which is a common issue in composites and coating materials. For biomedical applications, the capsules should be biocompatible and possess functional groups on the surface to lower nonspecific interactions with the biological environment and/or to engineer specific interactions for drug delivery devices. The functionalization of the polymer capsules are performed through post-modifications of the interior void space and/or the exterior shell surfaces. On the one hand, the functionalization of the core of hollow nanocapsules can be achieved by encapsulating foreign guest materials or by installing various chemical functionalities in the capsule interior. The previously mentioned yolk-shell hybrid capsules are typical examples of the core functionalization where they include semiconductor nanoparticles as the guest core material for facilitating identification of different capsules, magnetic particles for allowing the hybrid capsules in a magnetic field, and noble metal nanoparticles for enhanced catalytic performances. One typical example of a core interior decorated with various chemical functional groups was reported by Liu and Basu [117] (Figure 10.20). The disulfide exchange reaction was utilized to impart, in the capsule interior, various chemical groups, such as thiol, allyl, amine, ferrocene and carboxylic acids. The groups in the core impart diverse functionalities to the capsules, which is exemplified here by the selective extraction of dyes. On the other hand, the exterior surface modification by the covalent attachment of functional chemicals, including biomolecules, can be achieved by various coupling reactions, such as amine/epoxide, amine/glutaraldehyde, thiol/maleimide, carbodiimide, and click chemistry. Among these reactions, click chemistry has recently been explored for the functionalization of polymer capsules because it proceeds under mild reaction conditions and results in high yields without unwanted side reactions. Using the azide-alkyne click chemistry, the surface functionalization of poly(N-vinylpyrrolidone) capsules with antibodies that are specific to colorectal cancer cells was recently reported by Caruso *et al.* [118]. Using thiol-ene click

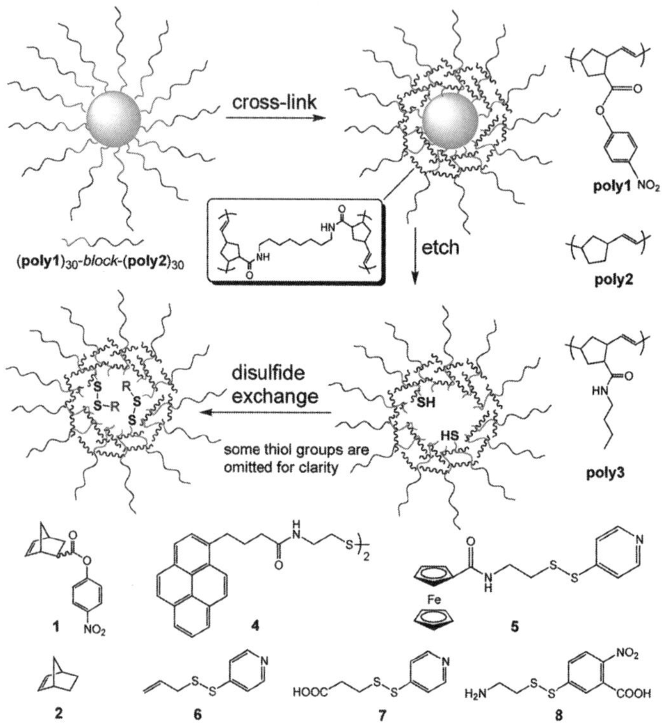

Figure 10.20 Template-based nanocapsule synthesis followed by core functionalization [117].

chemistry, the surface functionalization of metal/polymer yolk-shell particles with hairy functional polymers (polyethyleneglycol or poly(N-isopropylacrylamide)) was reported by Kang *et al.* [119].

10.9 Conclusions

Polymer capsules with dimensions in the nano- to micrometer region possess great potential for encapsulation of chemical molecules into their empty core domains. The utility of the polymer capsules for any given application is determined primarily by the release profile of the active ingredient. For a given capsule-containing system, the release profile is determined by the morphological features of the capsule, the properties of the capsule wall, primarily its thickness and permeability, and its environment. Thus, the need to obtain the optimum capsule features for good control over the time-release profile, for both sustained release and targeted release applications, is a primary driving force for the continued development of new polymer capsules.

Several promising approaches for the preparation of polymer capsules, each of them having its own strength and weakness with regard to the exact control over the particle morphology and loading/release behavior, were reviewed and summarized in Table 10.1. On the one hand, the possibility of precise control of shell properties provided by the layer-by-layer deposition technique allows applications of polymer capsules in the targeted drug delivery system. However, the tedious and time-consuming fabrication process is an obvious obstacle for scaling up the production of the polymer capsules. On the other hand, the heterophase polymerization method, e.g., interfacially-confined miniemulsion polymerization method, allows a scaling up of the production of mechanically robust and already loaded polymer capsules. However, the method does not provide any possibility to control and manipulate the shell properties in a nanometer precision. Therefore, the combination of the advantages of the two fabrication methods is a matter of future intensive research. With regard to polymer shell materials, control of the time-release profile and trigger responsiveness are the key issues for their tailored applications in biomedical and self-healing materials. In addition, multiple-time response characteristics should be implemented in the capsules for the ideal self-healing materials with longer lifetimes. Thus, new chemistries such as click chemistry, self-immolative reaction chemistry and controlled radical polymerization have been explored to prepare an ideal polymer capsule system. In conclusion, it is obvious that polymer capsules containing active chemical molecules inside will create tremendous opportunities in many research and industrial fields such as medicine, functional coatings and self-healing materials.

References

1. F. Guillemot, A. Brunet-Bruneau, E. Bourgeat-Lami, T. Gacoin, E. Barthel, J-P. Boilot. *Chem. Mater.* 2010, 22, 2822.
2. S.W. Kim, M. Kim M, W.Y. Lee, T. Hyeon. *J. Am. Chem. Soc.* 2002, 124, 7642.
3. J.M. Park. *J. Ind. Eng. Chem.* 2001, 7(1), 11.
4. B.E. Yoldas, M.J. Annen, J. Bostaph. *Chem. Mater.* 2000, 12, 2475.
5. X.W. Lou, Y. Wang, C. Yuan, J.Y. Lee, L.A. Archer. *Adv. Mater.* 2006, 18, 2325.
6. V. Kozlovskaya, E. Kharlampieva, I. Drachuk, D. Cheng, V.V. Tsukruk. *Soft Matter*, 2010, 6, 3596.

7. C.J. Martinez, B. Hockey, C.B. Montgomery, S. Semancik. *Langmuir* 2005, 21, 7937.
8. Z. Liqun, Z. Wei, L. Feng. *J. Mater. Sci.* 2004, 39, 495.
9. J.F. Su, L.X. Wang, L. Ren. *J. Appl. Polym. Sci.* 2005, 97, 1755.
10. V. Mailander, K. Landfester. *Biomacromolecules* 2009, 10, 2379.
11. E.N. Brown, S.R. White, N.R. Sottos. *J. Mater. Sci.* 2004, 39, 1703.
12. H. Choi, Y.K. Song, K.Y. Kim, J.M. Park. *Surf. Coat. Technol.* 2012, 206, 2354.
13. S. De Koker, R. Hoogenboom, B.G. De Geest. *Chem. Soc. Rev.* 2012, 41, 2867.
14. O.D. Velev, K. Furusawa, K. Nagayama. *Langmuir* 1996, 12, 2374.
15. A.D. Dinsmore, M.F. Hsu, M.G. Nikolaides, M. Marquez, D.A. Weitz. *Science* 2002, 298, 1006.
16. J.I. Amalvy, G. Unali, Y.T. Li, S. Granger-Bevan, S.P. Armes, B.P. Binks, J.A. Rodrigues, C.P. Whitby. *Langmuir* 2004, 20, 4345.
17. E.S. Read, S. Fujii, J.I. Amalvy, D.P. Randall, S.P. Armes. *Langmuir* 2004, 20, 7422.
18. E.S. Read, S. Fujii, J.I. Amalvy, D.P. Randall, S.P. Armes. *Langmuir* 2005, 21, 1662.
19. M.F. Hsu, M.G. Nikolaides, A.D. Dinsmore, A.R. Bausch, V.D. Gordon, X. Chen, J.W. Hutchinson, D.A. Weitz, M. Marquez. *Langmuir* 2005, 21, 2963.
20. S. Laib, A.F. Routh. *J. Colloid Interface Sci.* 2008, 317, 121.
21. O.J. Cayre, P.F. Noble, V.N. Paunov. *J. Mater. Chem.* 2004, 14, 3351.
22. D. Lee, D.A. Weitz. *Adv. Mater.* 2008, 20, 3498.
23. D.B. Lawrence, T. Cai, Z. Hu, M. Marquez, A.D. Dinsmore. *Langmuir* 2007, 23, 395.
24. S. Berger, H. Zhang, A. Pich. *Adv. Funct. Mater.* 2009, 19, 554.
25. A. San Miguel, J. Scrimgeour, J.E. Curtis, S.H. Behrens. *Soft Matter* 2010, 6, 3163.
26. H. Duan, D. Wang, N.S. Sobal, M. Giersig, D.G. Kurth, H. Möhwald. *Nano Lett.* 2005, 5, 949.
27. A.G. Skirtach, A.M. Javier, O. Kreft, K. Köhler, A.P. Alberola, H. Möhwald, W.J. Parak, W.B. Sukhorukov. *Angew. Chem. Int. Ed.* 2006, 45, 4612.
28. F. Tiarks, K. Landfester, M. Antonietti. *Langmuir* 2001, 17, 908.
29. A. Loxley, B. Vincent. *J. Colloid Interface Sci.* 1998, 208, 49.
30. A. Shulkin, H.D.H. Stöver. *Macromolecules* 2003, 36, 9836.
31. R. Atkin, P. Davies, J. Hardy, B. Vincent. *Macromolecules* 2004, 37, 7979.
32. N. Zydowicz, E. Nzimba-Ganyanad, N. Zydowicz. *Polym. Bull.* 2002, 47, 457.
33. E. Lorenceau, A.S. Utada, D.R. Link, G. Cristobal, M. Joanicot, D.A. Weitz. *Langmuir* 2005, 21, 9183.
34. R.C. Hayward, A.S. Utada, N. Dan, D.A. Weitz. *Langmuir* 2006, 22, 4457.
35. H. Aranda-Espinoza, H. Bermudez, F.S. Bates, D.E. Discher. *Phys. Rev. Lett.* 2001, 8720, 20801.
36. X. Yu, Z. Zhao, W. Nie, R. Deng, S. Liu, R. Liang, J. Zhu, X. Ji. *Langmuir* 2011, 27, 10265.
37. U. Paiphansiri, P. Tangboriboonrat, K. Landfester. *Macromol. Biosci.* 2006, 6, 33.
38. Y. Cao, B. You, L. Wu. *Langmuir* 2010, 26, 6115.
39. J. Han, G. Song, R. Guo. *J. Polym. Sci. Polym. Chem. Ed.* 2007, 45, 2638.

40. D.J. Adams, S. Adams, D. Atkins, M.F. Butler, S. Furzeland. *J. Controlled Release* 2008, 128, 165.
41. F. Meng, C. Hiemstra, G.H.M. Engbers, J. Feijen, *Macromolecules* 2003, 36, 3004.
42. A.S. Utada, E. Lorenceau, D.R. Link, P.D. Kaplan, H.A. Stone, D.A. Weitz. *Science* 2005, 308, 537.
43. J. Du, Y. Tang, A.L. Lewis, S.P. Armes. *J. Am. Chem. Soc.* 2005, 127, 17982.
44. J. Ding, G. Liu. *Macromolecules* 1997, 30, 655.
45. M. Maskos, J.R. Harris. *Macromol. Rapid Commun.* 2001, 22, 271.
46. C. Nardin, T. Hirt, J. Leukel, W. Meier. *Langmuir* 2000, 16, 1035.
47. H. Zhu, Q.C. Liu, Y.M. Chen. *Langmuir* 2007, 23, 790.
48. J.Z. Du, Y.M. Chen, Y.H. Zhang, C.C. Han, K. Fischer. *J. Am. Chem. Soc.* 2003, 125, 14710.
49. J. Hotz, W. Meier. *Adv. Mater.* 1998, 10, 1387.
50. F. Cuomo, F. Lopez, M.G. Miguel, B. Lindman. *Langmuir* 2010, 26, 10555.
51. S.I. Ali, J.P.A. Heuts, A.M. van Herk. *Langmuir* 2010, 26, 7848.
52. S.I. Ali, J.P.A. Heuts, A.M. van Herk. *Soft Matter* 2011, 7, 5382.
53. S. Stewart, G.J. Liu. *Chem. Mater.* 1999, 11, 1048.
54. E. Donath, G.B. Sukhorukov, F. Caruso, S.A. Davis, H. Möhwald. *Angew. Chem., Int. Ed.* 1998, 37, 2201.
55. G.B. Sukhorukov, E. Donath, S. Moya, A.S. Susha, A. Voigt, J. Hartmann, H. Möhwald. *J. Microencaps.* 2000, 17, 177.
56. C. Tedeschi, F. Caruso, H. Möhwald, S. Kirstein. *J. Am. Chem. Soc.* 2000, 122, 5841.
57. F. Caruso, R.A. Caruso, and H. Möhwald. *Science* 1998, 282, 1111.
58. Y. Zhang, Y. Guan, S. Yang, J. Xu, C.C. Han. *Adv. Mater.* 2003, 15, 832.
59. V. Kozlovskaya, S. Ok, A. Sousa, M. Libera, S. Sukhishvili. *Macromolecules* 2003, 36, 8590.
60. G.K. Such, A.P.R. Johnston, K. Liang, F. Caruso. *Prog. Polym. Sci.* 2012, 37, 985.
61. D.O. Grigoriev, T. Bukreeva, H. Möhwald, D.G. Shchukin. *Langmuir* 2008, 24, 999.
62. J.F.G.A. Jansen, D.A.F.J. van Boxtel, E.M.M. de Brabander-van den Berg, E.W. Meijer. *J. Am. Chem. Soc.* 1995, 117, 4417.
63. C.R. Newkome, C.N. Moorefield, G.R. Baker, M.J. Saunders, S.H. Grossman. *Angew. Chem., Int. Ed.* 1991, 30, 1178.
64. A. Sunder, M. Krämer, R. Hanselmann, R. Mühlhaupt, and H. Frey. *Angew. Chem., Int. Ed.*, 1999, 38, 3552.
65. M.S. Wendland, S.C. Zimmerman. *J. Am. Chem. Soc.*, 1999, 121, 1389.
66. K. Ishizu, J. Park, K. Tanimure, S. Uchida. *J Mater. Sci.* 2004, 39, 4353.
67. P. Cao, R. Zhao, L. Li, W. Yang, F. Cheng, Y. Chen, C. Lu, S. Jiang. *J. Polym. Sci. Polym. Chem. Ed.* 2012, 50, 227.
68. W. Tao, Y. Liu, B. Jiang, S. Yu, W. Huang, Y. Zhou, D. Yan. *J. Am. Chem. Soc.* 2012, 134, 762.
69. D. Kim, E. Kim, J. Kim, K.M. Park, K. Baek, M. Jung, Y.H. Ko, W. Sung, H.S. Kim, J.H. Suh, C.G. Park, O.S. Na, D. Lee, K.E. Lee, S.S. Han, K. Kim, *Angew. Chem. Int. Ed.* 2007, 46, 3471.
70. U.S. Patent 3,839,253 (1968).
71. D. Sarkar, J. El-Khoury, S.T. Lopina, J. Hu. *Macromolecules* 2005, 38, 8603.

72. C. Scott, D. Wu, C. Ho, C.C. Co. *J. Am. Chem. Soc.* 2005, 127, 4160.
73. C. Chen, Z. Chen, X. Zeng, X. Fang, Z. Zhang. *Colloid Polym. Sci.* 2012, 290, 307.
74. Z. Cao, Z. Shan. *J. Polym. Sci. Polym. Chem. Ed.* 2009, 47, 1522.
75. F. Lu, Y. Luo, B. Li. *Macromol. Rapid Commun.* 2007, 28, 868.
76. C.J. McDonald, M.J. Devon. *Adv. Colloid Interface Sci.* 2002, 99, 181.
77. J.H. Park, K.Y. Kim, J.M. Park. *Polymer* 2010, 51, 3014.
78. M. Okubo, A. Ito, A. Hashiba. *Colloid Polym. Sci.* 1996, 274, 428.
79. M. Okubo, H. Mori, A. Ito. *Colloid Polym. Sci.* 2000, 278, 358.
80. M. Okubo, H. Mori, A. Ito. *Colloid Polym. Sci.* 1999, 277, 589.
81. M. Okubo, H. Minami. *Colloid Polym. Sci.* 1996, 274, 433.
82. M. Okubo, H. Minami. *Colloid Polym. Sci.* 1997, 275, 992.
83. S.H. Im, U. Jeong, Y. Xia. *Nat. Mater.* 2005, 4, 671.
84. P. Van Der Voort, E.F. Vansant. *J. Liq. Chromatogr. Relat. Technol.* 1996, 19, 2723.
85. D. Hoffmann, K. Landfester, M. Antonietti. *Magnetohydrodynamics* 2001, 37, 217.
86. K. Yoshinaga, T. Yokoyama, T. Kito. *Polym. Adv. Technol.* 1993, 4, 38.
87. E. Bourgeat-Lami, P. Espiard, A. Guyot. *Polymer* 1995, 36, 4385.
88. P. Espiard, A. Guyot. *Polymer* 1995, 36, 4391.
89. P. Liu, G. Liu, W. Zhang, F. Jiang. *Nanotechnology* 2010, 21, 015603.
90. C. Thies. Microencapsulation. In *Encyclopedia of polymer sceince and technology*. 2nd ed. John Wiley & Sons, Inc., 2005, Vol. 9, 724–745.
91. S.H. Cho, S.R. White, P.V. Braun. *Adv. Mater.* 2009, 21, 645.
92. A. Shulkin, H. Stöver. *J. Membrane Sci.* 2002, 209, 421.
93. M.M. Caruso, B.J. Blaiszik, H. Jin, S.R. Schelkopf, D.S. Stradley, N.R. Sottos, S.R. White, J.S. Moore. *ACS Appl. Mater. & Interface* 2010, 2, 1195.
94. M. Kobaslijia, D.T. McQuade. *Macromolecules* 2006, 39, 6371.
95. H. Skai, K. Tanaka, H. Fukushima, K. Tsuchiya, K. Sakai, T. Kondo, M. Abe. *Colloids and Surfaces B* 2008, 66(2), 287.
96. A. Jackson, B.J. Blaiszik, D.McIlroy, N.R. Sottos, P.V. Braun. *Polymer Preprints* 2008, 49, 968.
97. J. Cui, Y. Wang, A. Postma, J. Hao, L. Hosta-Rigau, F. Caruso. *Adv. Funct. Mater.* 2010, 20, 1625.
98. Y.H. Bae. *Handbook of pharmaceutical controlled release technology*. D.L. Wise, ed. CRC Press: New York, 2001; pp 553–554.
99. B.J. Blaiszik, N.R. Sottos, S.R. White. *Composites Sci. and Technol.* 2008, 68, 978.
100. V. Kozlovskaya, W. Higgins, J. Chen, E. Kharlampieva. *Chem. Commun.* 2011, 47, 8352.
101. P. Paika, Y. Zhang. *Nanoscale* 2011, 3, 2215.
102. Y. Zhao, H.C. Shum, L.L.A. Adams, B. Sun, C. Holtze, Z. Gu, D.A. Weitz. *Langmuir* 2011, 27, 13988.
103. B. Samanta, D. Patra, C. Subramani, Y. Ofir, G. Yesilbag, A. Sanyal, V.M. Rotello. *Small* 2009, 5, 685.
104. Z. Wei, M. Wan. *Adv. Mater.* 2002, 14,1314.
105. J. Fei, Y. Cui, X. Yan, Y. Yang, K. Wang, J. Li. *ACS Nano* 2009, 3, 3714.
106. M. Zhang, Y. Lan, D. Wang, R. Yan, S. Wang, L. Yang, W. Zhang. *Macromolecules* 2011, 44, 842.
107. J.K. Oh, J.M. Park. *Prog. Polym. Sci.* 2011, 36, 168.

108. L.B. Chen, F. Zhang, C.C. Wang. *Small* 2009, 5, 621.
109. E. Mathiowitz, M.D. Cohen. *J. Membr. Sci.* 1989, 40, 27.
110. A. Shulkin, H.D.H. Stöver. *J. Membr. Sci.* 2002, 209, 433.
111. Y. Wang, F. Caruso. *Chem. Mater.* 2006, 18, 4089.
112. A.L. Becker, A.N. Zelikin, A.P.R. Johnston, F. Caruso. *Langmuir* 2009, 25, 14079.
113. A.S. Angelatos, B. Radt, F. Caruso. *J. Phys. Chem. B* 2005, 109, 3071.
114. X. Tao, J.B. Li, H. Möhwald. *Chem.–Eur. J.* 2004, 10, 3397.
115. N. Fomina, C. McFearin, M. Sermsakdi, O. Edigin, A. Almutairi. *J. Am. Chem. Soc.* 2010, 132, 9540.
116. A. Fery, R. Weinkamer. *Polymer* 2007, 48, 7221.
117. X. Liu, A. Basu. *J. Am. Chem. Soc.* 2009, 131, 5718.
118. M.M.J. Kamphuis, A.P.R. Johnston, G.K. Such, H.H. Dam, R.A. Evans, A.M. Scott, E.C. Nice, J.K. Heath, F. Caruso. *J. Am. Chem. Soc.* 2010, 132, 15881.
119. G.L. Li, L.Q. Xu, K.G. Neoh, E.T. Kang. *Macromolecules* 2011, 44, 2365.

11

Protic Ionic Liquids Confinement in Macro, Meso and Microporous Materials for Proton Conduction

A. Eguizábal and M.P. Pina

Chemical Engineering Department, Nanoscience Institute of Aragón (INA), Zaragoza, Spain

Abstract

This chapter describes the potentialities of encapsulated ionic liquids within porous moieties in the proton exchange membranes field. For such application, two different approaches have been carefully studied. The first one relies on the IL immobilization in large pore zeolites, which are further deployed as inorganic fillers to the polymeric membrane casting solution. In this case, ammonium- and imidazolium-based protic ionic liquids imbibed within the microporous framework of hydrophilic FAU and BEA zeolites have been fully characterized to illustrate the proton conduction performance of the composites. The second approach is based on the membrane pores filling concept. In this case, pre-existing macroporous and mesoporous (organic or inorganic) supports are deployed as containers for the liquid salts. Special emphasis has been devoted to porous polybenzimidazol films because of its well-known properties for high-temperature PEMFCs. Particularly, different pore morphology, pore size, coordination number and overall porosity values have been studied to underline the presence of different proton conduction pathways contributing to conduction phenomena over heterogeneous media. Finally, new research pathways for future development based on polymerizable ionic liquids to alleviate the protic ionic liquid dragging with time on stream are briefly presented

Keywords: Protic ionic liquids, pore confinement, zeolite host, porous membranes, proton transport, conduction mechanism, high temperature PEMFCs

Vikas Mittal (ed.) Encapsulation Nanotechnologies, (347–390) © 2013 Scrivener Publishing LLC

11.1 Introduction

Ionic Liquids (ILs) are organic salts commonly encountered as liquids at room conditions or below 25°C. ILs are fluids at ambient temperatures primarily due to the large size and asymmetry of the cations, combined with resonance stabilized anions. Many ILs are liquids over a wide temperature range with some having melting points as low as −96°C and some liquid ranges in excess of 300°C. They exhibit unique physicochemical properties such as non-volatility, non-flammability, high thermal stability, and tunable electrochemical and ion conduction. Unlike traditional organic media, IL's properties can be adjusted via chemical alteration of the cation or anion to produce application specific compounds. Low symmetry organic cations such as ammonium, sulfonium or imidazole anions are usually combined with poly- or mononuclear anions. As a matter of fact, these organic salts have been the subject of many experimental and theoretical investigations over the past decade [1–3]. Among their potentialities for industrial applications [4–5], gas separation [1, 6–8], catalysis [9–13] and electrochemistry [14–15] are the most outstanding.

According to the published literature, the encapsulation of ionic liquids within porous media in powder form has been scarcely explored either for catalytic or energy applications. De Castro *et al.* [16] have immobilized a mixture of 1-butyl-3-methyl-imidazolium chloride and $AlCl_3$ (AL-IL) within macro-, meso- and microporous materials (SiO_2, Al_2O_3, TiO_2, ZrO_2 and H-BEA zeolite) in order to prepare catalysts for the alkylation reactions of aromatic compounds. The immobilization was carried out by addition of the IL to the previously dried and calcined porous support until its appearance changed from a dry to wet powder. The excess of the ionic liquid was removed by Soxhlet extraction. Higher IL uptake values were observed by SiO_2 and Al_2O_3 supports due to the formation of covalent bonds between surface hydroxyl groups and Al atoms from the AL-IL. In the case of HBEA zeolite, the crystalline structure collapse observed by XRD was attributed to the formation of hydrochloric acid.

The direct addition of the IL to the porous support by the so called "incipient wetness" method has been studied by Valkenberg *et al* [17] for the immobilization of the ionic liquids in porous SiO_2 to prepare Lewis acid catalysts for Friedel-Crafts reaction. The obtained materials were analyzed using ICP-AES, CHN-analysis, XRD, DRIFT and MAS-NMR. ^{29}Si MAS NMR measurements revealed the formation of covalent bonds between the Lewis acid and surface silanol groups from the support.

Unlike previous works, Pietschmann *et al.* [18] impregnated BEA zeolite and mesoporous silica with a solution of 1-ethyl-3-methylimidazolium tetrafluoroborate ([$EMIM^+$][BF_4^-]) and methanol as solvent. After mixing under vigorous stirring for several hours, the crystals were separated from the suspension using filtration and any excess of IL was removed by Soxhlet extraction. BET measurements showed significant decrease of the BET surface area due the IL encapsulation. The amount of immobilized IL before and after Soxhlet extraction was 4–8% wt and 0.6–1.3 wt %, respectively. ^{13}C VACP/MAS-NMR measurements substantiated the immobilization of imidazolium cations within the microporous BEA cavities.

The inmobilization of IL inside porous solids could be also carried out by "grafting method" of ionic liquid precursors on hydroxyl groups at the support surface. This method has been extensively used during the last decades for functionalization purposes, i.e., mesoporous silica [19, 20], by means of organosilanes as coupling agents. This method has proven to be of great importance due to the extensive applications of the obtained materials in chromatography, biochemistry, catalysis, etc. For the particular case of IL anchoring on mesoporous silica cavities, there are no related publications; but the approach will be right straightforward. Thus, the organic halide containing the cation of the ionic liquid would be "grafted" to the silica surface in a first step. After the addition of the lithium salt containing the anion of the ionic liquid, the ion exchange reaction would lead to the "ship in a bottle" synthesis of IL.

Porous polymer matrices have been traditionally used as containers for active liquid species in supported liquid membranes applied to gas and liquid separation processes [21]. Based on that, supported ionic liquid membranes (SILMs) have been extensively studied over the past decade [22]. By far, CO_2 has been the most successful separation due to the fact that the quadrupole moment of the CO_2 interacts with the electrical charge of the ILs [8, 23–25]. This specific interaction provides an enhancement in the CO_2 solubility over other gases such as N_2 or CH_4.

Particularly in the PEMFCs field, several authors [26, 27] have proposed the deployment of ionic liquids as electrolytes. In this way, promising results have been reported by Lojoiu *et al.* [28], who studied the performance of Nafion membranes post-impregnated with two protic ionic liquids (triflate triethylammonium, methane sulfonate triethylammonium). Conducting polybenzimidazole-based systems containing ILs have been already reported by dissolving the polymer and IL in a common solvent and casting the film [29–31]. The pioneering work of Greenbaum *et al.* [29] demonstrated the feasibility of anhydrous proton solvent H_3PO_4, the protic ionic liquid 1-propyl-3-methylimidazolium dihydrogen phosphate and PBI for operation up to 150°C. Under completely anhydrous conditions, these novel membranes exhibited conductivities up to 2.04 $mS{\cdot}cm^{-1}$ at 150°C. In a step further [31], composite membranes were prepared from a fluorine-containing PBI with 1-hexyl-3-methylimidazolium trifluoromethanesulfonate. The ionic liquid-based composite membranes showed a significant improvement in thermal stability compared to the H_3PO_4/PBI system, and ionic conductivities up to 16 $mS{\cdot}cm^{-1}$ at 250°C under anhydrous conditions. Lee *et al.* [32] tested sulphonated polyimide/diethylmethylammonium trifluoromethanesulfonate composite membranes with conductivity values higher than 10 $mS{\cdot}cm^{-1}$ at 120°C.

In spite of the exhibited benefits in terms of conduction properties, the number of publications dealing with ionic liquids as intrinsic conductors in PEM is scarce, and the ionic liquids tested are limited to a few. In fact, the main challenge hindering the extended use of ionic liquids as proton conductor in PEMFCs is the phase separation process that takes place between the polymer phase and the ionic liquid during the casting process resulting in inhomogeneous dense membranes. One alternative could rely on the use of porous polymeric membranes as ionic liquid containers, similarly to the supported ionic liquid membrane approach commonly used for gas separations. Thus, 2D nanoporous polymer matrices have already been used for PEM by Yamaguchi's group [33–37] in the so-called "pore filling membrane" concept where a non-ordered porous support is filled with a conducting polymer.

Summarizing, the main goal of this work is to demonstrate the potentialities of encapsulated ionic liquids within porous moieties in the proton exchange membrane field. For such application, two different approaches have been fully studied. The first one relies on the IL immobilization in large pore zeolites, which are further deployed as inorganic fillers to the polymer casting solution [38]. In particular, the encapsulation procedures for different ammonium- and imidazolium-based protic ionic liquids within the microporous framework of hydrophilic FAU and BEA zeolites are deeply studied [39]. The second approach is based on the Yamuguchi concept.

Thus, our electrolyte membrane approach implies a porous polybenzimidazol film (with macro- and/or mesoporous voids) [40] where ionic liquid molecules should be confined [41]. In order to avoid the IL leakage/dragging with time on stream by water reaction molecules, zeolite coating could be deployed as diffusional barriers over supported protic ionic liquid membranes.

After a description of the main physico-chemical properties of the starting materials (i.e., protic ionic liquids, large pore microporous zeolites and macro- mesoporous PBI membranes) in Section 11.2, the encapsulation procedures will be presented, discussed and selected on the basis of proton conduction performance in Section 11.3. To conclude, new research pathways for future development will be briefly introduced in Section 11.4.

11.2 Structure and Properties of Materials for Proton Conduction

For low temperature applications, proton transport properties are mainly attributed to the presence of acid sites and/or water molecules, which, in fact, are controlled by chemical composition, structure and morphology. Understanding how all these properties affect proton conductivity is crucial to develop ad-hoc materials for conduction applications.

Grotthuss mechanism [42] and vehicle mechanism [43] are the most extended postulated mechanisms for conduction phenomena. According to the Grotthuss or Hopping mechanism, protons tunnel from one water molecule to the next via hydrogen bonding. The process consists of two steps, the proton translation from an oxonium ion to a water molecule by tunneling in a hydrogen bond, and subsequent reorientation (rotation) of the released water molecule thus formed, ready for the next H^+ uptake. In contrast, vehicle mechanism involves the presence of mobile carrier such as H_2O or NH_3 molecules to ensure protons migration such as H_3O^+, NH_4^+.

11.2.1 Protic Ionic Liquids

On the basis of the postulated mechanisms for H^+ transport, the family of protic ionic liquids (PILs) appears to be a very attractive set of intrinsic conductors. PILs include those containing at least one H-bond donor site supported either by the cation or the anion.

So, PILs could be systematically synthesized by mixing of Brönsted acid and base [4, 44]. The involved proton transfer is highly exothermic. So, the original acid is not easily regenerated because organic salts are firstly decomposed by heating [44]. Thus, the presence of a mobile proton able to migrate through the PIL donor-acceptor proton network allows conduction under anhydrous and high temperature conditions [45]. For this reason, proton exchangecon membranes (PEMs) based on PILs would not suffer from the common problems encountered at high temperature operation [46, 47]; conditions which are unavoidable to increase FC performance.

In this study, four protic ionic liquids have been used for encapsulation in porous supports: ammonium-based such as ((2-hydromethyl) trimethylammoniun dimethyl phosphate (IL1) and N,N-dimethyl-N-(2-hydroxyethyl) ammonium bis(trifluoromethanesulfonyl)imide (IL2); and imidazolium-based such as: 1-H-3-methylimidazolium bis(trifluoromethanesulfonyl) imide (IL3)) and 1-ethyl-3-methylimidazolium ethyl-phosponate (IL4). The molecular size of IL1 and IL2 is around 6–8 Å; whereas for imidazolium counterparts (IL3, IL4) it exceeds 8 Å. Their main physico-chemical properties are listed in Table 11.1. The selected protic ionic liquids exhibiting decomposition temperatures above 200°C have revealed highly attractive possibilities, not only as embedded proton carriers in porous PBI due to its conductive properties (see Section 11.3.2), but also as guest molecules inside large pore zeolites to eventually improve the proton conduction properties of these microporous inorganic materials (see Section 11.3.1).

11.2.1.1 Basic Characterization of Ionic Liquids

TGA analyses, ATR-FTIR and proton conductive tests have been carried out for PILs characterization. In particular, the conductivity properties of imidazolium-based ionic liquids have been widely described in the published literature [48]. Table 11.1 compiles PILs decomposition temperature values T_d evaluated by TGA carried out from room temperature to 650°C under flowing Ar with a heating rate 5°C·min^{-1}. According to the exhibited values, the selected PILs could allow stable operation at temperatures below 200°C. Quite noteworthy is the decomposition temperature exhibited by IL3 (i.e., 420°C). FTIR spectra of PILs are depicted in Figure 11.1 within the region of 500 to 1500 cm^{-1}, where the main characteristic bands are located.

Before starting the PILs ionic conductivity experiments at 100% RH, the bottom of the autoclave-type electrochemical cell was filled

Table 11.1 Main physico-chemical properties of the protic ionic liquids used in this work.

Structure	Name-abbreviation		$T_d^{(1)}$	$T_m^{(2)}$	μ (25°C)	Supplier
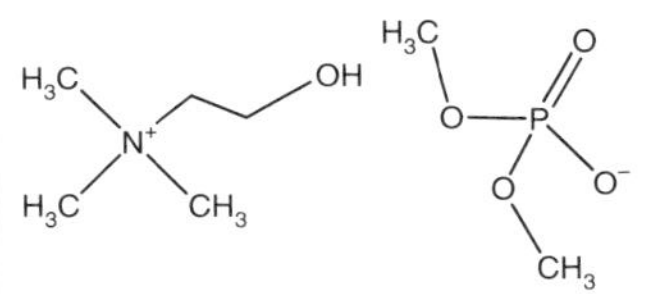	(2-hydroxymethyl) trimethylammonium dimethyl phosphate	IL1	225°C	40°C	-	Solvent Innovation GmbH
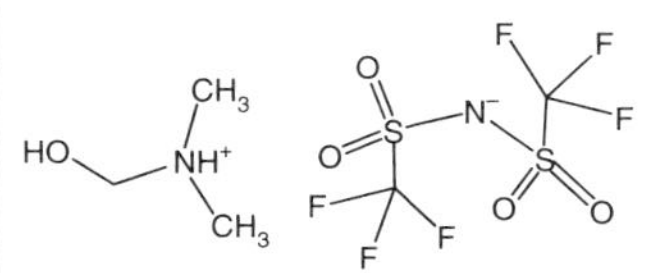	N,N-dimethyl-N-(2-hydroxyethyl) ammonium bis(trifluoromethanesulfonyl) imide	IL2	378°C	-	-	Solvionic(3)
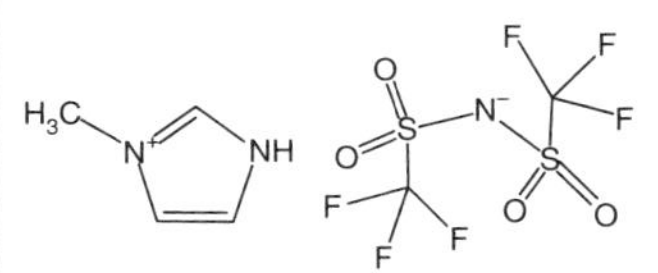	1-H-3-methylimidazolium bis(trifluoromethanesulfonyl) imide	IL3	420°C	9°C	81 cp	Solvionic(3)
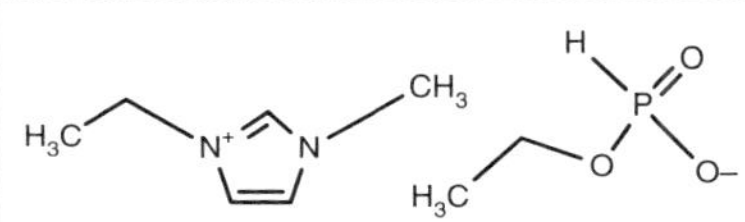	1-ethyl-3-methylimidazolium ethyl-phosphonate	IL4	275°C	-	140 cp	Solvionic(3)

(1) Decomposition Temperature; (2) Melting point; (3) http://en.solvionic.com/

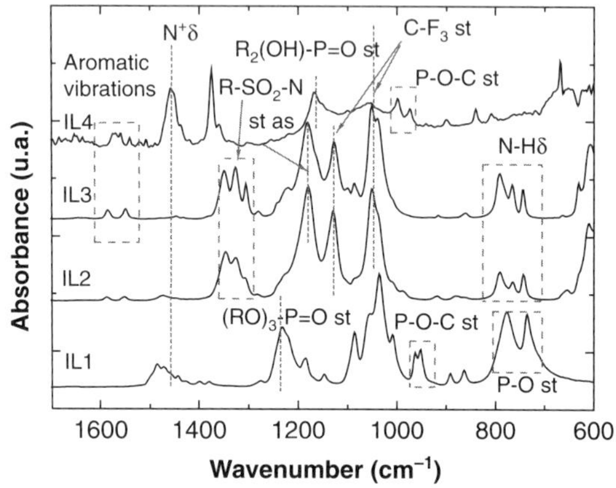

Figure 11.1 FTIR sprectra of studied PILs.

up with 100 cm^3 of distilled water DD to attain its vapor pressure once the chamber is closed. On the contrary, for dry conditions, the electrochemical cell previously stored at 80°C overnight was carefully assembled using dry inert gas to prevent water traces. Figure 11.2 shows PILs conductivity data versus temperature. In general, the conductivity values obtained at saturated conditions are higher due to the presence of water that provides additional pathways for H^+ transport. However, a distinct behavior between ammonium-based (IL1, IL2) and imidazolium-based (IL3, IL4) PILs could be ascertained on the basis of estimated Arrhenius activation energies (Table 11.2). In the case of ammonium-based PILs, the presence of water decreases the Ea values for H^+ transport due to the hydrophilicy/water solubility properties of IL1 and IL2. On the other hand, for the less hydrophilic imidazolium-based ionic liquids (IL3 and IL4), the Ea values for H^+ transport increase at saturated conditions. This behaviour is in agreement with the coexistence of hydrophilic and hydrophobic moieties within the electrolyte solution.

11.2.2 Porous Materials: Zeolites, PBI

11.2.2.1 Zeolites

Zeolites are perhaps the most widely employed group of silicon-based nanoporous solids. The term zeolites designate a variety of crystalline, hydrated aluminosilicates with framework structure. Their well defined pores of subnanometric size have earned them the name of molecular sieves, meaning that operation in the size

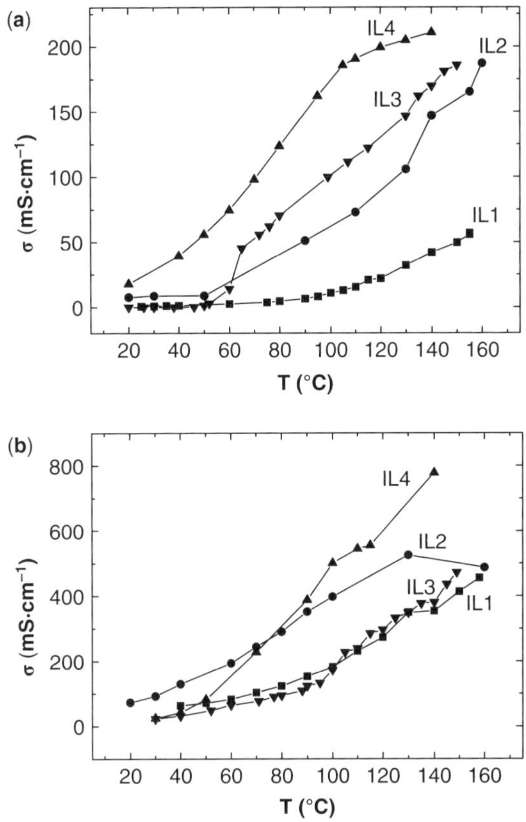

Figure 11.2 Conductivity performance of pure ionic liquids: a) dry conditions; b) saturated conditions.

Table 11.2 Arrhenius type activation energies for proton transport in the studied PILs.

PILs	Ea (kJ/mol)	
	Dry conditions	Saturated conditions
IL1	40.0	23.1
IL2	29.3	18.7
IL3	22.4	30.7
IL4	23.7	36.8

exclusion regime is possible by selecting, among over 200 structures available, the zeolite whose pores allow the desired molecule to pass, while keeping larger molecules outside. In addition, the adsorption properties of the zeolites can be fine-tuned by adjusting their Si/Al ratio (that determines to a large extent the hydrophobic/hydrophilic and polar/nonpolar character of the host-guest interactions between the zeolite and the fluid phase molecules) and their exchange cations [49]. Recently, zeolites were chosen as one of the top 10 runners-up to become the scientific breakthrough of 2011 [50], indicating that a large research effort will be focused on this field in the near future.

Zeolites and related microporous materials have been proposed as alternative materials in ionic conducting membranes for direct methanol fuel cells (DMFC) because of their regular micropores that provide selective separations based on adsorption properties, as well as molecular size and shape effects. Accordingly, they are quite appropriate to reduce fuel crossover phenomena. In addition, their tailored hydrophilic properties coupled to their excellent thermal resistance make them ideal fillers to improve the water uptake properties of ionomeric membranes at temperatures above 150°C for high temperature proton exchange membrane fuel cells (HTPEMFCs).

Zeolites do not exhibit electron conductivity due to their band gap of several eV. However, the extra-framework cations, electrostatically bound to the host lattice, are capable of ion transport [51]. In fact, previous studies assign zeolite conduction properties to compensation cation migration [52]. It is well known that in zeolite frameworks, every aluminum joined to oxygen generates a negative charge, which is compensated by mobile extra-framework cations. Thereby, proton transport by the Grotthus mechanism is possible when those cations are solvated by the presence of water (Figure 11.3). Thus, proton exchanged zeolites could be beneficial for proton conduction; but experimental conductivity values of H+ exchanged zeolites are two orders of magnitude lower than Na+ exchanged counterparts [53] due to the strong interactions between proton and T-O-T atoms (T=Si, Al). More noticeable is the water sorption behavior, capable of significantly increasing the ionic conductivity values up to 10^{-4} **S·cm^{-1}** [54].

The two previously described proton conduction mechanisms are also present in zeolites: i) vehicle-type mechanism (mainly assisted by water molecules as proton carriers), and; ii) Grotthus

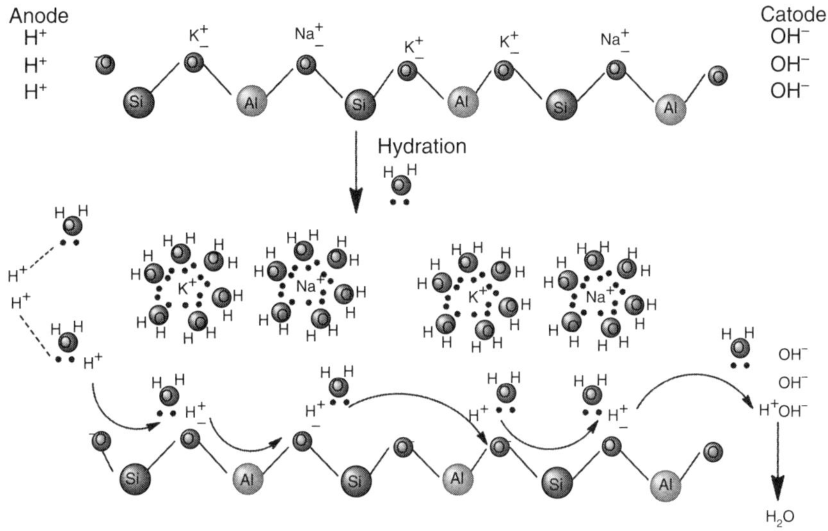

Figure 11.3 Proton transport mechanisms in zeolites and related materials.

mechanism involving proton hopping between neighboring equilibrium sites. Both proton conduction pathways are illustrated in Figure 11.3 for hydrated zeolites. In the hydrated state, the electrostatic forces between extra-framework cations and the zeolite lattice are weakened due to solvation. Depending on the zeolite, the physi- and chemisorbed water molecules sustain the ionic conductivity up to 200°–325°C [55].

The main features of the synthetic BEA and FAU large pore zeolites herein studied for PILs encapsulation are shown in the next section.

11.2.2.1.1 BEA type zeolite

Beta zeolite was discovered before Mobil began the "ZSM" naming sequence. As the name implies, it was the second in an earlier sequence. Its framework topology consists of an intergrowth of two distinct structures termed Polymorphs A and B with a three dimensional network of channels defined by 12 T (Al or Si) membered rings (Figure 11.4). The polymorphs grow as two-dimensional sheets randomly alternated [56]. The intergrowth of the polymorphs does not significantly affect the pores in two of the dimensions, but in the faulting direction it becomes tortuous. The unit cell is tetragonal ($P4_122$, a = 12.6Å, c = 26.2Å).

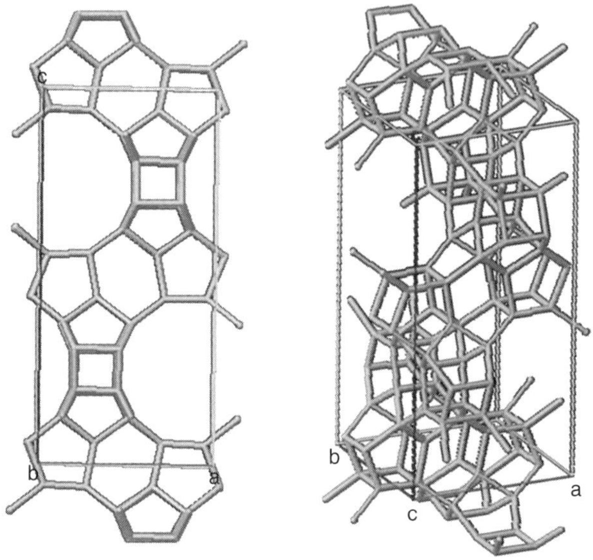

Figure 11.4 BEA framework (channel size: 6.6×6.7 – 5.6×5.6 Å) viewed along a) [010]; b) [111].

The Si/Al ratio of the commercial NH_4-BEA-type zeolite herein studied is 12.5. It favors proton transport due to: i) the higher proximity between electron deficient zones; and, ii) the higher concentration of compensation cations with solvation properties.

11.2.2.1.2 NaY type zeolite

NaY type zeolite exhibits the FAU (faujasite) structure. Its framework topology consists of a three-dimensional pore structure with pores running perpendicular to each other. The pore opening is defined by 12 T membered rings and leads into a larger β cavity (13 Å in diameter). The cavity is surrounded by ten sodalite cages (truncated octahedral) connected on their hexagonal faces (Figure 11.5). The unit cell is cubic (a = 24.7 Å) with Fd-3m symmetry.

The Si/Al ratio of the commercial NaY-type zeolite herein studied is 2.8; thus, more hydrophilic than the BEA counterpart.

Figure 11.6 shows conduction performance of pristine zeolites under saturation conditions [38, 57]. When zeolites are fully hydrated, vehicle mechanism is prevalent for H^+ transport. On the other hand, hopping mechanism is possible due to extra-framework

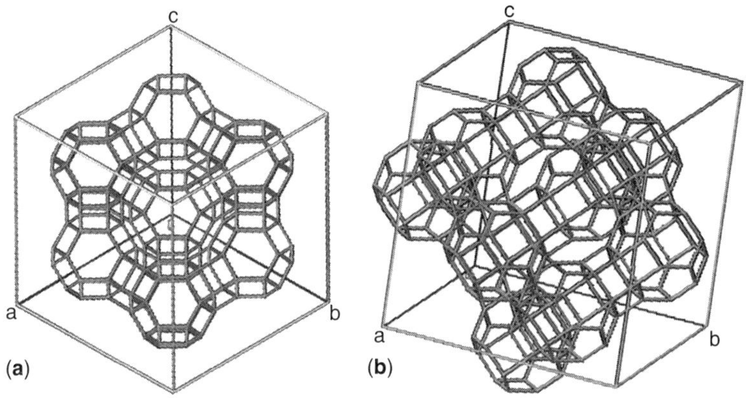

Figure 11.5 FAU framework (Channel size 7.4×7.4Å) viewed along: a) [110]; b) [111].

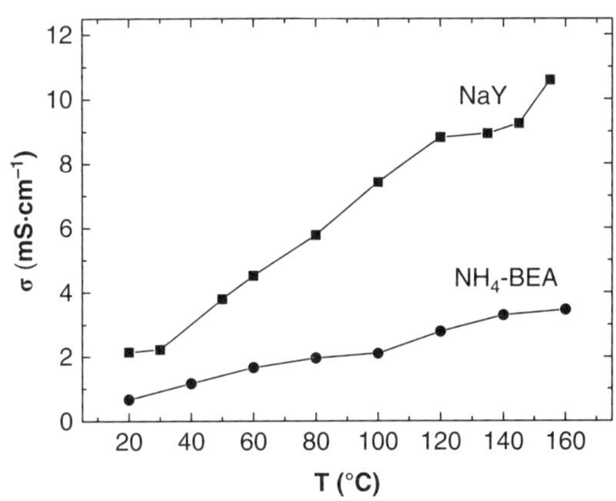

Figure 11.6 Conduction performance of pristine zeolites under saturated conditions.

cation solvation. The exhibited NaY conduction properties vs. BEA counterpart could be explained by the Na^+ solvation capability (vs. NH_4^+) and its hydrophilic nature.

11.2.2.2 Polybenzimidazol (PBI)

The Polybenzimidazol (PBI) polymer is well known for its excellent thermal and chemical stability and mechanical properties. It has a glass transition temperature of about 450°C and melting point of up to 600°C because of its all-aromatic structure (see Figure 11.7). Pure

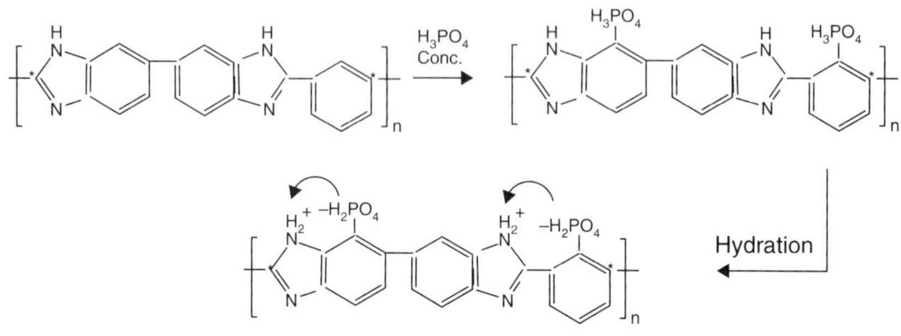

Figure 11.7 PBI (poly [2,2 - (m-phenylene) -5,5-bibenzimidazole]) structure before and after phosphoric acid doping.

PBI is an electronic and ionic insulator which becomes a very good ionic conductor when it is modified by acids under proper conditions. The benzimidazole group has a pKa of about 5.5 due to the presence of secondary amines with Lewis base properties [58, 59]. This fact facilitates mineral acids sorption. PBI has been doped with several acids, sulfuric and phosphoric being the most extensively used. Under standard conditions, the best results were obtained for the weaker phosphoric acid doping due to the fact that this acid is weaker facilitating proton donation to be accepted by secondary amines to generate NH^{+}-. Thus, proton conductivity significantly increases when the membrane is hydrated [60], becoming an acid-based membrane able to H^{+} transport by vehicle and hopping mechanisms [61]. However, degradation and durability issues of phosphoric acid doped PBI membranes remain unsolved at temperatures above 140°C due to oligomerization and acid leaching.

All the PBI-based membranes studied in this work were prepared from commercial Fumion® APH polymer (purchased to FuMA-Tech GmbH) with average molecular weight and inherent viscosity values of 59–62 kDa and 91–95 $cm^{3}\cdot g^{-1}$, respectively.

11.2.2.2.1 Porous Membranes Preparation

Porous polymeric membranes with a controlled thickness (15–90 μm), porosity (60%–85% values and nominal pore sizes below 5 μm) and mechanical, chemical and thermal stability up to 200°C, are required for high temperature PEMFC applications according to the approach herein considered. For such purposes two different types of preparation routes were studied: i) the inverse phase separation method, and ii) the leaching of a porogen.

11.2.2.2.1.1 Delayed Demixing Method

The phase separation of the PBI solution is performed by a two-step coagulation process to avoid a rapid demixing resulting in macrovoid formation. Poly[2,2-(m-phenylene)-5,5-bibenzimidazole] powder has been dissolved in N-methyl-2-Pyrrolidone (NMP) at 160°C for 24 h to obtain 18 %wt of solids in polymer solution. The addition of LiCl as stabilizing agent (2 %wt) was necessary to avoid the reversible phasing out of the polymer after two week's storage at room temperature. High- and low-molecular PVP (K 90 (Mw = 360 kDa) K 30 (Mw = 40 kDa)) were deployed as weak solvents to promote macrovoid suppression during the phase separation process. The nominal composition solution is PBI (12%) / PVP K30 (2%) / PVP K90 (2%) / NMP (82%) / LiCl (2%). Before use, the PBI solution is filtered by pressurized air through metal filter (25 μm in pore size) to remove insoluble solids from the starting PBI powder.

The membrane casting was performed at 20°C over the surface of glass plates by using a 0.1 μm casting knife, and immediately placed in the coagulation bath. Firstly, the cast polymer solution is immersed in NMP/Water (50/50) mixture during 30 minutes [62]. Subsequently, the membrane formation is completed in a second coagulation bath containing DD water for 1 h. Finally, the membrane is immersed in DD water to rinse out the last traces of solvent and stored in pure water. The most remarkable feature is that no macrovoids are identified along and across the membrane confirming the viability of the preparation procedure. The so-obtained wet porous PBI membranes are subjected to successive washing steps from less polar (ethanol) to nonpolar (hexane) solvents to avoid membrane collapse, and finally were dried under vacuum at 200°C for 4 h before use.

11.2.2.2.1.2 Porogen Leaching Method

PBI membranes are obtained by casting from a polymer solution (5 wt% in DMAc) containing the porogen agent (dibutyl phthalate (DBP) or triphenyl phosphate (TPP)) on a glass plate support [40].

Poly[2,2-(m-phenylene)-5,5-bibenzimidazole] powder has been dissolved in N-N dimethylacetamide (DMAc) under autogenous pressure at 240°C for 24 h to obtain 5 %wt of solids in polymer solution. Porous proton-conducting membranes were obtained by solution casting from a polymer solution using DMAc as solvent.

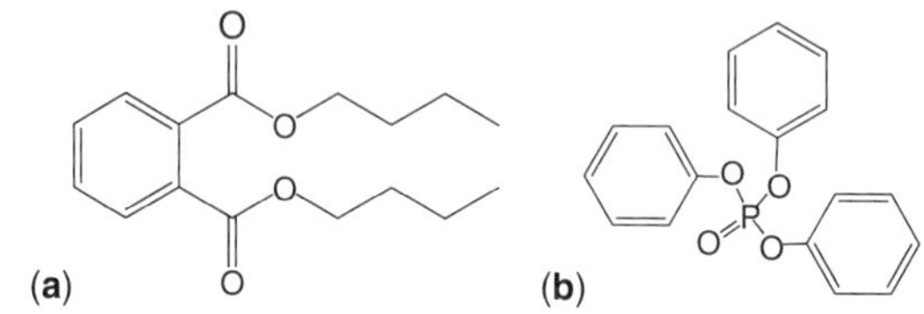

Figure 11.8 Porogen molecules used in this work: a) DBP y b) TPP.

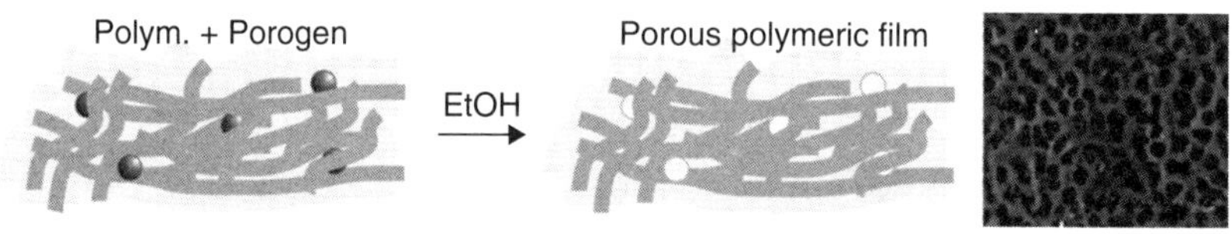

Figure 11.9 Schematic representation of the porous PBI films formation by porogen leaching using ethanol as solvent.

Appropiate amounts of DBP or TPP (Figure 11.8.) as porogen, molecules were added to prepare PBI membranes 45, 60 and 75% in porosity. The films were dried on a heating plate for 1 h at room temperature, 2 h at 80°C, 4 h at 120°C and finally 2 h at 180°C. The polymer film was separated from the glass plate support by immersion in water. Afterwards, porous polybenzimidazole films were obtained by leaching out the low-molecular-weight porogen compound using ethanol/methanol as selective solvents. For such purposes, all the membranes were washed three-fold in ethanol at 50°C for one hour. The schematic representation of the porosity release process is depicted in Figure 11.9.

11.2.2.2.2 Morphological Characterization of Randomly Porous PBI Films

Because the polymer membrane architecture plays the key role to ensure proton transport through heterogeneous media, the morphology of the so-obtained porous PBI films was systematically characterized by SEM. Porosity, average pore size and thickness values of the porous PBI films studied in this work are summarized in Table 11.3.

Figures 11.10, 11.11 and 11.12 show the SEM images of the as-prepared porous membranes prepared for this work. As it can be observed, different porous structure morphologies (size, shape and coordination number) are provided for each of the studied

Table 11.3 PBI porous films studied in this work.

<table>
<tr><th>Membrane</th><th colspan="2">Method</th><th>Porosity (%)</th><th>Pore size (μm)</th><th>thickness (μm)</th></tr>
<tr><td>PBI_60DBP</td><td>Porogen</td><td>DBP</td><td>60</td><td>2–5</td><td rowspan="4">60–90</td></tr>
<tr><td>PBI_75DBP</td><td>Porogen</td><td>DBP</td><td>75</td><td>2–5</td></tr>
<tr><td>PBI_60TTP</td><td>Porogen</td><td>TPP</td><td>60</td><td>< 1; 2–5</td></tr>
<tr><td>PBI_75TTP</td><td>Porogen</td><td>TPP</td><td>75</td><td>2–5</td></tr>
<tr><td>PBI_65DM</td><td colspan="2">Delayed de-mixing</td><td>65</td><td>< 1</td><td rowspan="2">15–25</td></tr>
<tr><td>PBI_85DM</td><td colspan="2">Delayed de-mixing</td><td>85</td><td>< 1</td></tr>
</table>

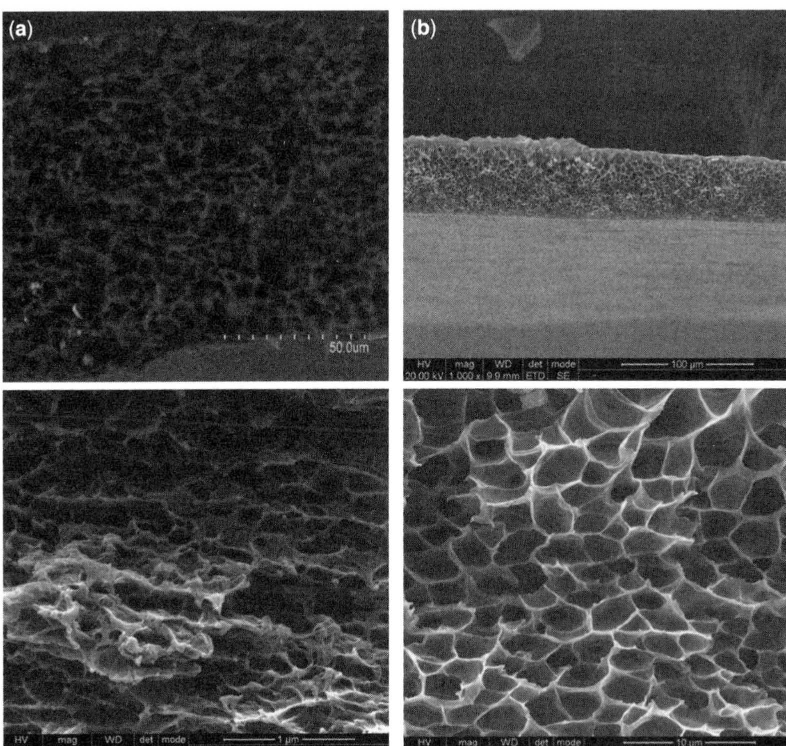

Figure 11.10 SEM analyses of the cross section of porous PBI films prepared by leaching DBP porogen: a) 60 % in porosity; b) 75 % in porosity.

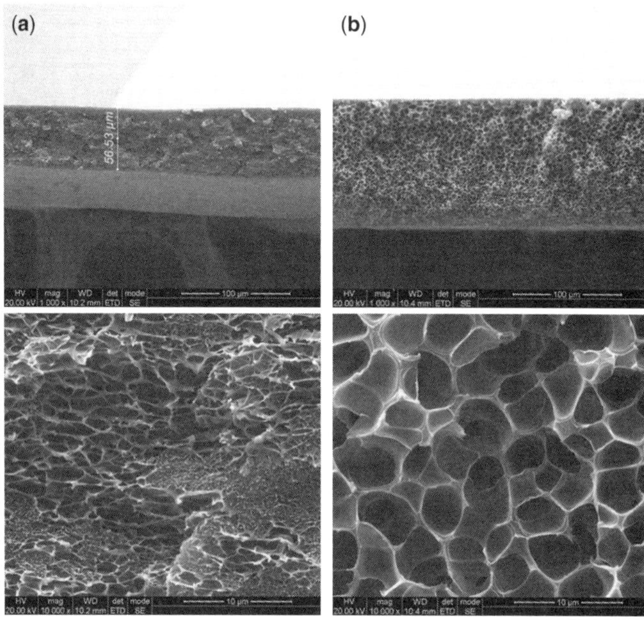

Figure 11.11 SEM analyses of the cross section of porous PBI films prepared by leaching TPP porogen: a) 60 % in porosity; b) 75 % in porosity.

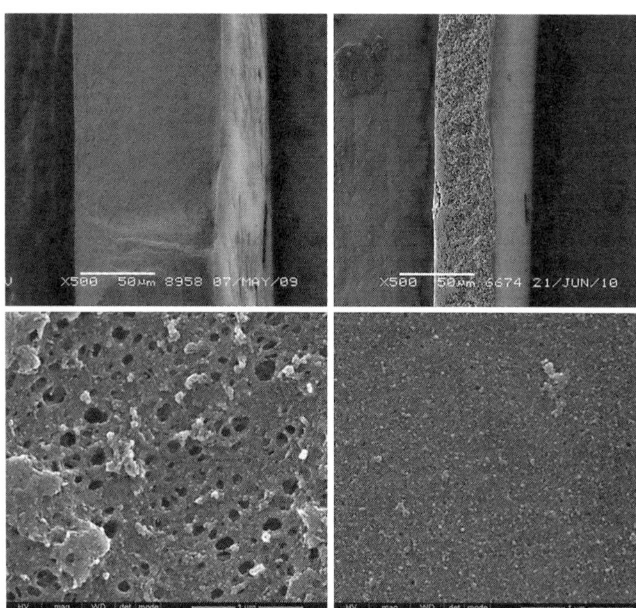

Figure 11.12 SEM analyses of porous PBI films prepared by delayed-demixing method: top side) cross section view for 65% (left) and 85% (right) in porosity; botton side) top section views for 85% in porosity.

methodologies. In general, the porogen method allows control over the macroporosity level (the higher the porogen content, the higher pore size and total pore volume) and the morphology by adjusting the porogen/PBI ratio and the chemical nature of the porogen [40].

In this work, the addition of DBP porogen in a 75 %wt referred to the polymer, on one hand provides interconnected pores with an irregular shape of 2–10 μm (see Figure 11.10), well-suited to attain uninterrupted proton conduction pathways after PILs encapsulation; but, on the other hand, durability issues related to the PIL dragging are likely to occur. By changing the porogen-type molecule, from DBP to the aromatic TPP, smaller and less interconnected pores are obtained; although these differences become less notorious with the porogen content (Figure 11.11).

The most remarkable feature for porous PBI films prepared by delayed demixing is that no macrovoids are identified along and across the membrane thickness (Figure 11.12) whatever the porosity level; confirming the viability of the preparation procedure. SEM micrographs of both external porous PBI surfaces are shown in Figure 11.12 for 85% porosity membrane. Pore size values around 200 nm and 40 nm could be identified on the top (air side) and bottom (glass side), respectively.

11.3 Encapsulation Procedures and Proton Conduction Performance

11.3.1 Encapsulation in Zeolite-Type Materials

11.3.1.1 Encapsulation Procedures

The synthesized Protic Ionic Liquids exhibiting decomposition temperatures above 200°C have revealed highly attractive possibilities as guest molecules inside large pore zeolites to eventually improve the proton conduction properties of these microporous inorganic materials. For such purposes, two different "wet impregnation" methods (i.e., Method 1 and Method 2) for outgassed zeolite powders with PILs solutions have been deeply studied to define the best encapsulation procedure.

These PIL-zeolite composites could be further deployed as fillers to the casting solution of conventional high temperature PEM to improve membrane performance. Furthermore, the encapsulation of PILs inside microporous cavities could alleviate or eventually suppress the PIL dragging phenomena in presence of water reaction molecules with time on stream. Thus, the as-conceived membranes could maintain a satisfactory extended PEMFC operation at temperatures above 100°C without gases humidification to accomplish power density requirements.

In a step further, these membranes might be able to operate in absence of mineral acids after adequate membrane activation processes, or by fine tuning temperature and humidity conditions within the stack. The final aim is the controlled PILs delivery from the internal microporous cavities to the external surface of zeolite crystals, to provide donor-acceptor sites for proton hopping through the membrane thickness [38]. According to this approach, the higher PIL-zeolite composite loading, the higher the number of intrinsic conductor reservoirs to ensure stable operation.

11.3.1.1.1 Method 1

Method 1 involves the following steps: i) zeolite evacuation step at 100°C at 1 mm Hg for 20 min to remove physisorbed species; ii) preparation of IL solution in a nonpolar solvent such as dichloroethane with a 1:9 wt. ratio; iii) zeolite addition to the IL solution at 1:1 IL-Z wt ratio; iv) vigorous stirring at room temperature for 24 hours; v) Sohxlet extraction to remove the IL excess from the surface at solvent reflux temperature (85°C) for 2 hours; and vi) final drying at 100°C overnight in an oven.

11.3.1.1.2 Method 2

Similarly, for those samples prepared according to Method 2, the following procedure has been used: i) zeolite crystals outgassing for ~24 hrs at 300°C under vacuum; ii) IL solution in methanol (99.9%); iii) zeolite addition to the IL solution at 1:1 IL-Z wt ratio; iv) heating of the suspension at 90°C overnight for solvent evaporation; and v) final drying at 130°C for ~8 hrs. The entire procedure was carried out in a glove bag filled with Ar. In order to remove the excess of the ionic liquid, Soxhlet extraction with methanol at solvent reflux temperature (65°C) was also performed in some samples (denoted as Method 2 + soxhlet).

11.3.1.2 Characterization

The as-prepared PIL-zeolite composites, similarly to PILs, have been characterized by ATR-FTIR and TGA analyses. On the contrary, the proton conductivity measurements at 100% relative humidity have

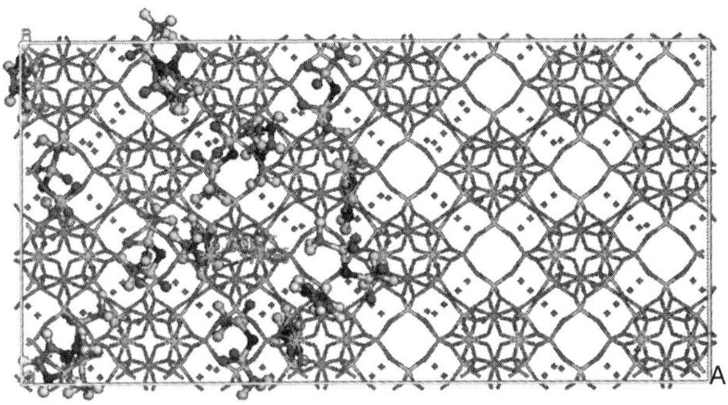

Figure 11.13 Super-cell structure constituted of two adjacent faujasite unit cells in NaY type zeolite, one of which (left) was initially full of IL3 protic ionic liquid, while the other one (right) was initially empty.

been performed following the protocol used for pristine zeolites. In addition, conduction tests at typical water partial pressure values in PEMFC y_{H_2O}=5%, using N_2 as carrier gas, have also been carried out.

In the case of NaY-type zeolite, molecular dynamics simulations [63] show that the protic ionic liquids fit energetically inside the faujasite cells and their ions are mobile within the zeolite framework [64] (Figure 11.13).

11.3.1.2.1 ATR-FTIR Analyses

ATR-FTIR analyses (VERTEX 70 equipment with microscope slide MKII Golden Gate ATR from 4000 to 600 cm^{-1}, 256 scans and resolution of 0.05 cm^{-1}) were performed over NaY- (Figure 11.14) and NH_4BEA-based (Figure 11.15) composites, respectively. The starting zeolites and PILs have also been depicted for comparison purposes. The obtained spectra reveal the existence of the protic ionic liquids in all the composites prepared with independence of the preparation conditions. This observation is also corroborated by FT-Raman spectroscopy studies carried out in previous works [39, 63, 65]. In general, no relevant changes can be observed in the Raman spectra of composite samples in comparison with pristine PILs, although variations in the relative intensities are identified in agreement either with conformational changes of the voluminous ions inside the zeolite cavities or with extra-framework cation exchange processes.

As was expected, the characteristic PILs FTIR assignments are more pronounced for those samples not exposed to the final Sohxlet extraction step to remove the PIL excess.

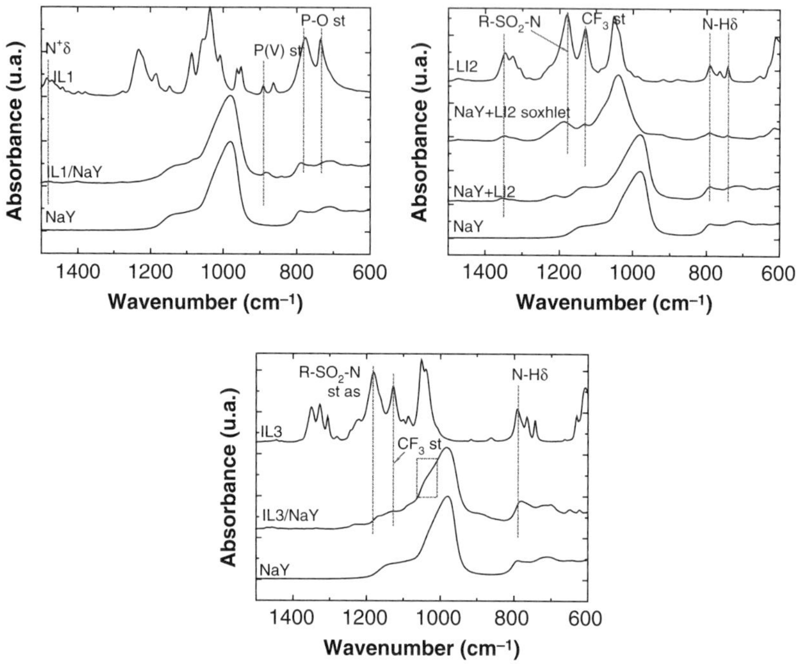

Figure 11.14 ATR-FTIR analyses of PIL-NaY based composites: (top left) IL1/NaY; (top right) IL2/NaY; (bottom) IL3/NaY.

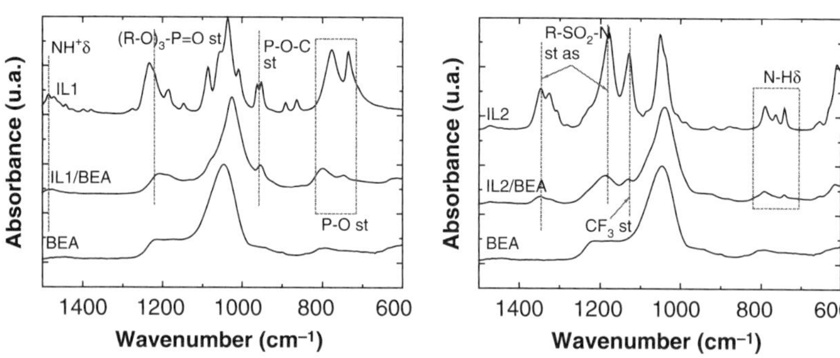

Figure 11.15 ATR-FTIR analysis of ammonium PIL-BEA type zeolite composites: (left) IL1/BEA; (right) IL2/BEA.

11.3.1.2.1 Thermogravimetric Analyses

The final amount of PIL entrapped onto the zeolite host has been determined by TGA analyses for quantification purposes (Table 11.4). The differential thermograms have also been depicted to illustrate the water and IL thermal events (Figure 11.16). It is also

Table 11.4 Estimated composition of the PIL-zeolite composites prepared in this work by TGA analyses.

Sample	Method 1		Method 2	
	PIL (wt %)	H_2O (wt %)	PIL (wt %)	H_2O (wt %)
IL1/NaY	29.3	5.3	33.2	3.9
IL2/NaY	17.0	8.6	21.5	9.3
IL2/NaY	-	-	15.1*	8.3*
IL3/NaY	17.5	3.5	-	-
IL1/BEA	28.8	8.4	36.3	4.4
IL2/BEA	5.0	2.1	31.7	1.0

*Prepared by Method 2 + soxhlet.

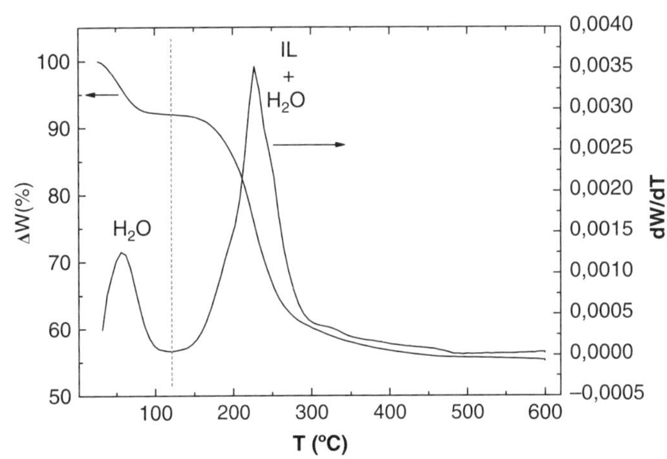

Figure 11.16 TGA analysis of IL1/BEA prepared by method 1.

noticeable that ILs decompose in the same temperature range (circa 225–255°C for IL1) when encapsulated. For Method 1 (PIL solution in a nonpolar solvent) and a given zeolite host, the IL1 loadings are always higher than their IL2 counterparts (29.3% wt vs. 17% wt for NaY composites), in agreement with the lower molecular size of dimethyl phosphate anion. Among the tested, the lower encapsulation percentage is registered for IL3 due to its minor hydrophilicity in comparison with ammonium counterparts.

The microporous zeolite framework seems to have no influence in the case of IL1 (29.3% wt for NaY vs. 28.8% wt for BEA composites), but it is relevant for IL2 (17% wt for NaY vs. 5% wt for BEA composites) where steric factors and diffusional limitations in BEA structure could be rate controlling.

According to TGA results, Method 2 (PIL solution in a polar solvent) seems to provide higher encapsulation values whatever the zeolite composite formulation. This observation could be explained by preferential PIL-zeolite interactions over solvent-PIL/solvent-zeolite interactions and/or the absence of the final Soxhlet extraction step. The exhibited behavior by IL2/NaY sample prepared by Method 2 underlines the importance of PIL excess removal whatever the solvent used. As can be observed, Method 1 and Method 2 yield to similar PIL loadings (17.0 vs. 15.1 for IL2/NaY) when identical washing procedures are carried out.

Summarizing, both methods are suitable to encapsulate the PILs while preserving the zeolite framework. In spite of the higher IL loadings attained without Soxhlet extraction, this last preparation step is highly recommended for stability and reproducibility issues.

11.3.1.2.3 Conduction Performance

Unlike pristine materials, the PIL-zeolite composites show a gradual increase of conductivity up to a maximum followed by a decrease with temperature (Figures 11.18, 11.20). Synergic-inhibition effects between both proton conductors (i.e., encapsulated protic ionic liquids and H_2O vapor molecules) coupled to

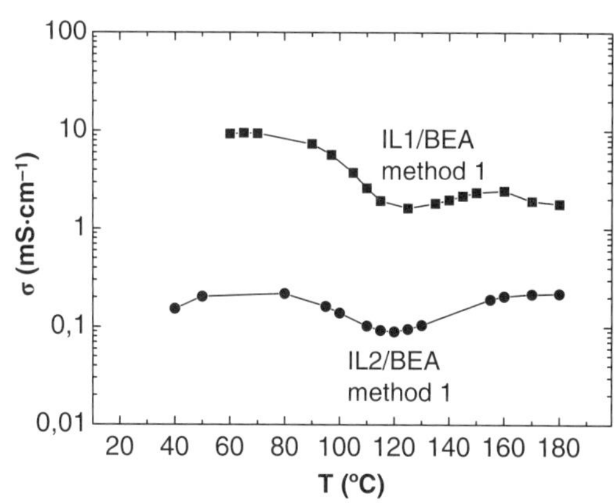

Figure 11.17 Conductivity performance in presence of 5% RH for materials based on BEA composites.

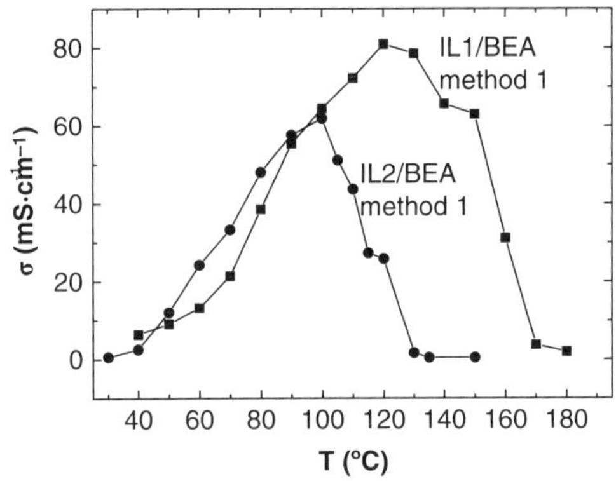

Figure 11.18 Conductivity performance in presence of 100% RH for materials based on BEA composites.

protic ionic liquid dragging from micropores by water desorption, could explain the observed behavior. The maximum location depends on the hydrophilicity, not only of the zeolitic host but also on the ionic liquid itself. Once physisorbed water molecules have been completely removed from the composites, a gradual increase of conductivity (Arrhenius dependence) due to the remaning PILs molecules should be observed unless PIL decomposition occurs.

The conduction performance at saturated conditions of NaY-based composites prepared following Methods 1 and 2 is shown in Figure 11.20. For a given composite, Method 2 provides with lower conductivity properties in the medium temperature region (19 mS·cm^{-1} vs. 42.8 mS·cm^{-1} for IL2/NaY y 9.9 mS·cm^{-1} vs. 17.5 mS·cm^{-1} for IL1/NaY at 110°C). Accordingly, Method 1 has been systematically used for the remaining conductivity measurements. At 100% relative humidity, IL3/NaY composite seems to be the most adequate for proton transport among those tested. For this sample, the controlling steps for proton transport are clearly affected by temperature. The initial conductivity increase with temperature up to the exhibited maximum at 100°C (78 mS·cm^{-1}) is mainly attributed to the presence of continuos PIL channels inside micropores due to its relative low water solubility. Vehicle mechanism assisted by water and hopping mechanism through PIL network are synergistically combined. Then, conductivity starts to decrease up to exhibited minimum at 120°C (30 mS·cm^{-1}). This decay could be explained by PILs

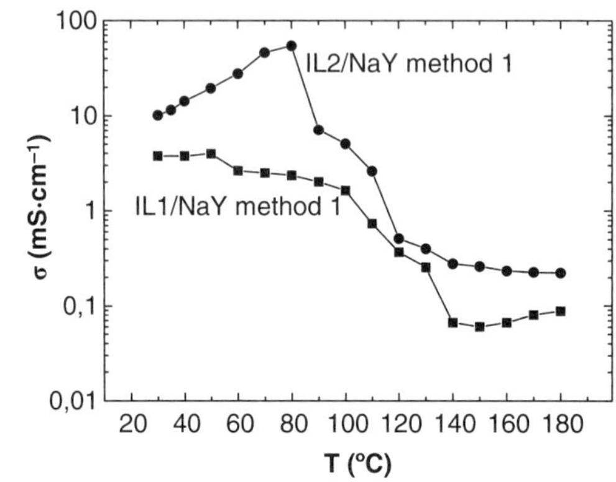

Figure 11.19 Conductivity performance in presence of 5 % RH for materials based on NaY composites.

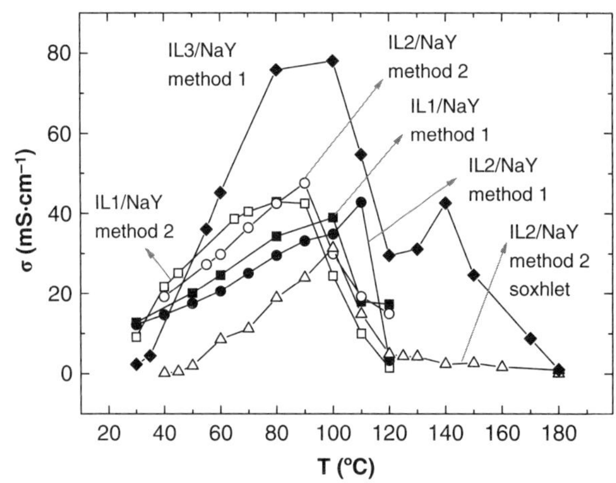

Figure 11.20 Conductivity performance in presence of 100% RH for materials based on NaY composites.

replacement from microporous cavities by less conducting water molecules due to the highly hydrophilic nature of NaY-type zeolite (Si/Al ratio=2.8). Afterwards, conductivity increases again (45 mS·cm^{-1} 140°C) due to the activated proton transport assisted by PILs molecules on the external crystals surface. Under saturated conditions, further temperature increase (above 140°C) leads to physisorbed water desorption coupled to PILs dragging from the solid. Accordingly, proton conductivity starts to decay due to proton conductor losses.

When comparing IL1/NaY vs. IL2/NaY under typical water partial pressures in a PEMFC (y_{H_2O}=5%), the observed behaviour is somewhat different (Figure 11.19). These results indicate that conduction performance in the low-medium temperature region is not only due to the IL molecules trapped inside the zeolite framework; and competition effects between zeolite and IL for water molecules take place hindering, in some cases, the protons migration. For IL1, the less hydrophilic material, a beneficial water effect (either as proton vehicle or to promote compensation-cation solvation) is prevalent (i.e., 2.4 $mS{\cdot}cm^{-1}$ vs. 34 $mS{\cdot}cm^{-1}$ at 80°C and 5% and 100% RH, respectively). In a different way, for the hydrophilic and more voluminous IL2, the water inhibition effects are quite notorious (i.e., 52.1 $mS{\cdot}cm^{-1}$ vs. 28.5 $mS{\cdot}cm^{-1}$ at 80°C for 5% and 100% RH, respectively). In this case, not only the IL2-encapsulated molecules but also the acid zeolite sites are competing for water adsorption inside the heavily-trafficked zeolite framework, hindering the proton motion through either the solvated IL2 acid-base network or the zeolite framework.

The conduction performance of BEA-based composites at 100% RH and y_{H_2O}=5% is shown in Figures 11.18 and 11.17, respectively. One of the most remarkable features is that the conductivity drops occur at temperature slightly higher (up to 130°C for IL2/BEA at 100% RH), probably due to the less hydrophilic nature of BEA zeolite (Si/Al ratio=12.5).

Under saturated conditions, the IL2/BEA composites outperform IL1-based counterparts in the medium temperature region (46.5 $mS{\cdot}cm^{-1}$ vs. 36.3 $mS{\cdot}cm^{-1}$ at 80°C). On the contrary, at temperatures above 100°C the behavior is just the opposite (0.43 $mS{\cdot}cm^{-1}$ vs. 61 $mS{\cdot}cm^{-1}$ at 150°C). These observations are in agreement with the low IL2 loading values (around 5% wt), which are not enough to form a continuous percolating path for proton conduction. In the low–medium temperature region, this effect is hindered by the beneficial water adsorption; but becomes more noticeable as temperature increases. It is worthwhile to mention that under saturated conditions, IL2/BEA composites perform similarly to IL3/NaY. However, the second maximum is not observed for IL2/BEA composite due to the less conductive properties of the ammonium-based PIL.

When the water partial pressure decreases up to 4.2 kPa (y_{H_2O}~5%), the IL contribution to the proton conduction is higher and therefore the filling of the zeolite pores by IL is crucial (9 $mS \cdot cm^{-1}$ vs. 0.2 $mS \cdot cm^{-1}$ at 80°C for IL1/BEA and IL2/BEA, respectively). The amount of IL2 incorporated might be too low to ensure a continuous pathway of IL inside the porous framework. Therefore, the proton IL network is somewhere interrupted and mainly the IL2 molecules are playing the role of zeolite competitors for water adsorption, inhibiting the solvation of extra-framework cations.

Summarizing, for ammonium-based PILs, BEA composites outperform NaY counterparts under saturated conditions. In principle, this result could seem a bit contradictory due to the hydrophilic properties of NaY host, but it could be fairly understood when proton conductor molecules trapped in the zeolite cavities are in competition for water adsorption with the zeolite framework. Accounting from the results obtained at 4.2 kPa water partial pressure, it could be concluded that IL1/BEA arises at the most adequate for HT PEMFCs applications; whereas IL3/NaY composite is the most promising at temperatures below 100°C.

11.3.2 Encapsulation in Membrane Materials

The conduction properties of bulky protic ionic liquids coupled to their physical and chemical properties have been the main factors that motivated the study of supported protic ionic liquid membranes. The development of experimental procedures (assisted by vacuum and/or temperature) to achieve a complete filling of the porous supports by protic ionic liquids and avoid its leakage, is one of the main challenges for this dual system. Table 11.5 shows the main textural properties of the inorganic (commercial anodized alumina) and organic (PBI) containers studied in this work. Hence, the required protic ionic liquid amount to fill the membrane porosity could be estimated.

The proton conduction over SILMs based on porous PBI, unlike phosphoric acid doped porous PBI membranes, primarily depends not only on support porosity but also on pore connectivity (coordination number denoted as z) as revealed by modelling studies (Figure 11.21). In general, the conductivity values of heterogeneous media increase markedly with porosity for values above the percolation threshold. Therefore, the conduction performance of the SILMs herein studied has been somewhat limited due to the availability of adequate PBI porous supports.

Table 11.5 Textural properties of the porous membranes used as containers for ionic liquids.

	Track-etched membranes	Randomly porous membranes		
	APA	PBI		
	Anodisk	DBP	DM	
Porosity	0.7	0.60	0.65	0.85
Bulk Density ($g{\cdot}mL^{-1}$)	1.51	0.54	0.75	0.43
Skeletal Density ($g{\cdot}mL^{-1}$)	2.74	1.62	2.14	2.89
Estimated IL loading ($g{\cdot}g^{-1}$) by gravimetric	1	1.43	1.30	-
Estimated IL loading ($g{\cdot}g^{-1}$) by TGA	0.70	1	3.16	11.5

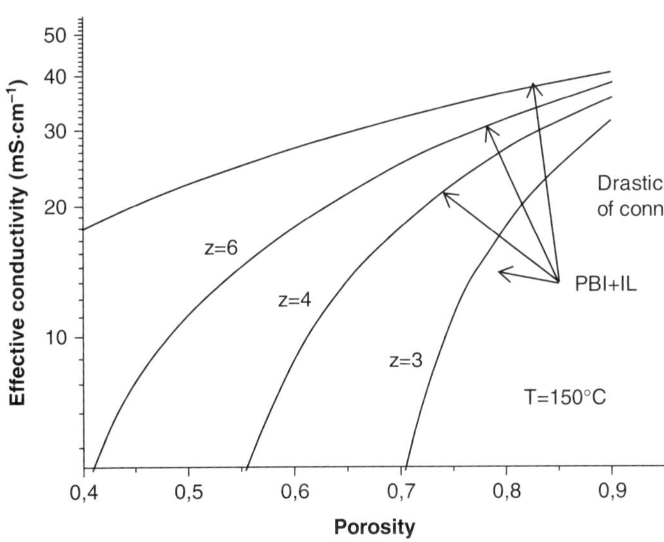

Figure 11.21 Modelling results of conduction performance on porous media by Effective Medium Theory.

11.3.2.1 *Optimization of Encapsulation Process In Membranes*

Due to the high melting point and viscosity values of the selected imidazolioum protic ionic liquids (Table 11.1), the use of vacuum and high temperature were required to ensure the ionic liquid embedding within the porous membranes. To accomplish this (Figure 11.22), a

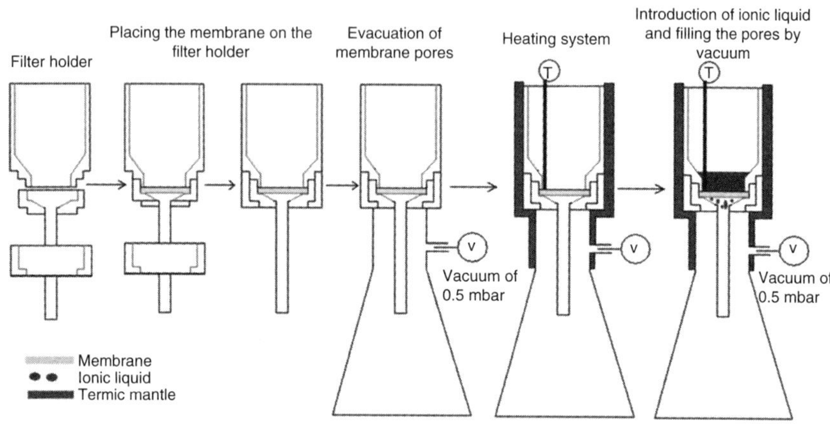

Figure 11.22 Scheme of general procedure to immobilize ionic liquids into porous membranes.

Pall filter holder 25 mm in diameter wrapped with a heating tape was used. The filtration procedure is kept at the fixed temperature for 8 h under vacuum until most of the PIL passes through the membrane ensuring that the PBI pores are filled with it. The resulted embedded membranes were dried at room temperature for 3 hours. PIL loadings have been quantified by differential gravimetry and/or TG analyses.

From the general procedure described above, some parameters were further studied to ensure that the percolation threshold value was achieved. Among them, the operating temperature, the number of filtration cycles, the membrane allocation in the holder and the final wetting stages of both top surfaces revealed as key issues.

11.3.2.2 *Supported Protic Ionic Liquid Membranes on APA Filters*

Commercial track-etched APA (anodized porous alumina) membranes supplied by Whatman® (see Figure 11.23) were firstly used for a proper evaluation of the immobilization scheme. Thus, APA membranes were impregnated at 120°C with the imidazolium-based ionic liquids (IL3 and IL4) according to the procedure described in Figure 11.22.

At 4.2 kPa water partial pressure, the conductivity-temperature dependence shown by supported IL4 on APA is rather similar to that exhibited by PIL-zeolite composites. In particular, for IL4 embedded in APA membrane, the conductivity starts to decrease above 135°C (Figure 11.24a) in agreement with the PIL removal from the

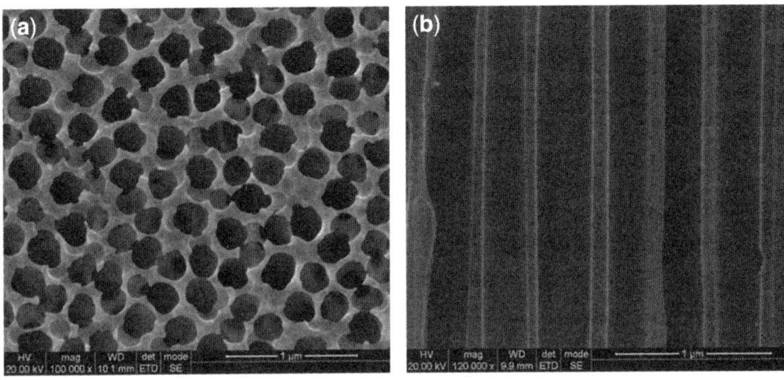

Figure 11.23 SEM Image of track-etched anodized porous alumina Anodisc™ from Whatman®.

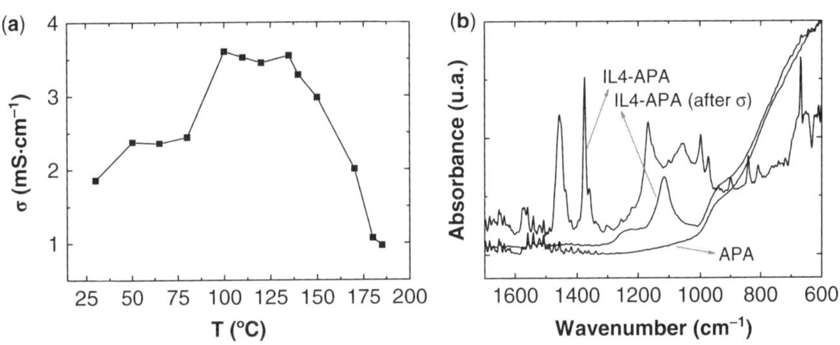

Figure 11.24 (A) Conductivity measurements at y_{H_2O} = 5 % for SLIMs based on IL4-APA; (B) Assessment about IL4 removal from APA by FTIR analyses over SLIMs before and after conductivity tests.

porous network evidenced by FTIR analyses (Figure 11.24b). On the contrary, a large amount of the initially embedded IL3 remains stable (up to 190°C) within the APA membrane due to its relative low water solubility as is demonstrated by FTIR analyses (Figure 11.25).

As a result, the IL3-APA SLIM was used for the optimization of the impregnation procedure in terms of IL loadings and conduction properties. IL immobilization was studied at temperatures from 120°C to 170°C; whereas the impregnation was carried out by simple diffusion or successive vacuum-assisted filtration cycles. Moreover, membrane treatments before the impregnation step (pore evacuation), or after the impregnation step (final soaking of the membrane in the IL), were also analyzed to improve the electrical contact at the interface (Figure 11.26).

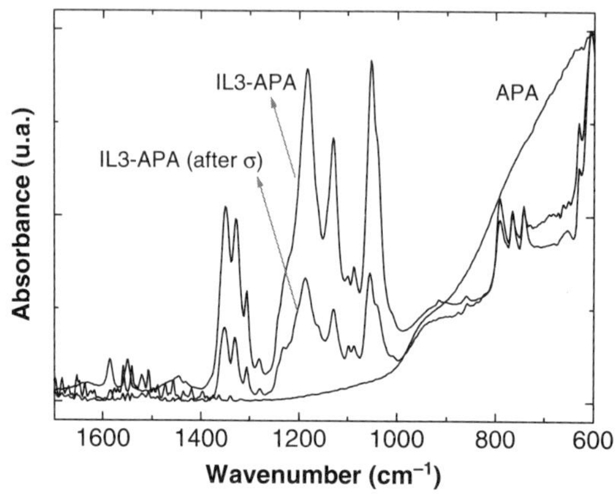

Figure 11.25 Assessment about IL3 removal from APA by FTIR analyses over SLIMs before and after conduction tests.

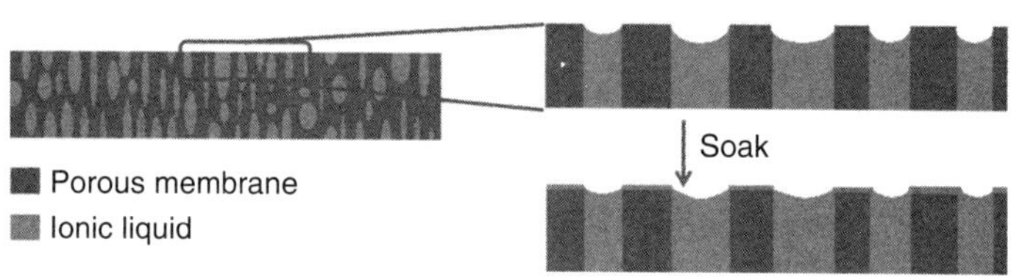

Figure 11.26 PIL meniscus shape inside APA pores (100-200 nm in diameter).

Figure 11.27 summarizes the conductivity results of APA membranes subjected to different IL3 immobilization conditions. From the depicted results, the vacuum-assisted filtration at 170°C followed by a final soaking of the membrane in the IL seems to be the most adequate.

To check endurance properties of the as-prepared SLIMs, durability experiments were also carried out. Figure 11.28 shows the time on stream conductivity values for IL3/APA membranes at 120°C. According to the depicted results, conductivity values remain constant at 22 mS·cm^{-1} for at least 180 h. Therefore, no PILs losses are observed under the tested experimental conditions indicating the suitability of the as-prepared SLIMs for PEMFC applications. Nevertheless, the recommended working temperature should be lower than PIL immobilization temperature (i.e., 170°C) to avoid unsteadiness by PILs dragging. In fact, the discrepancies observed between conductivity values at steady-state conditions (22 mS·cm^{-1}) with those previously attained in the standard conductivity test up to 180°C (i.e., 38 mS·cm^{-1}) registered in Figure 11.27 are attributed to this effect.

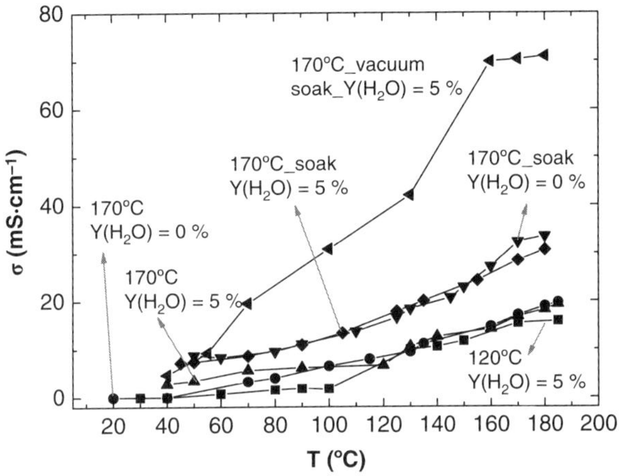

Figure 11.27 Conduction Performance of IL3-APA membranes prepared in this work .

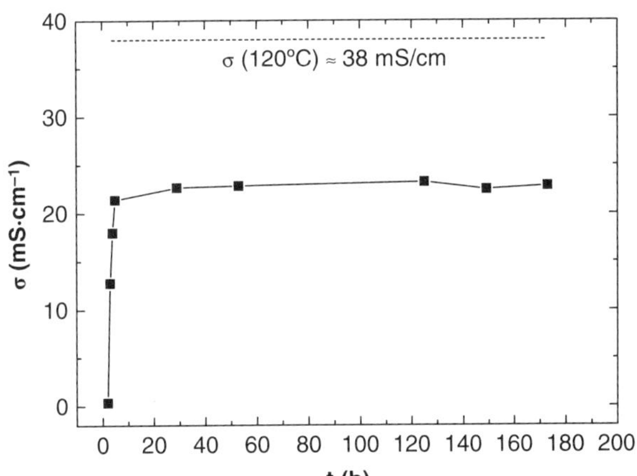

Figure 11.28 Time on stream conductivity measurements at 120°C and at y_{H_2O} = 5 % for SLIMs based on IL3-APA.

11.3.2.3 Supported Protic Ionic Liquid Membranes on Porous PBI

Different SLIMs based on IL3 and randomly porous PBI supports (described in Section 11.2.2.2) prepared following the optimized PIL embedding process described above, are herein studied. Their conduction properties are shown in Figure 11.29. The improved performance of SLIMs based on PBI supports prepared by delayed demixing method is partly attributed to the higher IL loading

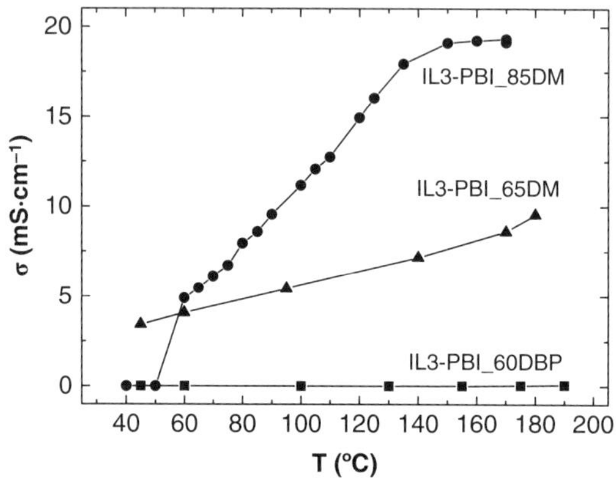

Figure 11.29 Conduction Performance of SLIMs based on IL3 and randomly porous PBI containers at y_{H_2O}=5%.

estimated by TGA analyses (Figure 11.31). Moreover, for a given porosity value (i.e., 60–65%), the PILs loading and conductivity values are clearly lower for porous PBI prepared by porogen leaching. The explanation relies on the porous architecture, in particular, the tortuosity and pore connectivity of porogen-based membranes which should be clearly improved (study of new porogens or dual porogen systems) for confinement purposes.

PBI containers prepared by delayed-demixing method show PIL loadings in agreement with their porosity values (Figure 11.31). Unlike recently published results [62], the higher conductivity values herein reported (Figure 11.29) are attributed to the PIL confinement procedure.

It is clearly outstanding the thermal stability of these SLIMs due to no thermal events are registered at temperatures below 250°C. This feature is clearly advantageous for the high temperature systems application here envisioned. Moreover, the beneficial effects of porosity on proton conductivity are quite noticeable. In fact, IL3-PBI_85DM·membrane shows the best conductivity values even when normalized per mass of IL3 (Figure 11.30). Thus, higher porosity values enhance pores connectivity (coordination number); and consequently conduction phenomena through heterogeneous media is facilitated (Figure 11.21).

Considering the differences between the pore morphologies of PBI membranes prepared either by porogen leaching or by delayed demixing; the analysis of the apparent activation energies for proton transport (estimated from Arrhenius type fitting) could be

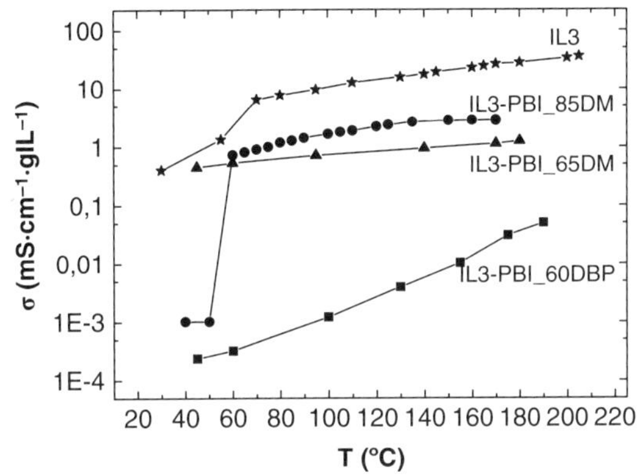

Figure 11.30 Conductivity values expressed in mS•cm^{-1}•gPIL^{-1} for SLIMs based on IL3 and randomly porous PBI containers at y_{H_2O}=5%.

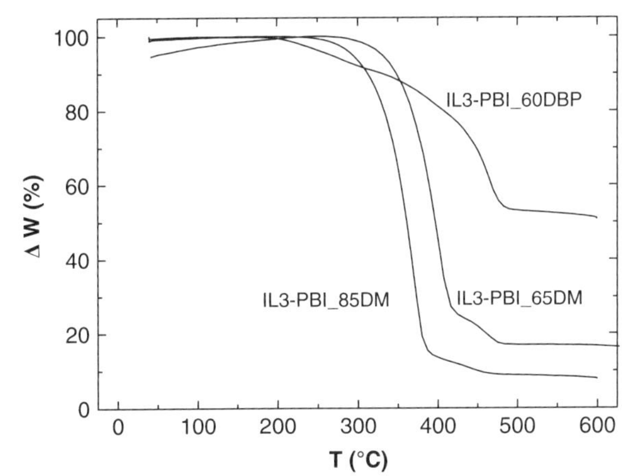

Figure 11.31 Thermogravimetric analyses for SLIMs based on IL3 and randomly porous PBI containers.

really clarifying (Figure 11.32). As was expected, similar activation energy values are found for bulky IL3 and SLIMs based on delayed demixing support 85% in porosity. On the other hand, the scarce degree of pore connectivity for PBI_DBP supports makes the activation energy required for proton hopping three-fold higher.

Time on stream (up to 150 h) conductivity properties at 150°C for the outperforming PBI_85DM are shown in Figure 11.33. After the initial performance decay, conductivity value remains almost constant at 6 mS·cm^{-1}. Considering the successful UV-assisted polymerization of monomers protic ionic liquids prepared from IL3,

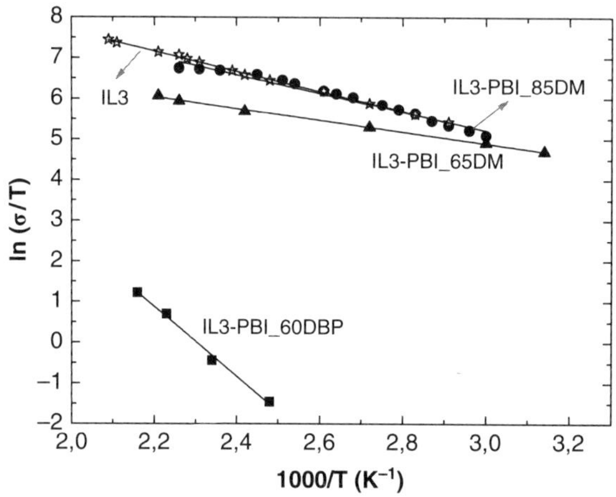

Samples	E_a (kJ/mol)
IL3-PBI_60DBP	85,2
IL3-PBI_65DM	14,3
IL3-PBI_85DM	22,8
IL3	24,6

Figure 11.32 Arrhenius type activation energy for proton transport on SLIMs based on IL3 and randomly porous PBI containers. The analysis of bulk IL3 is also depicted for comparison purposes.

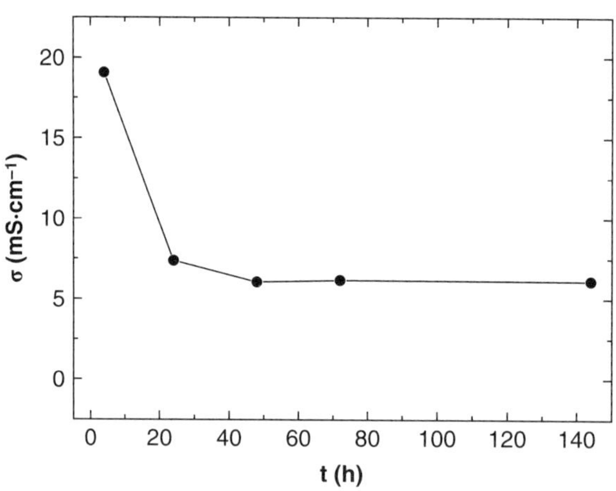

Figure 11.33 Time on stream conductivity measurements at 150°C and y_{H_2O}=5%for IL3-PBI_85DM membrane.

polymeric protic ionic liquid-based membranes have been recently developed [65] with the final aim to improve endurance properties of SLIMs membranes.

Summarizing, Figure 11.34 shows a comparison of the conductivity properties of the outperforming SLIMs membranes based on IL3 (i.e., IL3-APA and IL3-PBI_85DM) studied in this work. As the amount of ionic liquid encapsulated is not comparable due to the pore volume differences (Table 11.5), the intrinsic proton

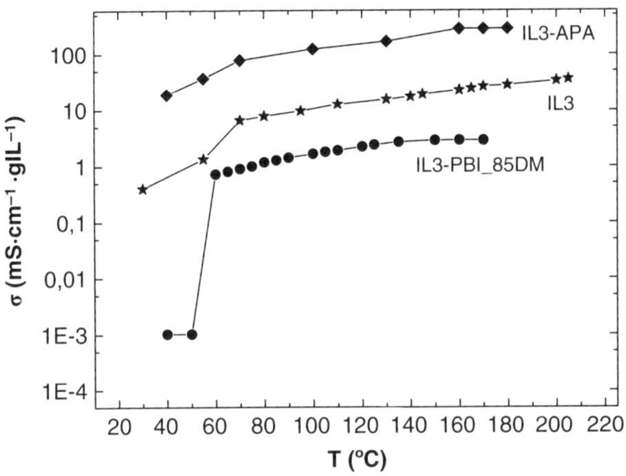

Figure 11.34 Conductivity values expressed in mS•cm^{-1}•gPIL^{-1} for the outperforming SLIMs based on IL3 studied in this work at y_{H_2O}=5%..

conductivity (i.e., normalized per IL3 mass) has been plotted on the y axis. As can be observed, pores connectivity (coordination number) is the key parameter controlling the conduction phenomena. As was expected, higher values are attained by using track-etched supports because the proton diffusion pathways are shorter. According to these observations, a potential pathway for future development would be the fabrication of straight pore PBI membranes by low-cost technologies for their deployment as inert supports for PIL encapsulation [64].

11.4 New Activities and Development Trends

The protic ionic liquids herein studied have demonstrated highly attractive possibilities, not only as guest molecules inside large-pore zeolites but also as embedded proton carriers in porous supports, to enhance the transport properties of these systems.

The deployment of composite membranes based on undoped PBI and PILs-zeolite composite fillers as electrolyte membranes for HT PEMFCs [38] could alleviate or eventually suppress commonly encountered problems in this field (phosphoric acid catalyst poisoning, conductivity losses due to dehydration, acid oligorimerization...).

Protic ionic liquid supported membranes have been successfully prepared by vacuum-assisted filtration at 170°C, for highly viscous PILs, followed by a final soaking of the porous container in the PIL.

The best performances of SILMs based on PBI correspond to those prepared from delayed demixing of porous supports. Moreover, the upper limit for working temperature should be lower than PIL immobilization temperature values to avoid unsteadiness by PILs dragging. One possible solution could rely on the immobilization of monomeric protic ionic liquids within porous PBI followed by *in situ* polymerization by UV radiation [66] (Figure 11.35). As an example of potential candidates for the preparation of such supported polymeric protic ionic liquid membranes, Figure 11.36 shows the conductivity properties of the vinyl derivate from the IL3 monomer herein studied.

For a given intrinsic conductor, SLIMs conductivity primarily depends not only on support porosity but also on pore connectivity (coordination number). Thus, the conduction performance of the SLIMs has been somewhat limited due to the availability of adequate porous containers. Several authors have proposed the deployment of straight-pores membranes [67] to enhance conduction by shortening proton pathways. Accordingly, a potential pathway for future development in the PEMFC field would be the fabrication of straight-pores PBI membranes by low-cost technologies (i.e., microtransfer molding) for their deployment as inert supports for PIL encapsulation [64] (Figures 11.37, 11.38).

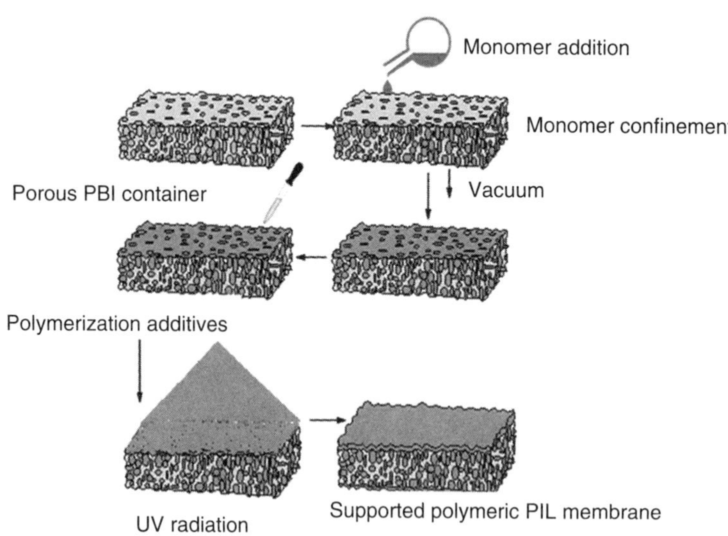

Figure 11.35 Preparation scheme for Supported Polymeric Protic Ionic Liquids Membranes on porous PBI containers.

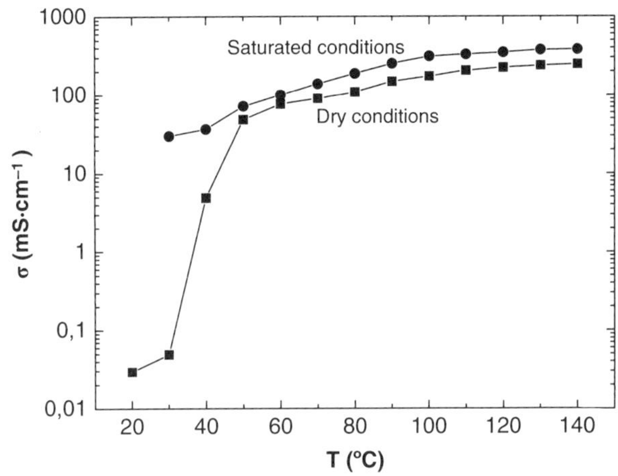

Figure 11.36 P Conduction performance of the monomeric 1-H-3-vinylimidazolium bis(trifluoromethanesulfonyl)imide derivate from the IL3 used in this work.

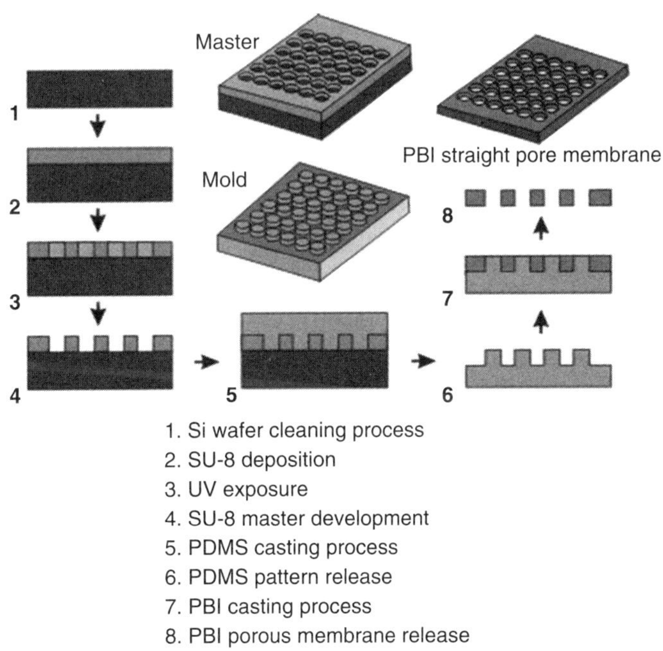

Figure 11.37 Microtransfer moulding approach to prepare PBI containers with straight pores.

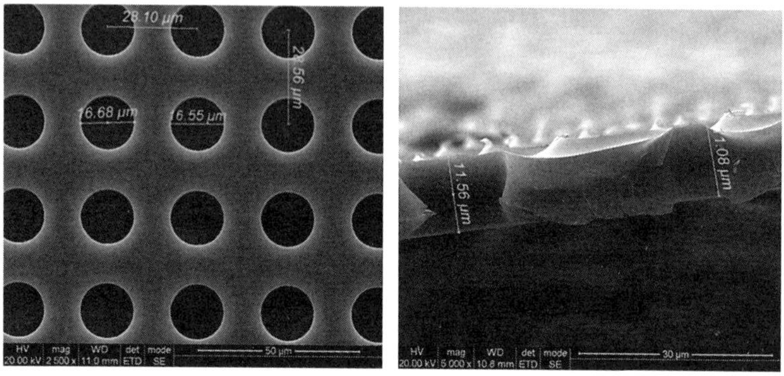

Figure 11.38 SEM micrographs of PBI containers with straight pores prepared by micro transfer-moulding technique.

References

1. P. Wasserscheid, and T. Welton. *Ionic liquids in synthesis*. Ed. M. Wiley-VCH. 2003.
2. J.F. Wishart, and E.W. Castner, Jr. The physical chemistry of ionic liquids. *Journal of Physical Chemistry B* 2007. 111(18): p. 4639–4640.
3. M. Deetlefs, and K.R. Seddon. Ionic liquids: Fact and fiction. *Chimica Oggi-Chemistry Today* 2006. 24(2): p. 16-+.
4. T.L. Greaves, and C.J. Drummond. Protic ionic liquids: Properties and applications. *Chemical Reviews* 2008. 108(1): p. 206–237.
5. N.V. Plechkova, and K.R. Seddon. Applications of ionic liquids in the chemical industry. *Chemical Society Reviews* 2008. 37(1): p. 123–150.
6. L.A. Blanchard, et al. Green processing using ionic liquids and CO2. *Nature* 1999. 399(6731): p. 28–29.
7. R.D. Noble, and D.L. Gin. Perspective on ionic liquids and ionic liquid membranes. *Journal of Membrane Science* 2011. 369(1–2): p. 1–4.
8. J.E. Bara, et al. Guide to CO2 separations in imidazolium-based room-temperature ionic liquids. *Industrial & Engineering Chemistry Research* 2009. 48(6): p. 2739–2751.
9. D. Zhan, and J.B. Fenn. Gas phase hydration of electrospray ions from small peptides. *International Journal of Mass Spectrometry* 2002. 219(1): p. 1–10.
10. H. Olivier-Bourbigou, L. Magna, and D. Morvan. Ionic liquids and catalysis: Recent progress from knowledge to applications. *Applied Catalysis A: General* 2010. 373(1–2): p. 1–56.
11. D. Zhao, et al. Ionic liquids: Applications in catalysis. *Catalysis Today* 2002. 74(1–2): p. 157–189.
12. M. Iglesias, et al. Bronsted ionic liquids: Study of physico-chemical properties and catalytic activity in aldol condensations. *Chemical Engineering Journal* 2010. 162(2): p. 802–808.
13. P. Kubisa. Ionic liquids as solvents for polymerization processes: Progress and challenges. *Progress in Polymer Science* 2009. 34(12): p. 1333–1347.

14. H. Ohno. *Electrochemical aspects of ionic liquids*. 2005: John Wiley & Sons, Inc.
15. H. Ohno, et al. The first samarium(II)-mediated aryl radical cyclization onto an aromatic ring. *ChemInform* 2005. 36(10).
16. C. DeCastro, et al. Immobilised ionic liquids as Lewis acid catalysts for the alkylation of aromatic compounds with dodecene. *Journal of Catalysis* 2000. 196(1): p. 86–94.
17. M.H. Valkenberg, C. deCastro, and W.F. Holderich. Immobilisation of ionic liquids on solid supports. *Green Chemistry* 2002. 4(2): p. 88–93.
18. B. Pietschmann, et al. Immobilization of ionic liquids within micro- and mesoporous materials. In *Studies in surface science and catalysis*. 2008. p. 325–328.
19. J. Blumel. Reactions of ethoxysilanes with silica -a solid-state NMR-study. *Journal of the American Chemical Society* 1995. 117(7): p. 2112–2113.
20. D. Brunel, et al. Preferential grafting of alkoxysilane coupling agents on the hydrophobic portion of the surface of micelle-templated silica. *New Journal of Chemistry* 2000. 24(10): p. 807–813.
21. V. Kislik. *Liquid membranes: Principles and applications in chemical separations and wastewater treatment*. 2010: Elsevier B.V.
22. D.Y. Takigawa. The effect of porous support composition and operating parameters on the performance of supported liquid membranes. *Separation Science and Technology* 1992. 27(3): p. 325–339.
23. J.E. Bara, et al. Room-temperature ionic liquids and composite materials: platform technologies for CO2 capture. *Accounts of Chemical Research* 2009. 43(1): p. 152–159.
24. T.K. Carlisle. et al. Main-chain imidazolium polymer membranes for CO2 separations: An initial study of a new ionic liquid-inspired platform. *Journal of Membrane Science* 2010. 359(1–2): p. 37–43.
25. P. Cserjési, N. Nemestóthy, and K. Bélafi-Bakó. Gas separation properties of supported liquid membranes prepared with unconventional ionic liquids. *Journal of Membrane Science* 2010. 349(1–2): p. 6–11.
26. A. Noda, et al. Brönsted acid and base ionic liquids as proton-conducting nonaqueous electrolytes. *The Journal of Physical Chemistry B* 2003. 107(17): p. 4024–4033.
27. M. Galinski, A. Lewandowski, and I. Statmpniak. Ionic liquids as electrolytes. *Electrochimica Acta* 2006. 51(26): p. 5567–5580.
28. C. Iojoiu, et al. PILs-based Nafion membranes: a route to high-temperature PEFMCs dedicated to electric and hybrid vehicles. *Polymers for Advanced Technologies* 2008. 19(10): p. 1406–1414.
29. H. Ye, et al. New membranes based on ionic liquids for PEM fuel cells at elevated temperatures. *Journal of Power Sources* 2008. 178(2): p. 651–660.
30. J. Schauer, et al. Ion-conductive polymer membranes containing 1-butyl-3-methylimidazolium trifluoromethanesulfonate and 1-ethylimidazolium trifluoromethanesulfonate. *Journal of Membrane Science* 2011. 367(1–2): p. 332–339.
31. J.T.-W. Wang, and S.L.-C. Hsu. Enhanced high-temperature polymer electrolyte membrane for fuel cells based on polybenzimidazole and ionic liquids. *Electrochimica Acta* 2011. 56(7): p. 2842–2846.
32. S.Y. Lee, T. Yasuda, and M. Watanabe. Fabrication of protic ionic liquid/sulfonated polyimide composite membranes for non-humidified fuel cells. *Journal of Power Sources* 2010. 195(18): p. 5909–5914.

33. T. Yamaguchi, H. Kuroki, and F. Miyata. DMFC performances using a pore-filling polymer electrolyte membrane for portable usages. *Electrochemistry Communications* 2005. 7: p. 730–734.
34. T. Yamaguchi et al. A pore-filling electrolyte membrane-electrode integrated system for direct methanol fuel cell application. *J. Electrochem. Soc.* 2002. 149(11): p. 1448–1453.
35. T. Yamaguchi, et al. Plasma-graft pore-filling electrolyte membranes using a porous poly(tetrafluoroethylene) substrate. *Electrochemistry* 2002. 70(12): p. 950–952.
36. H. Nishimura, and T. Yamaguchi. Performance of a pore-filling electrolyte membrane in hydrogen-oxygen PEFC. *Electrochemical and Solid State Letters* 2004. 7(11): p. A385-A388.
37. T. Yamaguchi, F. Miyata, and S. Nakao. Pore-filling type polymer electrolyte membranes for a direct methanol fuel cell. *Journal of Membrane Science* 2003. 214: p. 283–292.
38. A. Eguizábal, J. Lemus, and M.P. Pina. On the incorporation of protic ionic liquids imbibed in large pore zeolites to polybenzimidazole membranes for high temperature proton exchange membrane fuel cells. *Journal of Power Sources* 2013. 222(0): p. 483–492.
39. A. Eguizábal. et al. Ammonium based ionic liquids immobilized in large pore zeolites: Encapsulation procedures and proton conduction performance. *Journal of Power Sources* 2011. 196(9): p. 4314–4323.
40. D. Mecerreyes, et al. Porous polybenzimidazole membranes doped with phosphoric acid: Highly proton-conducting solid electrolytes. *Chemistry of Materials* 2004. 16(4): p. 604–607.
41. A. Eguizábal, et al. Nanostructured electrolyte membranes based on zeotypes, protic ionic liquids and porous PBI membranes: Preparation, characterization and MEA testing. *International Journal of Hydrogen Energy* 2012. 37(8): p. 7221–7234.
42. K.D. Kreuer. Proton conductivity: Materials and applications. *Chemistry of Materials* 1996. 8(3): p. 610–641.
43. K.D. Kreuer, A. Rabenau, and W. Weppner. Vehicle mechanism, a new model for the interpretation of the conductivity of fast proton conductors. *Angewandte Chemie-International Edition in English* 1982. 21(3): p. 208–209.
44. C.A. Angell, et al. *Physical chemistry of ionic liquids, inorganic and organic, protic and aprotic, in electrochemical aspects of ionic liquids.* 2005, John Wiley & Sons, Inc. p. 5–23.
45. C. Laberty-Robert, et al. Design and properties of functional hybrid organic-inorganic membranes for fuel cells. *Chemical Society Reviews* 40(2): p. 961–1005.
46. M.A.B.H. Susan, et al. Bronsted acid-base ionic liquids and their use as new materials for anhydrous proton conductors. *Chemical Communications* 2003(8): p. 938–939.
47. H. Nakamoto, and M. Watanabe. Bronsted acid-base ionic liquids for fuel cell electrolytes. *Chemical Communications* 2007(24): p. 2539–2541.
48. K.D. Kreuer, et al. Imidazole and pyrazole-based proton conducting polymers and liquids. *Electrochimica Acta* 1998. 43(10–11): p. 1281–1288.
49. M.S. Auerbach, K.A. Carrado, and P.K. Dutta, eds. *Handbook of zeolite science and technology.* CRC Press. 2003.

50. Breakthrough of the year. The runners-up. *Science* 2011. 334: p. 1629–1535.
51. U. Simon, and M.E. Franke. Electrical properties of nanoscaled host/guest compounds. *Microporous and Mesoporous Materials* 2000. 41(1–3): p. 1–36.
52. D.C. Freeman, and D.N. Stamires. Electrical conductivity of synthetic crystalline zeolites. *Journal of Chemical Physics* 1961. 35(3): p. 799.
53. A. Abdoulaye, et al. Polarization conductivity in dehydrated zeolites NaY and HY. *Microporous Materials* 1997. 8(1–2): p. 63–68.
54. D.N. Stamires. Effect of adsorbed phases on the electrical conductivity of synthetic crystalline zeolites. *Journal of Chemical Physics* 1962. 36(12): p. 3174.
55. U. Simon, et al. The effect of NH3 on the ionic conductivity of dehydrated zeolites Na beta and H beta. *Microporous and Mesoporous Materials* 1998. 21: p. 111–116.
56. International Zeolite Association. Available from: www.iza-structures.org.
57. T. Sancho, et al. Zeolites and zeotype materials as efficient barriers for methanol cross-over in DMFCs. *Microporous and Mesoporous Materials* 2008. 115(1–2): p. 206–213.
58. E.J. Powers, and G.A. Serad. *History and development of polybenzimidazoles*. 1986.
59. S.M. Aharoni, and M.H. Litt. Synthesis and some properties of poly-(2,5-trimethylene benzimidazole) and poly-(2,5-trimethylene benzimidazole hydrochloride). *Journal of Polymer Science: Polymer Chemistry Edition* 1974. 12(3): p. 639–650.
60. D.J. Jones, and J. Rozière. Recent advances in the functionalisation of polybenzimidazole and polyetherketone for fuel cell applications. *Journal of Membrane Science* 2001. 185(1): p. 41–58.
61. J.S. Wainright, et al. Acid-doped polybenzimidazoles: A new polymer electrolyte. *Journal of Electrochemical Society* 1995. 142(7): p. 121–123.
62. E. van de Ven, et al. Ionic liquid doped polybenzimidazole membranes for high temperature proton exchange membrane fuel cell applications. *Journal of Power Sources* 2013. 222(0): p. 202–209.
63. S. Ntais, et al. Preparation and ion transport properties of NaY zeolite-ionic liquid composites. *Journal of Power Sources* 2011. 196(4): p. 2202–2210.
64. http://cordis.europa.eu/documents/documentlibrary/117238781EN6.pdf.
65. S. Ntais, et al. Ionic liquid/zeolite composites: Synthesis and characterization using vibrational spectroscopy techniques. *ECS Transactions* 33(7): p. 41–47.
66. F.J. Lemus, A. Eguizábal, and M.P. Pina. Membranas reforzadas basadas en líquidos iónicos poliméricos para sus aplicación en procesos de transporte de iones y métodos de fabricación de dichas membranas. 2012, P201231812.
67. S. Bose, et al. Polymer membranes for high temperature proton exchange membrane fuel cell: Recent advances and challenges. *Progress in Polymer Science* 2011. 36(6): p. 813–843.

12

Encapsulation Methods with Supercritical Carbon Dioxide: Basis and Applications

Soraya Rodríguez-Rojo, Ángel Martín and María José Cocero

High Pressure Processes Group, Chemical Engineering and Environmental Technology Dept., School of Industrial Engineering, Valladolid, Spain

Abstract
Supercritical fluid techniques for particle engineering have attracted a lot of interest over recent years because they have been proposed as an alternative clean technology. These techniques allow for the improvement of product quality in terms of reduction of particle size and control of morphology and particle size distribution, without degradation or contamination of the product.

This chapter reviews the encapsulation and co-precipitation processes based on the use of supercritical fluids, i.e., carbon dioxide. These processes are classified according to the role of the carbon dioxide (solvent, antisolvent, solute or reaction medium). The focus is on the process mechanisms description, as well as on the evolution of the different techniques to overcome the challenges set according to the physical properties of the different processed materials.

Keywords: Particle formation, encapsulation, carbon dioxide, RESS, GAS, SAS, PGSS, impregnation, reaction

12.1 Introduction

The application of supercritical fluids (SFC), namely supercritical carbon dioxide (SC-CO_2), in particle engineering, i.e., production of particles, of pure compounds or in combination with a carrier material, whose physical characteristics (size, morphology, structure,

Vikas Mittal (ed.) Encapsulation Nanotechnologies, (391–424) © 2013 Scrivener Publishing LLC

physicochemical stability, etc.) are optimized, has attracted great attention over the last twenty years. The main advantages of processes based on SC-CO_2 are:

- mild processing temperatures, generally below 50°C;
- inert atmosphere, suitable to process unstable compounds;
- absence or reduced used of organic solvents; and in the latter case, residual levels below legal limits;
- high purity products, avoiding post processing steps, i.e., filtering and drying, of conventional crystallization/precipitation process.

Therefore, applications are largely focused in pharmaceutics, as well as in food and cosmetics, and have been extensively reviewed [1–9]. There are also developments in other areas of industrial chemistry, such as the manufacturing of catalysts or explosives.

The aim of this chapter is to provide, firstly, the fundamentals about SCF physical properties that make them a real alternative in particle engineering; and secondly, to give a broad overview of the main precipitation and encapsulation processes found in this technology including the basis, advantages and drawbacks, and some applications.

12.2 Supercritical Fluids – Properties

A supercritical fluid (SCF) is any substance above its critical temperature (T_c) and pressure (P_c), that is, its critical point (CP), as shown in Figure 12.1. In the supercritical region there is no longer equilibrium between the vapor and liquid state; therefore the physico-chemical properties of SCFs are intermediate between those of liquid and gases (Table 12.1): gas-like low viscosity and high diffusivity like gases that facilitate mass transfer, and liquid-like density that grants the solvent power of SCF. Moreover, the high compressibility of SCF, especially near the CP, allows tuning of the density, and consequently the solvent power, with small changes in operating pressure and temperature [10].

Although any fluid or substance can attain supercritical state above their CP, several factors have to be considered to choose the

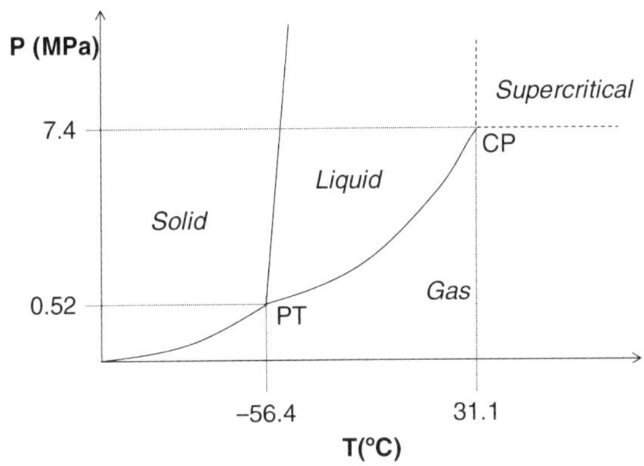

Figure 12.1 Phase diagram of a pure substance, particularized for CO2 values. CP: Critical Point. TP: Triple point.

Table 12.1 Typical values of density, diffusivity and viscosity for liquids, gases and supercritical fluids [11].

	Density (kg/m³)	Viscosity (μPa·s)	Diffusivity (mm²/s)
Gases	1	10	1–10
Supercritical Fluids	100–1000	50–100	0.01–0.1
Liquids	1000	500–1000	0.001

most suitable SCF for each application, regarding operating conditions of the materials to be processed, economics and safety.

Carbon dioxide (CO_2) is the most preferred since it has low T_c (31.1°C) and P_c (7.4MPa) allowing for mild operating conditions. Besides, it is cheap and available at different levels of purity, non-flammable, non-toxic and environmentally safe. From a chemical point of view, CO_2 has a low dielectric constant (1.1–1.5). Thus, it dissolves nonpolar or slightly polar compounds of low molecular weight (MW) [12]. Far from being a disadvantage, due to this property CO_2 can be used as selective solvent, as an antisolvent or as a solute, depending on the applications and the phase equilibrium between the CO_2 and the compound of interest.

Major industrial applications of SC-CO_2 are developed in the food industry [13] as solvent for low MW molecules, such as caffeine or vitamine E. However, despite the advantages of this technology, the industrial implementation of particle engineering and encapsulation applications with SCF is still very limited, which is likely due to the high cost of the equipment and the weak knowledge of this area [2].

12.3 Particle Engineering and Encapsulation with Supercritical Fluids

The precipitation mechanisms of precipitation and crystallization processes by supercritical fluids are essentially the same as in conventional ones: reduction in the solvent power of the solvent by changes in the operating conditions (pressure and temperature, instead of only temperature as in conventional "cooling crystallization" as the solvent power of SC-CO_2 is related to its density, as explained previously) or by the addition of an antisolvent, the SC-CO_2. Therefore, precipitation (or encapsulation when a coating material is involved) processes are classified according to the role of SC-CO_2 in respect to the materials to be processed: solvent or antisolvent. Although the basic mechanisms are the same as in conventional processes, in supercritical processes the supersaturation values are, in general, higher and achieved in a faster way, due to the possibility of drastically changing the properties of the SCF with changes in operating conditions, and to the favorable transport properties [4]. Hence, particle size can be reduced to the submicron or nanometer scale. Besides, it can be used as solute, propeller in atomization processes or as reaction media, as detailed in the following sections.

12.3.1 Supercritical Fluid as Solvent

12.3.1.1 Rapid Expansion of Supercritical Solution (RESS) and Related Processes

The RESS process consists of the rapid expansion of a solution of the compound of interest in the SCF, commonly SC-CO_2, through a nozzle into an atmospheric expansion chamber causing the precipitation of a product into very small particles free of solvent, since during the expansion the CO_2 passes from a dense supercritical phase to the gas phase. Depending on the nature of the substance

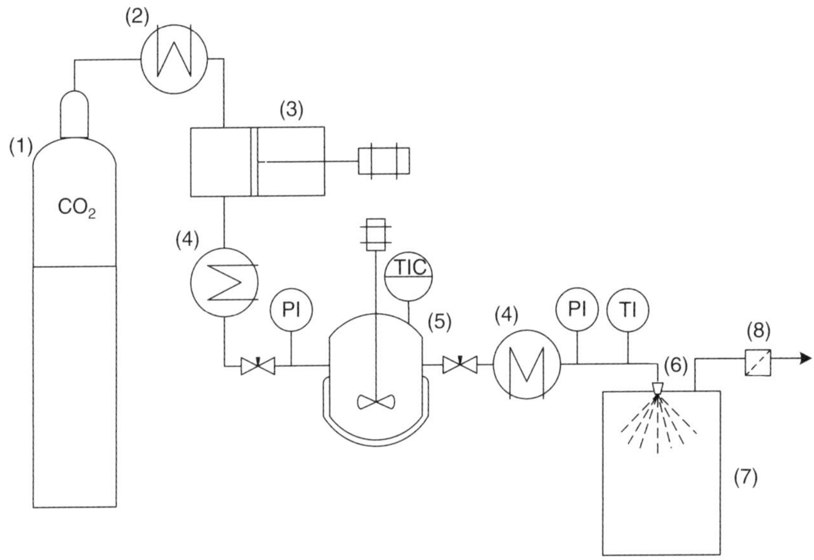

Figure 12.2 Typical RESS experimental set-up: (1) CO_2 cylinder, (2) chiller, (3) High pressure liquid pump, (4) Heater, (5) High pressure vessel – saturator, (6) Nozzle, (7) Ambient pressure vessel for particle recovery and (8) Filter in CO_2-exhaust line to safe place or for re-use.

fibers can also be formed [14]. In some applications, the expansion chamber is substituted by a flat surface, where additionally a high voltage can be applied, as well as to the nozzle, to uniformly coat the surface [14, 15].

In Figure 12.2, a typical flowchart of a semi-continuous RESS apparatus is presented. The dissolution of the compound in the SCF can be carried out in a high-pressure stirred vessel or in an extraction column. The nozzle should be heated to avoid clogging, since an intense cooling is produced during the expansion due to the Joule-Thompson effect.

The fast depressurization (10^{-5}s) of the solution causes an extremely high supersaturation (10^5 to 10^8) due to the sudden decrease in density of the solvent, and thus, high nucleation rates (up to 10^{26} cm^{-3} s^{-1}) are achieved, which enable the production of very fine particles (<1μm) with narrow size distribution. Nevertheless, as in any precipitation process, after nucleation, particles may grow by coagulation through the particles' collision, and by condensation of molecules on the particles surface [7].

The main process parameters are pre-expansion temperature, which is above the saturation value for the operating pressure, pre-expansion pressure, nozzle geometry and dimensions of the expansion vessel. Additionally, the pre-expansion temperature and pressure determins the solubility of the material in the SCF; a lower solubility value produces a decrease in particle size by coagulation since particle collision rate is directly proportional to the square of particle concentration [7]. Nevertheless, a lower solubility limit on the order of 10^{-4} molar fraction can be fixed to develop an economically viable process [2].

Pre-expansion pressure and nozzle geometry determine the solute-saturated CO_2 solution mass flow rate through the nozzle. An increase in any of them produce an increase in the flow rate, which decreases the residence time of the particles in the expansion chamber, resulting in a lower growth of particles, and hence, in smaller particles [7].

As mentioned before, the nozzle geometry is a key parameter of the process since it determines the fluid mechanics in the depressurization process, pressure variation along the process, and the time scale in which it takes place. During the depressurization through the nozzle, three regions have to be considered: the inlet region of the nozzle (I), the nozzle itself (II), and the expansion region, which in turn is divided in two zones: (III) and (IV). As shown in Figure 12.3, most of the pressure drop is produced at the supersonic free jet formed at the outlet of the nozzle, since the ratio

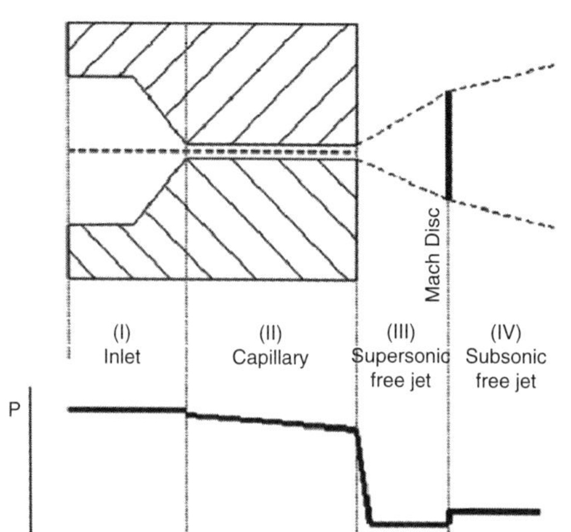

Figure 12.3 Schematic diagram of a RESS expansion device with approximate pressure profile [4].

between the pre-expansion and the post-expansion pressure is very high; pressure can even decrease below the bulk pressure of the expansion vessel. The supersonic jet ends at the Mach shock disc. Afterwards, the pressure increases up to that of surrounding ambient, accompanied by an increase in temperature [16].

Consequently, the RESS process is very attractive since small particles with narrow particle size distribution (PSD) are obtained in the absence of organic solvents, and the moderate temperatures (typically below 80°C) allow processing heat-sensitive materials. Unfortunately, its application is restricted due to the low solubility in SC-CO_2 of most organic compounds, and especially high molecular weight compounds such as polymers, which are an essential component in encapsulation processes. Nevertheless, short-chain alkenes such as paraffin, lipids such as lecithin, fluorinated polymers with application in electronics and siloxane polymers are quite soluble in SC- CO_2 [15]. Moreover, since CO_2 can form hydrogen-bonds, hydrocarbon-based copolymers that are CO_2-soluble, through site-specific solute–solvent interactions, can be designed [17].

To overcome low solubility, liquid cosolvents such as acetone or ethanol, can be used to modify the polarity of the solvent. Solubility can be commonly improved by 10^4- to 10^6-fold (defined as the measured solubility divided by the solubility in the SCF without cosolvent) [2]. However, the use of liquid cosolvents can be problematic during the expansion of the solution. If the P–T trajectory of the depressurization enters in the liquid–gas region of the solvent–CO_2 system, more agglomerated particles could be obtained, or particles could even be redissolved in the liquid [4]. Recently, a solid cosolvent, menthol, has been used to micronize Phenytoin, increasing the production rate by a factor of 400 with respect to simple RESS process [18]. This method seems to be more promising, since, besides the solubility enhancement, the solid cosolvent reduces particle growth and, in the case of menthol, can be easily removed by sublimation. Sometimes, different supercritical solvents such as trifluoromethane (CHF_3) are used to overcome low solubility problems in the SCF [7, 16].

Other drawbacks of the RESS process are the difficulties for the scale-up and nozzle design, as well as the energy cost associated with the recompression of CO_2 for its recirculation into the process.

In the following sections, different modifications of the RESS process are presented. All of them are focused in the production of micro- and nanocapsules, as well as in the reduction of agglomeration of the final product. The straight RESS process has already been used to produce fine capsules for the encapsulation of drugs (naproxene, phytosterol, pyren, lovastin) in biopolymers (L-PLA, DL-PLA or Eudragit) [7, 19]; the solute and the polymer are co-dissolved in SC-CO_2, producing through the expansion the simultaneous co-precipitation of both components. Depending on the process conditions and the phase behavior of each component, core-shell particles could be formed if one of them precipitates first and molecules of the other component (polymer) precipitates over them; also microspheres of both components together or separated could be obtained. Since the precipitation by RESS is extremely fast, the control of co-precipitates morphology and composition is very difficult. This, together with the limited solubility of polymers in SC-CO_2, may be the reason why co-precipitation has not been widely applied since it was presented in 1993 [19]. Therefore, some of these alternative RESS-based processes involve the precipitation of the carrier or coating material over previously formed microparticles of the active substance, making it easier to control the polymer coating thickness simply by manipulating the feed composition, as long as a homogeneous dispersion of the particles to be coated and the coating material is achieved in the precipitation chamber [5].

12.3.1.1.1 Fluidized Bed Coating by RESS

Conventional encapsulation in fluidized bed, the so called Wurster process, is a well established process in the industry [20]: a liquid solution of the coating material is sprayed on the core particles that are fluidized by hot air, or N_2, to evaporate the solvent. However, this process presents limitations to processing fine particles ($d_p < 100$ μm) and ultrafine particles ($d_p < 10$ μm) due to high cohesivity of small particles, i.e., electrostatic forces and van der Waals forces, which is increased by the formation of liquid bridges of solution between the particles leading to agglomeration of the product.

To solve this problem, Tsutsumi and collaborators in 1995 [21] proposed to make the expansion of the coating material solubilized in the SC-CO_2 into a bed of core particles fluidized by air at atmospheric conditions. Catalyst microparticles (50 μm) were coated with paraffin wax whose thickness was controlled by the concentration of wax in SC-CO_2.

Since fluidization of small particles ($d_p < 100$ μm) could be improved by the increase of pressure [22], the process evolved to

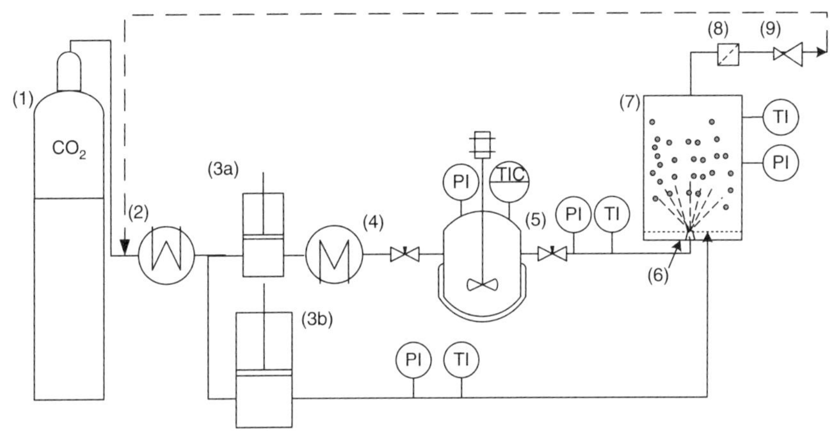

Figure 12.4 Typical experimental set-up for Fluidized Bed coupled with RESS: (1) CO_2 cylinder, (2) chiller, (3) High pressure CO_2 pump (a) for carrier saturation (b) for fluidization stream, (4) Heater, (5) High pressure vessel – saturator, (6) Nozzle, (7) High pressure fluidized bed vessel, (8) Filter and (9) Backpressure valve.

the use of high-pressure fluidized beds ($P > Pc$) [23, 24] according to the general flowchart shown in Figure 12.4. Since the CO_2 solution was not expanded to atmospheric pressure, the recirculation of CO_2 was quite common. The process was extensively studied by the research group of Prof. Brunner; they encapsulated materials with different morphology and surface properties (roughness, porosity and wettability: glass beads, lactose agglomerates, ceramic granules, potassium chloride crystals) with paraffins of different melting and glass transition temperatures [25]. They found that the glass transition of the coating material should be higher than the operating temperature in the pressurized fluidized bed to reduce agglomeration. Agglomeration is also related to particle surface, being that porous rough core particles are more prone to agglomeration during coating than nonporous and smooth ones. They also highlighted the importance of contact angle values of the system core particle–solute– SCF; values lower than 90° are necessary to get good wetting of particle surface, and hence, continuous and uniform coatings. However, such data are scarce.

Although paraffin is the most used material in RESS fluidized bed coating [25–27], other coating materials such as stearyl alcohol [28], stearyl stearate [23] or hydroxyl terminated polybutadiene (HTPB) [24] have been employed.

12.3.1.1.2 Rapid Expansion from Supercritical Solution with Nonsolvent (RESS-N)

This modification broadens the application of RESS process to the use of polymers with low solubility in SC-CO_2 (PEG, PMMA, PLA, PLGA, etc.) as coating materials. For that purpose, a cosolvent is used to enhance solubility of the polymer in the SCF. The cosolvent should be a nonsolvent for the polymer at atmospheric pressure, to avoid swelling of the polymer and agglomeration during expansion and particle formation. Common cosolvents are low molecular weight alcohols, such as ethanol, that highly increase the solubility in SC-CO_2 thanks to its hydrogen-bonding capacity. A typical application is the encapsulation of proteins, which are insoluble in SC-CO_2 [29]. Besides this, it has been further applied to the encapsulation of low MW drug, soluble in SC-CO_2 [7].

12.3.1.1.3 RES Suspensions

This variation attempts the coating or encapsulation of ultrafine particles, which is a major challenge due to the high surface area and high surface energy of such particles. It consists in the expansion of a suspension of the core particles, generally inorganic ones, in the solution of carrier material. The suspension is formed just before entering into the spray chamber. It proved to be successful for the coating of silica particles of 5 μm with paraffin [30]. A nanoscale paraffin layer was deposited on the surface of silica particles without significant agglomeration.

12.3.1.1.4 Rapid Expansion of Supercritical Solution into Liquid Solvent (RESOLV and RESSAS)

Although pristine particles from RESS formed in the supersonic jet are in the nanosize range, during the subsonic expansion they grow and agglomerate due to different collision mechanisms. In the RESOLV process the supercritical solution is expanded into a solution of a surfactant to avoid these two phenomena in the expansion jet, and therefore, to stabilize the particles in the nano range. If the solvent used is an aqueous solution, the process is called rapid expansion of supercritical solution into an aqueous solution (RESSAS). For these processes additional parameters should be taken into account in process optimization such as surfactant properties (surface tension and dynamic interfacial tension) or the solute solubility in the surfactant solution [7].

The stabilization agent can also produce the amorphization of the drug and modify its release profile, as a coating material of a dry powder. As an example, naproxen particle size was reduced from 0.8 μm by conventional RESS to 0.3 μm by RESSAS using PVP, a typical carrier material, as surfactant [31].

12.3.1.2 Impregnation Process

This process can be used to produce microcomposites, introducing an active compound in preformed particles of carrier material, but it cannot be considered strictly an encapsulation technique. Nevertheless, it is worth mentioning since it has several interesting applications.

Impregnation by supercritical fluids takes advantage of the relatively high solubility of low MW molecules or oils in SC-CO_2, and the ability of the SCF to diffuse through the carrier material [3, 10], which can be a powder or polymer with a preformed shape. Not only pressure and temperature of the impregnation step are important, but the depressurization rate is also a key parameter to avoid the deformation of the material during a fast depressurization if it swells by the effect of SC-CO_2 as happens to most of the polymers, and/or to avoid the extraction of the drug if the depressurization is too slow. Important applications are the impregnation with drugs of contact lenses [32] and scaffolds for tissue engineering [33], or the impregnation of starch with essentials oils [34].

12.3.2 Supercritical Fluid as Antisolvent and Related Techniques

These processes take advantage of the relatively low solubility of most organic solid compounds in SC-CO_2 compared to the high solubility of volatile organic solvents to overcome the limited applicability of the RESS process. The solute of interest is dissolved in a conventional organic solvent to form a solution which is pressurized and CO_2. Due to the antisolvent effect of CO_2 a fast increase in supersaturation is achieved, with the subsequent precipitation of particles by the simultaneous extraction of the solvent to the pressurized fluid, and saturation of the solvent with the pressurized CO_2.

From the point of view of the solution the process can be operated in batch or semi-continuous modes (Figure 12.5). In the batch process, the solute is solubilized in a conventional solvent, e.g., acetone, ethanol, DCM or DMSO. This solution is loaded in the high pressure precipitation vessel. Afterwards, the CO_2 is added into the

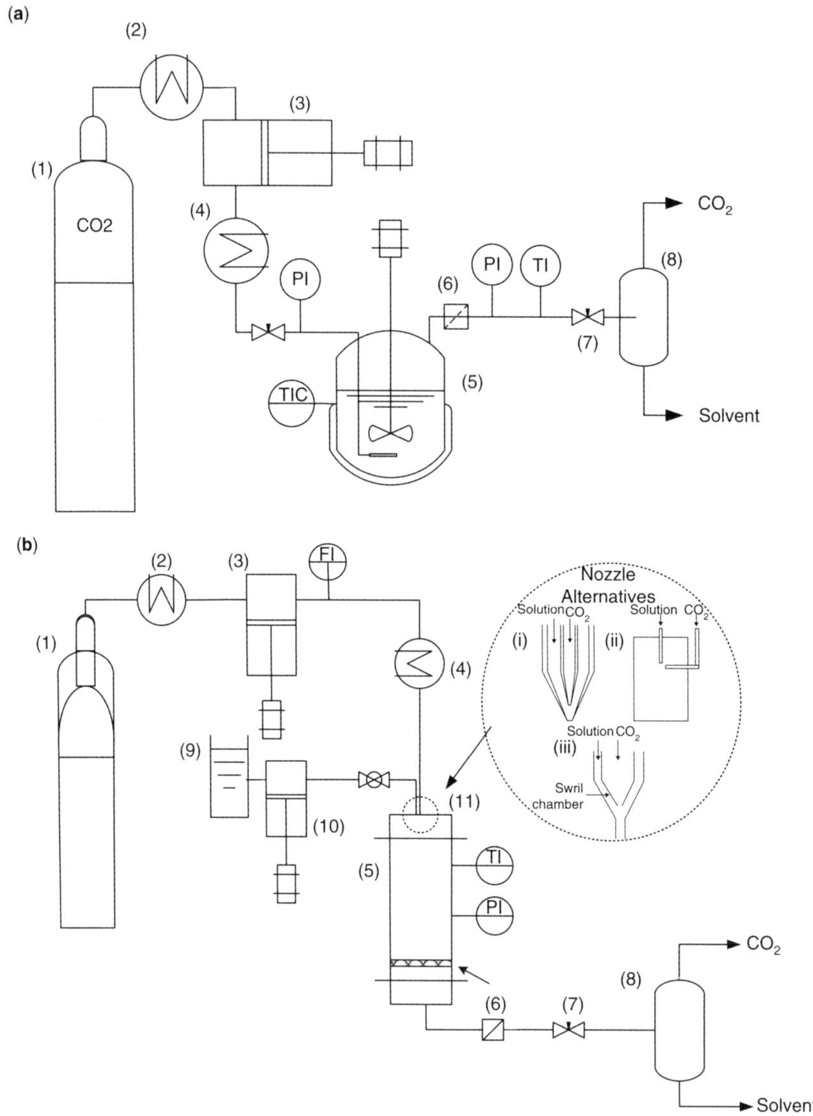

Figure 12.5 Experimental set-up for anti-solvent processes: (a) Batch method: (1) CO_2 cylinder, (2) chiller, (3) High pressure CO_2 pump (4) Heater, (5) High pressure vessel, (6) Filter, (7) Valve, (8) Flash at atmospheric pressure. (b) Semicontinuous method: (9) Organic solution vessel, (10) High pressure solution pump, (11) Solution-CO_2 injection system: independent or nozzle devices: (i) Concentric nozzle, SEDS process, (ii) impingent inlet, (iii) swirl nozzle.

precipitator and the pressure increases from atmospheric value to the desired final pressure at a certain rate. In the semi-continuous process, the liquid solution is also pumped simultaneously into the system at the selected operation temperature and pressure, so that the production capacity of the process is increased. In both cases, a drying cycle is performed at the end of particle precipitation in order to remove traces of unextracted solvent by passing an amount of SC-CO_2 at constant temperature and pressure equivalent to 2–3 times the volume of the precipitation vessel.

Commonly, the process is called gas antisolvent (GAS) when the mixture of carbon dioxide-organic solvent is in the two-phase region (Figure 12.6), i.e., below its critical pressure (P = 5 – 8 MPa) at a certain temperature, generally in the range from 25–55°C. When the mixture is in the miscible, i.e., one-phase region, the process is called supercritical antisolvent (SAS). Operating pressure is typically in the range of 9–15 MPa, depending on the selected organic solvent and operating temperature (35–55°C). The denomination of precipitation with compressed antisolvent (PCA) can be also used in a general way. Nevertheless, some researchers keep

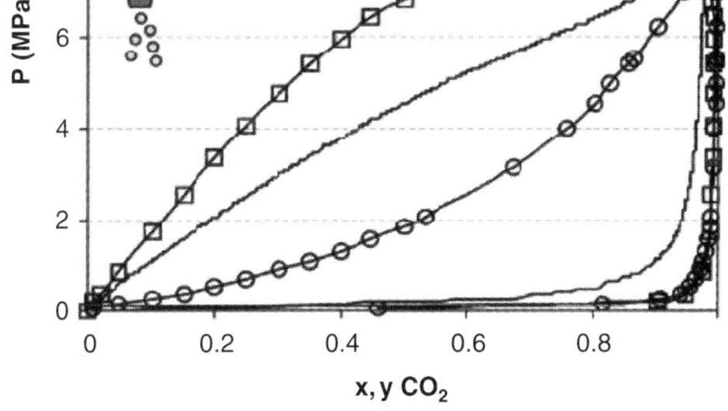

Figure 12.6 P–xy diagrams of CO_2–dichloromethane, CO_2– Ethanol and CO_2–ethyl acetate at 313 K, calculated with the Peng-Robinson EOS (from [4]).

the GAS denomination for the batch processes and SAS for the semi-continuous ones. As one of the main parameters influencing the process, as will be detailed later, is the mixing between the solution and the compressed CO_2, numerous patents with special focus on the design of the mixing device (coaxial nozzles, impinging systems, swirl nozzles, etc.) have been registered in the semi-continuous process giving rise to different processes with essentially the same basis, such as supercritical enhanced dispersion of solutions (SEDS) and aerosol solvent extraction system (ASES) [35].

12.3.2.1 Gas Antisolvent (GAS) Process

During the GAS process, CO_2 is transferred from the vapor phase to the solute-rich liquid phase, and vice versa, according to the phase equilibrium between the CO_2 and the organic solvent (Figure 12.6). The vapor-liquid equilibrium (VLE) of the CO_2-organic solvent mixture is normally not significantly affected by the presence of low molecular weight solutes, moreover because they are normally present at low concentrations. Thereupon, the solution is expanded, causing its solvent power to decrease and thus triggering solute precipitation. When the process is carried out in batch mode, the CO_2 is generally introduced at the bottom of the solution using diffusers to increase the mixing between the CO_2-phase and the liquid-phase, and additionally mechanical stirrers can be used (Figure 12.5a). If the process is carried out in the semi-continuous technique, the liquid solution will be disrupted into droplets as it get outs of the nozzle device, with typical size in the range of 50–100 microns. Following precipitation, excess organic solvent is removed by blowing additional CO_2 at constant pressure. Finally, the vessel is depressurized and the final product recovered [1, 4, 5, 35].

In the batch GAS method, the main parameter of the process is the specific CO_2 addition rate, defined as the ratio between the CO_2 flow rate and the initial amount of solution, as shown by Muhrer *et al.* [36]. They presented a comprehensive model of the batch GAS process which included a description of the solid–liquid–vapor equilibrium of the system, particle formation (primary and secondary nucleation) and particle growth. Their results confirmed their experimental observations showing three types of systems regarding the relative rate of secondary nucleation to primary homogenous nucleation (both depending on supersaturation), which depends on the selected solute-solvent system. If the secondary nucleation is slow, the final particle size distribution is unimodal and narrow, and the average particle size can be tuned over orders of magnitude by varying the CO_2 addition rate. This is the case for precipitation of L-asparagine from ethanol-water mixtures or paracetamol from acetone. On the contrary, when secondary nucleation is faster than primary nucleation, the final particle size distribution is unimodal but the average particle size is almost unaffected by the antisolvent addition rate, as it happens for the precipitation of amorphous lysozyme from DMSO. Finally, bimodal particle size distributions are obtained when primary and secondary nucleation rates are similar, i.e., recrystallization of ascorbic acid from ethanol.

Other parameters, such as initial solute concentration in the organic solution, temperature, and final pressure have a much lower influence on PSD of the product.

In the semi-continuous process, since CO_2 and organic solution are pumped at the same time the relative ratio between both of them, that is the mass or molar fraction of CO_2 in the mixture, is as important as the primary droplet size of the solution, therefore the interest in the nozzle design. As mathematically described by Werling and Debenedetti [37], the droplet formed in the spray first swells due to the dissolution of CO_2 in the organic solvent, and afterwards shrinks till the formation of the particle due to the extraction of the solvent in the CO_2-rich phase. Further, Martín *et al.* [38] developed a specific model to study the mass transfer during the supercritical drying of aqueous protein solutions with a mixture of SC-CO_2 and ethanol. They calculated the evolution of ethanol concentration in a water droplet and its diameter with time in the two different periods.

Besides previously described models, more empirical tools have been developed to choose appropriate operating conditions. Since the volume expansion caused by the dissolution of CO_2 in the solvent is the driving force of the precipitation in the GAS process, the knowledge of this expansion at different molar fraction of CO_2 values allows manipulation of supersaturation, and hence PSD of the product. Moreover, the definition of the volumetric expansion based on the variation of the partial molar volume of the solvent as proposed by De la Fuente *et al.* [39], allows selecting the combination of temperature, CO_2 mol fraction and solvent to achieve the maximal volume expansion for a given application.

In the next work [40] especially focused on batch GAS processes, they demonstrated that to obtain an adequate product with narrow

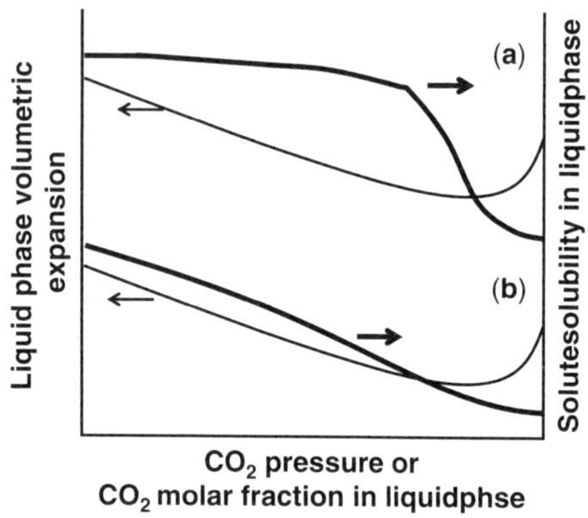

Figure 12.7 Volumetric expansion and solubility of solute in a gas antisolvent (GAS) system CO_2–organic solvent–solute: A. Successful precipitation. B. Unsuccessful precipitation: big particles and wide PSD. (Adapted from [40]).

PSD, the solute solubility in the mixture CO_2- solvent should decrease sharply (Figure 12.7a) to produce a fast and homogenous precipitation. If the solubility decreases slowly with the addition of CO_2 (Figure 12.7b), the precipitation will take place just after the introduction of $CO_{2,}$ continuously yielding bigger particles due to the lower supersaturation and having a broader PSD. In order to avoid this problem, semi-continuous processing is preferred since the solution is put into contact with CO_2 after stable operational pressure and temperature are achieved. There is also the possibility to carry out the process in batch mode by injecting the solution into a sufficient amount of CO_2 at certain temperature and pressure [41]. Nevertheless, this configuration is not widely used throughout the literature.

12.3.2.2 Supercritical Antisolvent Process

As pointed out previously, in supercritical antisolvent processes it is not the CO_2 itself that has to be at conditions above its critical point, but the mixture of CO_2-organic solvent (Figure 12.6), i.e., mixture critical point (MCP). It also should be noted that the process is generally carried out in semi-continuous mode and only this configuration will be referred along the section. Above the MCP, provided there is no influence of the solute that is aimed to be precipitated or recrystallized, the mixing between the organic solution and the CO_2 is faster and takes place without interface limitations since surface tension decreases to zero in a distance shorter than the characteristic break-up length of the spray. Therefore, distinct droplets of solution are never formed at supercritical conditions, and the jet spray forms a gaseous plume leading to the formation of smaller and less agglomerated particles [4]. There are many examples of compounds processed first by GAS and latter by SAS in order to improve product quality, i.e., reduce particle size and agglomeration (β-carotene [42], theophylline [43], itraconazole [44], etc.). Fusaro and collaborators [45] demonstrated that the difference in particle size of paracetamol precipitated from an acetone solution using CO_2 as antisolvent in batch GAS process (90–250 μm) and semi-continuous SAS (2 μm) is directly related to the difference of characteristic mass-transfer times (τ_{mt}) for both processes: 20s and 0.01s, respectively. Calculations were performed according to the GAS model previously presented [36] and the model proposed by Werling and Debenedetti [46] for mass transfer calculation in miscible conditions.

The influence of process parameters (pressure, temperature, solution flow rate and ratio to CO_2 flow rate, initial solution concentration, nozzle design) in product particle size and morphology is difficult to be analyzed in a general way, since all parameters are interconnected in the main physical phenomena leading to particle formation: thermodynamics (phase equilibrium), fluid-dynamics (mixing of organic solution and CO_2), mass transfer and crystallization kinetics. The model developed by Martin and Cocero [47] takes into account all these phenomena and uses the system β-carotene-DCM-CO_2 as benchmark. The model contributes to the understanding of the SAS process, scale-up and interpretation of experimental results in terms of the main process parameter, supersaturation. For instance, it justifies the "a priori" unexpected experimental observation of particle size reduction with increasing pressure when a pressure value of 15 MPa is exceeded: at higher pressures, the solubility of β-carotene in CO_2 is higher, but the solubility in the organic solvent is lower. Therefore, above this pressure value the increase of the supersaturation in the solvent-rich region balances the decrease in the CO_2-rich region. However, the model fails to predict the value of the mean particle size, since experimental values of certain physical properties, such as interfacial tension between the new solid phase and the fluid, are not available. Better particle size predictions are achieved if mixing of both streams, with special regard to the microscale, is included in the model as proposed by Sierra-Pallarés and coworkers [48] using the arbitrary Schmidt number approach.

They used different nozzle geometries to get an insight into the mixing process associated with each geometry and how mixing can be determinant in getting lower particle size.

Besides, the criteria that govern the final solid state, crystalline or amorphous, of the processed solute are not fully clear. There are systems that, depending on operating conditions (P,T), precipitate into amorphous or crystalline particles; moreover, different crystalline structures, i.e., polymorphs, can be obtained [49, 50] even in the homogenous supercritical phase. However, it has been observed that there are systems (solute-solvent-CO_2) that consistently precipitate into amorphous particles (yttrium acetate, YAc-dimethyl sulfoxide - CO_2), while others always form crystals (paracetamol, PCM-Ethanol-CO_2) [51]. The development of optical methods to visualize dynamic processes under high pressure, such as elastic and inelastic light scattering [52], gives rise to an explanation for the different morphologies of amorphous particles in terms of time for disappearance of the interface between the liquid and the fluid phase (liquid or SCF), and time for emergence of the new solid-fluid interface (particle precipitation at saturation mole fraction) during solution injection (liquid/fluid interface) into CO_2 in antisolvent processes. Therefore, it has been visually demonstrated that in amorphous systems, due to the influence of phase behavior on mass transfer times as described previously, nanoparticles are formed if particle formation takes place in a homogeneous supercritical phase; microparticles are obtained when the particle formation arises in a liquid phase of short lifetime; amorphous hollow microparticles or ballons are produced if precipitation occurs in a rather stable liquid phase of long lifetime, i.e., GAS process [51, 52]. Also, the use of previous optical techniques with Raman-scattering-based measurement technique allow for the imaging of supersaturation during the precipitation process, which is the driving force for particle precipitation [53].

Thanks to these visualization techniques, Rossmann and coworkers [54] have identified the saturation solubility of the solute in mixtures of solvents and antisolvents as indirect classification criterion to distinguish between amorphous precipitating and crystallizing SAS systems. They determined the supersaturation at the location of first particle generation during CO_2 antisolvent processing, and the saturation solubilities of the solutes in the mixtures organic solvent-CO_2 by *in situ* light scattering techniques in an optically accessible high-pressure vessel. They found that the supersaturation in the system producing amorphous particles (YAc/DMSO/CO_2)

was up to four orders of magnitude larger than for the SAS system producing crystals (PCM/EtOH/CO_2); this was in agreement with the saturation solubilities of the solutes which were found to be approximately four orders of magnitude larger for the PCM system than for the YAc system. This performance is equivalent to that of conventional particle generation in liquid phase, where precipitation is carried out under high supersaturation values and crystallization takes places at lower values, and the difference between the solubility of sparingly (high supersaturation) and slightly soluble solutes (low supersaturation) is some orders of magnitude.

They also confirmed that for the crystallizing SAS systems, crystals may be generated from either a supercritical or a liquid phase. Hence, if a normally crystallizing solute shall be micronized as an amorphous particle, the organic solvent has to be replaced by a different one that lowers the solubility of the solute in the solvent/antisolvent mixture.

However, there are not many available data for ternary systems solute-organic solvent-CO_2 and the selection of the solvent has to be done through screening experiments, or phase equilibrium modeling of the ternary systems from data of the binary systems CO_2-solvent, CO_2-solute and solute-solvent.

12.3.2.3 *Special Considerations Regarding Polymer Encapsulation and Co-Precipitation*

The Supercritical Antisolvent methods for encapsulation of compounds are performed essentially in the same way as previously presented processes. In this case a liquid solution containing both the active compound and the encapsulating material is prepared. Solvent mixtures can be used to achieve the desired concentration of both compounds or alternatively, each one can be dissolved in a different solvent and pumped independently but simultaneously into the high pressured vessel using, for instance, a three-coaxial-nozzle.

Regarding process parameters, in the case of co-precipitations the concentration of carrier material as well as the carrier/active compound ratio is a major parameter to be considered. As this ratio is varied, it is possible to establish, in some cases, whether the carrier solidifies before, simultaneously or after the active compound, and therefore to switch from microcomposites, which are the most typical morphology, to microcapsules [55].

The antisolvent process, either semi-continuous or batch, in one homogeneous supercritical phase or in the presence of a liquid phase, has been widely applied to the encapsulation with a wide variety of materials: lipids, carbohydrate materials and polymers.

The processing of lipid as encapsulating materials in CO_2-based antisolvent processing is mainly focused in the production of liposomes [56].

Concerning carbohydrates processing, there is a lot of work regarding cyclodextrines as encapsulating material for improving hydrophobic drug bioavalability [57] or taste masking of bitter drugs [58]. Usually they are precipitated into submicron amorphous particles from low concentration DMSO solutions (5–15 g/L) of both components in semi-continuous mode with CO_2 at 12–15 MPa and 35–40°C. Also, different morphologies of cyclodextrines, from amorphous microparticles and ballons to microcrystals, can be obtained by increasing solution concentration and varying operational conditions (P, T), including the two-phase region [59]. Cellulose derivatives, such as ethylcellulose, methylcellulose, hydroxipropilmethylcellulose or their mixtures are widely used, as well, to achieve control release profiles of aqueous soluble drugs [60, 61].

Polymer encapsulation by CO_2-antisolvent processes has been predominantly addressed and a wide variety of polymers have been successfully processed [5]; nevertheless, the interactions of CO_2 with the polymers and organic solvent/polymer mixtures can be unfavorable in some cases, as CO_2 can act as a cosolvent which is detrimental for the precipitation of the polymer [5, 62]. SC-CO_2 is highly soluble in amorphous polymers such as PLGA, DL-PLA or PVP, resulting in their swelling and a significant decrease of glass transition temperature (Tg) values. Similarly, in semicrystalline polymers such as PEG, L-PLA or PCL, CO_2 solubilization reduces both the melting temperature (Tm) and Tg values [63–66]. It should be noted that solubility of CO_2 is generally lower in semicrystalline than in amorphous polymers. As will be discussed later on, the interaction between CO_2 and the polymers is exploited in production microcomposites by solvent-free polymer processes (Section 12.3.3), in CO_2-assisted polymer extrusion [67], as well as in material processing for tissue engineering application as recently reviewed by Davis *et al.* [3].

This plasticization effect of dense CO_2 can be increased by the use of low molecular weight solvent, as typically used in CO_2 antisolvent processes, yielding a liquid–liquid phase split into a polymer-rich phase and a CO_2-solvent-rich one [5]. In such cases, CO_2 antisolvent processes leads to film products. This was observed in the encapsulation of β-carotene in PEG using DCM as solvent

[55] and tea extract into PCL using acetone as solvent [68]. In both works, the reduction of temperature from 35°C to temperatures in the range of 15–20°C at typical operating pressures of 9–10 MPa allows the formation of spherulitic microparticles with good encapsulation yields, although highly agglomerated due to the use of liquid CO_2. This issue was not encountered in the processing of Pluronic F-127 with ethanolic rosemary extract [69], despite having a similar melting point (ca. 50°C at ambient conditions) nor in the encapsulation with L-PLA [70, 71], although in this case the high melting temperature of the L-PLA (ca. 175°C) may be the reason preventing the formation of a liquid polymer-rich phase.

A similar behavior was found for amorphous materials with relatively low glass transition temperatures, such as DL-PLA (ca. 50°C), that has to be processed at temperatures below 20°C to avoid film formation [72]; whereas polymers with higher glass transition temperature can be satisfactorily processed by SAS processes. As an example, phenytoin has been encapsulated with PVP (Tg ca. 175°C) into amorphous submicron particles processed at 15 MPa and 40°C to improve its aqueous solubility [73]. Moreover, amorphous structure was proven to be stable after one year storage at room temperature.

12.3.2.4 Supercritical Fluid Extraction of Emulsions (SFEE)

The supercritical fluid extraction of emulsions (SFEE) process has been developed mainly to avoid the plasticization problems of certain polymers in SC-CO_2 atmosphere, as detailed previously, and to produce non-agglomerated uniform drug-loaded polymer nanoparticles [74].

Emulsions are prepared by ultrasounds or high-speed stirring according to conventional procedures for oil-in-water (O/W) emulsions using an emulsifier (eg., PLGA-Ketoprofen in ethyl acetate in water emulsion using PVA as surfactant). Water-in-oil-in water (W/O/W) emulsions can also be employed if a protein or other water soluble material is aiming to be encapsulated [75]. Alternatively, the encapsulating polymer can also be the surfactant as in the encapsulation with modified starches [76].

As in conventional precipitation processed from emulsions (solvent evaporation and emulsion diffusion), the emulsion provides a template for the formation of particles. The role of CO_2 is to diffuse through the water into the organic solvent droplets. Once these droplets are saturated with CO_2, the precipitation of the polymer and active compound takes places by antisolvent effect, as evidence by Mattea and coworkers [77]. Afterwards, the organic solvent is extracted from the droplets to the supercritical phase. Thus, a suspension of particles in water is obtained. The contact between the CO_2 and the solution is commonly carried out in continuous mode, although batch processes are also used [76]. In the continuous mode, both streams can be put into contact in a countercurrent high-pressure packed column [78], or by spraying them through a coaxial nozzle into a vessel at operational temperature and pressure, in the same way as semi-continuous antisolvent processes, with continuous removal of the water suspension.

The advantages of SFEE versus conventional processes to remove organic solvent from emulsions (solvent evaporation and emulsion diffusion) are faster extraction rates, higher production yields, no additional requirements of water, lower concentration of residual solvent (well below the legal limits), lower particle size of the final suspension and continuous operation [76, 78].

As general comment concerning all the techniques described in this section, it should be pointed out that, despite the use of organic solvents in CO_2-antisolvent techniques, their residual level in the final product is well below the requirements of ICH guideline for pharmaceutical products [79], as specifically stated in numerous works. Moreover, the applicability of these techniques thanks to the use of organics solvents is really wide. Besides the examples of precipitation and encapsulation of pharmaceuticals, natural substances and food additives, referred along the process description, superconductor precursors [49], metal complexes [80] and explosives [81] have been processed as well, thanks to the inert atmosphere provided by CO_2.

12.3.3 Supercritical Fluid as Solute

Particles from gas saturated solutions (PGSS™) process, also known as supercritical melt micronization, was patented in 1995 for the production of polymer coatings [82].

In the PGSS process, a SC-CO_2 saturated solution of the melted compound/s is expanded through a nozzle into a spray tower, generally at atmospheric conditions. Particles are formed after solidification of spray droplets due to the intense cooling produced by the expansion of the CO_2 (Joule-Thomson effect). Due to the fast solidification, the thermal stress is lower compared to the classic air drying process [83].

The PGSS process can be carried out in batch or semi-continuous mode. In the batch mode (Figure 12.8a), the molten material is saturated with CO_2 in a stirred vessel until the saturated molten

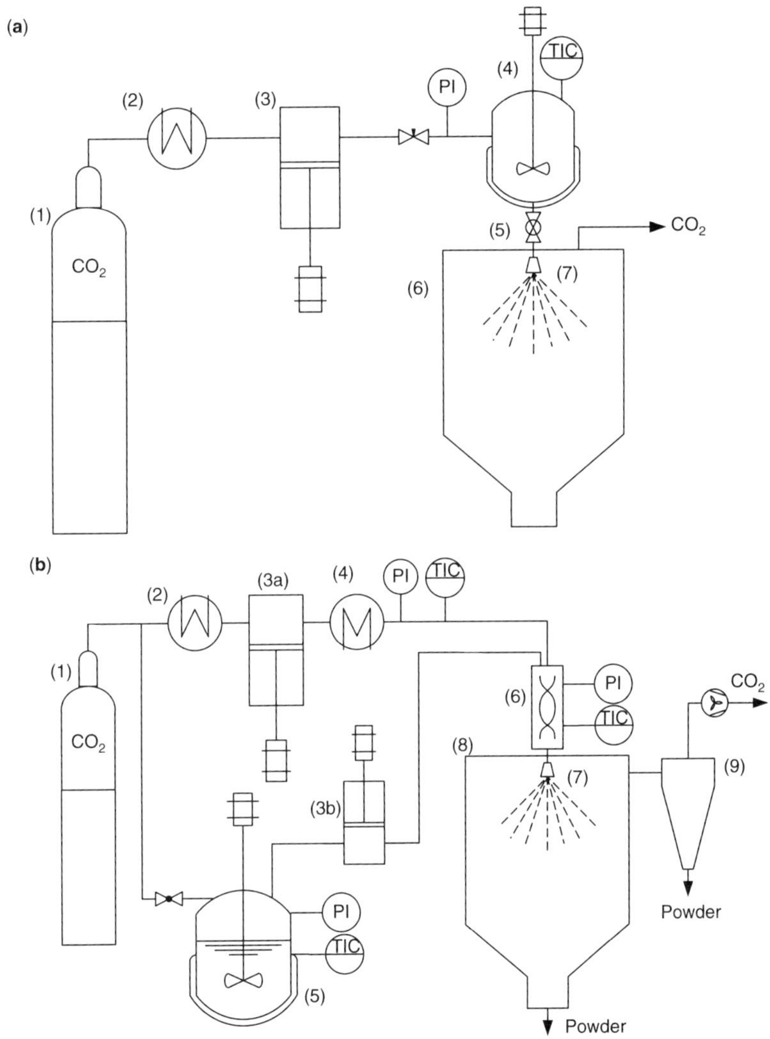

Figure 12.8 Usual experimental setup for PGSS process: (a) Batch system: (1) Gas cylinder (2) cryostate (3) High pressure CO_2 pump (4) Thermostated and stirred high pressure vessel (5) depressurization valve (6) ambient pressure recovery vessel (7) nozzle. (b) Continuous system: (1) Gas cylinder (2) cryostate (3a) High pressure CO_2 pump (3b) high pressure pump for polymer melt (4) heater (5) thermostated and stirred high pressure vessel for polymer melt (6) static mixer (7) nozzle (8) ambient pressure recovery vessel (9) cyclone for fine powder recovery.

is depressurized. In the semi-continuous mode (Figure 12.8b), the mixing is produced in a static mixer where CO_2 and molten streams are put into contact for a short period of time.

As mentioned before, solubility of polar compounds and high MW compounds in SC-CO_2 is very limited; this process takes advantage of the high solubility of SC-CO_2 in polymers or fats. It is also applicable to substances that are plasticized by SC-CO_2, such as small drug molecules like nifedipine [84]. In comparison with the processes previously explained in this chapter, the PGSS method has several advantages. No organic solvent is used, as well as in the RESS process and in contrast to antisolvent techniques. It can be applied to a wide range of substances, including mixtures for composites production, since the dissolution of substance in SC-CO_2 is not needed, contrary to RESS process, and the consumption of CO_2 is lower than in the RESS method by an order of magnitude of 10^3 [84]. Also, the SC-CO_2 is dissolved in the matrix reduce its glass transition (amorphous and semicrystalline compounds) and/or melting point (semicrystalline substances) as well as decrease the viscosity of the mixture. Therefore, it is especially suitable for polymer processing and encapsulation of labile substances and other materials that are not possible to process by conventional extrusion methods; moreover, energy cost is reduced. However, the particle size of the products is higher compared to products obtained by RESS or SAS, with mean particle sizes in the range of 10 to 100 μm depending on processing parameters [83].

Furthermore, to the best knowledge of the authors, this is the only supercritical fluid process for particle engineering already working on an industrial scale. Since the year 2000, Raps GbmH (Kulm, Germany) has had industrial equipment for the production of 200 kg/h of food additives [85].

CO_2 solubility and diffusivity in polymers, which is also exploited in supercritical impregnation process as shown in Section 12.3.1.2, are influenced by both the molecular structure (the interaction between CO_2 and molecular chains) and the morphology (crystalline or amorphous, related with free volume) of polymers. As CO_2 is incorporated in the matrix, a considerable increase of its-volume (swelling) is generally produced [3, 65]. As commented on in Section 12.3.2.3, the solubility of CO_2 as well as the consequent melting point depression, have been studied for different compounds commonly used as encapsulating agents, such us lipids [86], amorphous biodegradable polymers (PLGA and DL-PLA [65]) and semicrystalline ones (Poly(ethylene)glycol [63, 64], PCL [66]) and polysaccharides such as cyclodextrines [87].

Despite the simplicity of the process, the particle formation mechanism is relatively complex since it is controlled by the relative rates of atomization and solidification of the sprayed SC-CO_2 saturated solution. Therefore, powders with a wide variety of particle size and morphology can be obtained. Spherical particles are produced when the atomization precedes the solidification process, whereas fibers and more porous particles are obtained when the solidification is very fast [64, 83, 88, 89].

Atomization depends on nozzle design but is improved by the fast release of admixed and dissolved CO_2 breaking primary droplets into smaller secondary droplets (decompressive atomization). Also, the solubilization of CO_2 in the molten reduces its surface tension and viscosity, improving the atomization as well as the high pressure drop across the nozzle. The solidification depends on the heat transfer and heat conduction rates, which depends on CO_2 concentration in the molten (Joule-Thomson effect) and on particle size, which in turn depends on atomization. Therefore, pressure and temperature are identified as main process parameters, since SC-CO_2 solubility depends on them: At high pressure, large amounts of CO_2 are dissolved in the melt and higher pressure drop is produced across the nozzle improving the atomization into small droplets; also, more CO_2 gas bubbles are formed increasing the cooling rate (Joule-Thomson effect) which originate micro-foams and porous particles as the gas cannot diffuse out of the particles before particle solidification, perforating particle surface afterwards. On the contrary, as the temperature increased, the solubility of CO_2 decreased, allowing the formation of more spherical and closed structures since the slower solidification of the droplets facilitates the diffusion of CO_2 out of the particles [64, 83, 88, 89].

In addition, the performance of semi-continuous PGSS process can be modulated by the flow rates of CO_2. Similarly, high gas to product ratio (GTP), i.e., high SC-CO_2 to molten polymer ratio, improved the atomization and solidification rates producing smaller and more porous particles. The process was extensively studied by P. Kappler *et al.* in 2003 [88], and they proposed different correlations for particle size, shape factor and powder bulk density as function of operating parameters (pressure, temperature and GTP ratio) using PEG (MW: 6000 g/mol) as reference material.

As mentioned previously, viscosity of the polymer melt is a key factor in the atomization step; therefore, the higher the viscosity the bigger the obtained particles. Therefore, amorphous polymers, such as DL-PLA, are also difficult to process by PGSS since the molten CO_2-polymer solution is very viscous (2000 mPa·s vs 200 mPa·s for PEG) and fibrous material is obtained. Moreover, since amorphous materials do not really melt or solidify, spherical morphology is difficult to achieve. Hao and coworkers [89] proposed to recover the DL-PLA particles at 6.8 MPa back pressure of N_2 to decrease melt viscosity in a more gradual way, allowing the formation of spherical particles and reducing plasticization during particle formation.

In addition, the PGSS method allows the encapsulation of liquids. The PGSS process can also be used for generating fluid-filled particles. In general, oily liquids (rapeseed oil, lavandin essential oil) [90] are encapsulated in hydrophilic polymers, such as PEG, whereas aqueous solutions (liquor, extracts from plants) are encapsulated in fats (palm fat, castor fat) [85]. The idea is to form powderous w/o (water-in-oil) and o/w (oil-in-water) emulsions with liquid content up to 50%. The formation of particles with a liquid core again depends on the balance between the phase separation of the hydrophobic and hydrophilic material, and the rate of solidification of the solid material that would form the shell. If the solidification is faster, the core shell structure will be achieved; otherwise the liquid will be incorporated into the carrier by adsorption [85].

12.3.3.1 CO_2 as Solute and Propellant for Drying of Aqueous Solutions

As mentioned in Section 12.3.2, "Supercritical Fluid as Antisolvent," micronization of aqueous solutions is challenging due to the low solubility of water in SC-CO_2 [37]. The use of sc-CO_2 as solute and/or as a propellant in order to achieve an enhanced atomization of the solution improves the processing of such solutions since CO_2 is one of the most soluble gases in water (1.6 mole % at 63°C and 10 MPa).

In 1997, Sievers and Karst [91] patented the Carbon dioxide Assisted Nebulization with a Bubble Dry (CAN-BD) process. In this process, the aqueous solution containing the drug and any excipient or stabilizer is pumped (0.3–0.5 mL/min) at room temperature and mixed in a low volume tee with a stream of near critical

CO_2 (1–3 mL/min), typically, at room temperature and pressures slightly above the critical value, to generate a gas-liquid emulsion. The two-phase stream is expanded into a drying chamber (50–80°C) at atmospheric pressure where an additional stream of the heated nitrogen (15–30 L/min) is introduced to dry the particles. The inventors claim that CAN-BD does not belong to the gas-saturated solution processes due to the short residence time in the mixing device. The rapid expansion of the gas-liquid emulsion caused vaporization of the liquid and nebulizing fluid, forming a fine aerosol of microbubbles and microdroplets that dry faster and at lower temperatures than aerosols formed in conventional methods. This process has been applied for the encapsulation of vaccines, drugs and proteins with carbohydrates (trehalose, lactose) from aqueous solutions, or suspensions for pulmonary drug delivery since the aerodynamic diameter of the particles is consistently below 5 microns. Also, ethanol and water-ethanol solutions have been processed.

The supercritical assisted atomization (SAA) developed by Reverchon [92], can be considered as a modification of CAN-BD since the main difference is the increase of the contact time between the liquid solution (4–5 mL/min) and the CO_2 up to 4–5 min to ensure saturation of the solution with the dense gas in a packed high-pressure vessel to enlarge the contact surface. Also, CO_2 is always mixed in supercritical state (10 MPa and 80°C). Therefore, the enhanced atomization is due not only to the pneumatic atomization, but to the massive expansion of dissolved CO_2 in the primary droplets, forming smaller secondary droplets (decompressive atomization). This process has been applied to precipitation and encapsulation of drugs from aqueous solutions, i.e., encapsulation of amphicilin in chitosan [93], and from organic solutions (acetone, DCM) for the precipitation of L-PLA or PMMA [94]. In the latter case, the temperature in the precipitation chamber is reduced to 50–60°C.

Finally, in the PGSS drying process, the preheated N_2 stream is eliminated, while the SC-CO_2 flow rate is increased (gas flow rate to solution flow rate ratio: 15–40). Also, the temperature in the static mixer is increased (100–130°C). Nevertheless, since the residence time is decreased to a few seconds, thermal degradation of the compounds is avoided. The drying chamber is operated at ambient pressure and temperatures slightly above room conditions (40–60°C). This technique has been applied to dry aqueous green tea extracts [95] and soybean lecithin emulsions to encapsulate essential oil [96] and β-carotene [97].

To sum up, techniques using carbon dioxide as propellant and solute can be considered as an alternative to spray drying, with the advantages of lower processing temperatures and smaller and controlled particle size, and the disadvantage of requiring some high pressure equipment.

12.3.4 Supercritical Fluid as Reaction Media

Generally, processes that involve a reaction in SC-CO_2 or CO_2 mixtures with short chain alcohols leading to particle formation are used to synthesize ceramics and metal oxides, commonly in the nanoscale, via thermal decomposition of an organic precursor [98]. These nanoparticles can be deposited into microparticles to form core-shell structures. As an example, Pessey and collaborators [99] coated $SmCo_5$ microparticles with copper by decomposition of copper-hexafluoroacetylacetonate in CO_2/ethanol mixture (80:20) at 19 MPa and 200 °C. Copper particles are deposited onto the surface of $SmCo_5$ particles, whereas the organic product of the decomposition, which is soluble in the supercritical solvent, is recovered at the outlet of the system after expansion, thereby avoiding contamination of the particles.

Silanization of porous aggregates of nanoparticles to confer hydrophobic surface properties is another process with improved performance when it is carried out in SC-CO_2. Thanks to the enhanced mass transfer in SC-CO_2, inner mesopores are also processed as demonstrated by Loste *et al.* [100]. They coated the surface of two types of nanoparticles, hydroxyapatite and titanium dioxide, by trialkoxysilane-methacryloxypropyltrimethoxysilane in a one-step process in SC-CO_2 medium.

Similarly, SC-CO_2 can be used to manufacture catalyst. Aspromonte *et al.* [101] uniformly deposited nanoparticles of cobalt oxide over the inner surface of mesoporous supports (MCM-41), after thermal decomposition of the organometallic precursor previously solubilized in the SC-CO_2.

In addition, inorganic and organic particles can be coated by *in situ* polymerization in carbon dioxide [1]. Core particles are uniformly coated since they provide a heterogeneous nucleus for polymer precipitation after reaction. Polymerization in SC-CO_2 has been widely studied for the production of polycarbonates, polyesters (PLC, PLA, etc.) and polyamides [102]. The use of CO_2 reduces the viscosity of the polymer during processing resulting in higher conversions since the resistance to mass transfer is lower in comparison to conventional melt synthesis.

Acronyms

CAN-BD	Carbon dioxide Assisted Nebulization with a Bubble Dry
DCM	dichloromethane
DMSO	dimethyl-sulfoxide
GAS	Gas Antisolvent
GTP	gas to product ratio
MW	molecular weight
P	pressure (MPa)
PCL	polycaprolactone
PEG	poly(ethylenglycol)
PGSS	Particles from Gas Saturated Solution
PLA	poly-lactic acid (DL, mixture of enantiomers), L-PLA (from enantiopure L-lactide)
PLGA	poly(lactic-co-glycolic acid)
PMMA	Poly(methyl methacrylate)
PSD	particle size distribution
PVP	Polyvinylpyrrolidone
RESS	Rapid Expansion of Supercritical Solution
SAA	Supercritical Antisolvent Atomization
SAS	Supercritical Antisolvent
SC	supercritical
SCF	supercritical fluid
T	temperature (°C)
VLE	vapor-liquid equilibrium

References

1. M. Bahrami, and S. Ranjbarian. *J. of Supercritical Fluids* Vol. 40, pp. 263–283, 2007.
2. I. Pasquali, R. Bettini, and F. Giordano. *Advanced Drug Delivery Reviews* Vol. 60, pp. 399–410, 2008.
3. O.R. Davies, A.L. Lewis, M.J. Whitaker, H. Tai, K.M. Shakesheff, and S.M. Howdle. *Advanced Drug Delivery Reviews* Vol. 60, pp. 373–387, 2008.
4. A. Martín, and M.J. Cocero. *Advanced Drug Delivery Reviews* Vol. 60, pp. 339–350, 2008.

5. M.J. Cocero, Á. Martín, F. Mattea, and S. Varona. *J. of Supercritical Fluids* Vol. 47, pp. 546–555, 2009.
6. A.V.M. Nunes, and C.M.M. Duarte. *Materials* Vol. 4, pp. 2017–2041, 2011.
7. M. Türk. *J. of Supercritical Fluids* Vol. 47, pp. 537–545, 2009.
8. A. Tabernero, E.M. Martín del Valle, and M.A. Galán. *Chemical Engineering and Processing* Vol. 60, pp. 9–25, 2012.
9. E. Elizondo, J. Veciana, and N. Ventosa. *Nanomedicine* Vol. 7, pp. 1391–1408, 2012.
10. G. Brunner. *Gas extraction. An introduction to fundamentals of supercritical fluids and the application to separation processes.* Darmstadt: New York, N.Y.: Steinkopff, Springer, 1994.
11. F.P. Lucien, and N.R. Foster. Phase behaviour and solubility. In *Chemical synthesis using supercritical fluids,* P.G. Jessop and W. Leitner, eds. Wiley –VCH, p. 38, 1999.
12. E.J. Beckman. *J. of Supercritical Fluids* Vol. 28, pp. 121–191, 2004.
13. G. Brunner. *J. of Food Engineering* Vol. 67, pp. 21–33, 2005.
14. D.W.Matson, J.L. Fulton, R.C. Petersen, and R.D. Smith. *Industrial and Engineering Chemistry Research* Vol. 26, pp. 2298–2306, 1987.
15. J.L. Fulton, G.S. Deverman, C.R. Yonker, J.W. Grate, J. De Young, and J.B. McClain. *Polymer* Vol. 44, pp. 3627–3632, 2003.
16. B. Helfgen, M. Türk, K. Schaber. *J. Supercritical Fluids* Vol. 26, pp. 225–242, 2003.
17. T. Sarbu, T. Styranec, and E.J. Beckman. *Nature* Vol. 405, pp. 165–168, 2000.
18. R. Thakur, and R.B. Gupta. *International J. of Pharmaceutics* Vol. 308, pp. 190–199, 2006.
19. P.G. Debenedetti , J.W. Tom, X. Kwauk, and S.-D. Yeo. *Fluid Phase Equilibria* Vol. 82, pp. 311–321, 1993
20. E. Teunou, and D. Poncelet. *J. Food Engineering* Vol. 53, pp. 325–340, 2002.
21. A. Tsutsumi, S. Nakamoto, T. Mineo, and K. Yoshida. *Powder Technology* Vol. 85, pp. 275–278, 1995.
22. Marzocchella, and P. Salatino. *AIChE Symposium Series* Vol. 92, pp. 25–30, 1996.
23. M. Niehaus, U. Teipel, H. Krause, and W. Weisweiler. Coating of particles in a fluidized bed using supercritical carbon dioxide. In *Proceedings of the 5th meeting on supercritical fluids.* Nice, France, 1998.
24. A.K. Sunol, J. Kosky, M. Murphy, E. Hansen, J. Jones, B. Mierau, and S. Sunol. Supercritical fluid aided encapsulation of particles in a fluidised bed environment. In *Proceedings of the 5th meeting on supercritical fluids.* Nice, France, 1998.
25. R. Schreiber, B. Reinke, C. Vogt, J. Werther, and G. Brunner. *J. Supercritical Fluids* Vol. 138, pp. 31–38, 2003.
26. S. Rodríguez-Rojo, J. Marienfeld, and M.J. Cocero. *Chemical Engineering J.* Vol. 144, pp. 531–539, 2008.
27. K. Rosenkranz, M.M. Kasper, J. Werther, and G. Brunner. *J. of Supercritical Fluids* Vol. 46, pp. 351–357, 2008.
28. H. Kröber, and U. Teipel. *Chemical Engineering and Processing* Vol. 44, pp. 215–219, 2005.
29. K. Mishima, K. Matsuyama, D. Tanabe, and S. Yamauchi. *AIChE J.* Vol. 46, pp. 857–865, 2000.

30. A. Tsutsumi, M. Ikeda, W. Chen, and J. Iwatsuki. *Powder Technology* Vol. 138, pp. 211–215, 2003.
31. M. Türk, and D. Bolten. *J. of Supercritical Fluids* Vol. 55, pp. 778–785, 2010.
32. H.C. de Sousa, M.H.M. Gil, E.O.B. Leite, C.M.M. Duarte, and A.R.C. Duarte. Methods for preparing sustained-release therapeutic ophthalmic articles using compressed fluids for impregnation of drugs. EP Patent 1611877A1, January 4, 2006.
33. A.R.C. Duarte, J.F. Mano, and R.L. Reis. *European Polymer J.* Vol. 45, pp. 141–148, 2009.
34. S. Varona, S. Rodríguez-Rojo, A. Martín, M.J. Cocero, and C.M.M. Duarte. *J. of Supercritical Fluids* Vol. 58, pp. 313–319, 2011.
35. A. Martín, and M.J. Cocero. *Recent Patents on Engineering* Vol. 2, pp. 2–20, 2008.
36. G. Muhrer, C. Lin, and M. Mazzotti. *Industrial and Engineering Chemistry Research* Vol. 41, pp. 3566–3579, 2002.
37. J.O. Werling, and P.G. Debenedetti. *J. of Supercritical Fluids* Vol. 16, pp. 167–181, 1999.
38. A. Martín, A. Bouchard, G.W. Hofland, G.-J. Witkamp, and M.J. Cocero. *J. of Supercritical Fluids* Vol. 41, pp. 126–137, 2007.
39. J.C. De la Fuente, C.J. Peters, and J. de Swaan Arons. *J. of Supercritical Fluids* Vol. 17, pp. 13–23, 2000.
40. J.C. de la Fuente, A. Shariati, and C.J. Peters. *J. of Supercritical Fluids* Vol. 32, pp. 55–61, 2004.
41. W.J. Schmitt. Finely divided solid crystalline powders via precipitation into an antisolvent. US Patent 5707634, 1998.
42. M.J. Cocero, S. Ferrero, and F. Miguel. Crystallization of β-carotene by continuous gas process. Effect of mixer on crystals formation. In *4th International symposium on high pressure process technology and chemical engineering*, Venice, Italy, 2002.
43. C. Roy, A. Vega-González, and P. Subra-Paternault. *International J. of Pharmaceutics* Vol. 343, pp. 79–89, 2007.
44. A.M. Barrett, F. Dehghani, and N.R. Foster. *Pharmaceutical Research* Vol. 25, pp. 1274–89, 2008.
45. F. Fusaro, M. Hanchen, M. Mazzotti, G. Muhrer, and B. Subramaniam. *Industrial and Engineering Chemistry Research* Vol. 44, pp. 1502–1509, 2005.
46. J.O. Werling, and P.G. Debenedetti. *J.of Supercritical Fluids* Vol. 18, pp. 11–24, 2000.
47. A. Martín, and M.J. Cocero. *J. of Supercritical Fluids* Vol. 32, pp. 203–219, 2004.
48. J. Sierra-Pallares, D.L. Marchisio, M.T. Parra-Santos, J. García-Serna, F. Castro, and M.J. Cocero. *AIChE J.* Vol. 58, pp. 385–98, 2012.
49. Á. Martín, K. Scholle, F. Mattea, D. Meterc, and M.J. Cocero. *Crystal Growth and Design* Vol. 9, pp. 2504–2511, 2009.
50. G. Weber-Brun, Á. Martín, E. Cassel, R.M. Figueiró Vargas, and M.J. Cocero. *Crystal Growth and Design* Vol. 12, pp. 1943–1951, 2012.
51. E. Reverchon, E. Torino, S. Dowy, A. Braeuer, and A. Leipertz. *Chemical Engineering J.* Vol. 156, pp. 446–458, 2010.
52. A. Braeuer, S. Dowy, E. Torino, M. Rossmann, S.K. Luther, E. Schluecker, A. Leipertz, and E. Reverchon. *Chemical Engineering J.* Vol. 173, pp. 258–66, 2011.

53. S. Dowy, E. Torino, S.K. Luther, M. Rossmann, and A. Braeuer. *Chemical Engineering J.* Vol. 168, pp. 896–902, 2011.
54. M. Rossmann, A. Braeuer, S. Dowy, T.G. Gallinger, A. Leipertz, and E. Schluecker. *J. of Supercritical Fluids* Vol. 66, pp. 350–358, 2012.
55. F. Mattea, A. Martín, and M.J. Cocero. *Ind. Eng. Chem. Res.* 47 (2008) 3900–3906
56. C.C. Beh, R. Mammucari, and N.R. Foster. *Chemical Engineering J.* Vol. 188, pp. 1–14, 2012.
57. S.W. Jun, M.-S Kim, J.-S. Kim, H. J. Park, S. Lee, J.-S. Woo, and S.-J Hwang. *European J. of Pharmaceutics and Biopharmaceutics* Vol. 66, pp. 413–421, 2007.
58. C.-W. Lee, S.-J. Kim, Y.-S. Youn, E. Widjojokusumo, Y.-H. Lee, J. Kim, Y.-W Lee, and R.R. Tjandrawinata. *J. of Supercritical Fluids* Vol. 55, pp. 348–357, 2010.
59. I. De Marco, and E. Reverchon. *Powder Technology* Vol. 183, pp. 239–246, 2008.
60. A.R.C. Duarte, M.D. Gordillo, M.M. Cardoso, A.L. Simplício, and C.M.M. Duarte. *International J. of Pharmaceutics* Vol. 311, pp. 50–54, 2006.
61. A. Montes, M.D. Gordillo, C. Pereyra, and E.J. Martínez de la Ossa. *J. of Supercritical Fluids* Vol. 63, pp. 92–98, 2012.
62. A. Martín, F. Mattea, L. Gutiérrez, F. Miguel, and M.J. Cocero. *J. of Supercritical Fluids* Vol. 41, pp. 138–147, 2007.
63. E. Weidner, V. Wiesmet, Ž. Knez, and M. Skerget. *J. of Supercritical Fluids* Vol. 10, pp. 139–147, 1997.
64. J. Hao, M.J. Whitaker, G. Serhatkulu, K.M. Shakesheff, and S. M. Howdle. *J. of Materials Chemistry* Vol. 15, pp. 1148–1153, 2005.
65. R. Pini, G. Storti, M. Mazzotti, H. Tai, K.M. Shakesheff, and S.M. Howdle. *J. of Polymer Science: Part B: Polymer Physics* Vol. 46, pp. 483–496, 2008.
66. E. de Paz, A. Martín, S. Rodríguez-Rojo, J. Herreras, and M.J. Cocero. *J. of Chemical and Engineering Data* Vol. 55, pp. 2781–2785, 2010.
67. M. Sauceau, J. Fages, A. Common, C. Nikitine, and E. Rodier. *Progress in Polymer Science* Vol. 36, pp. 749–766, 2011.
68. M.V. Sosa, S. Rodríguez-Rojo, F. Mattea, M. Cismondi, and M.J. Cocero. *J. of Supercritical Fluids* Vol. 56, pp. 304–311, 2011.
69. A. Visentin, S. Rodríguez-Rojo, A. Navarrete, D. Maestri, and M.J. Cocero. *J. of Food Engineering* Vol. 109, pp. 9–15, 2012.
70. S. Taki, E. Badens, and G. Charbit. *J. of Supercritical Fluids* Vol. 21, pp. 61–70, 2001.
71. N. Elvassore, A. Bertucco, and P. Caliceti. *J. of Pharmaceutical Sciences* Vol. 90, pp. 1628–1636, 2001.
72. F. Miguel, A. Martín, F. Mattea, and M.J. Cocero. *Chemical Engineering and Processing* Vol. 47, pp. 1594–1602, 2008.
73. J. Kluge, F. Fusaro, G. Muhrer, R. Thakur, and M. Mazzotti. *J. of Supercritical Fluids* Vol. 48, pp. 176–182, 2009.
74. P. Chattopadhyay, R. Huff, and B.Y. Shekunov. *J. of Pharmaceutical Sciences* Vol. 95, pp. 667–679, 2006.
75. J. Kluge, F. Fusaro, N. Casas, M. Mazzotti, and G. Muhrer. *J. of Supercritical Fluids* Vol. 50, pp. 327–335, 2009.
76. F. Mattea, Á. Martín, A. Matías-Gago, and M.J. Cocero. *J. of Supercritical Fluids* Vol. 51, pp. 238–247, 2009.
77. F. Mattea, Á. Martín, C. Schulz, P. Jaeger, R. Eggers, and M.J. Cocero. *AIChE J.* Vol. 56, pp. 1184–1195, 2010.

78. R. Campardelli, G. Della Porta, and E. Reverchon. *J. of Supercritical Fluids* Vol. 70, pp. 100–105, 2012.
79. ICH harmonised tripartite guideline. Impurities: Guideline for residual solvents Q3C(R5). *International Conference on Harmonisation of Technical Requirements for Registration of Pharmaceuticals for Human Use*, Geneva, Switzerland, 2011.
80. J.G. Nguyen, C.A. Johnson, S. Sharma, B. Subramaniam, and A.S. Borovik. Green methods for processing and utilizing metal complexes. In *Gas-expanded liquids and near-critical media*, K.W. Hutchenson, A.M. Scurto, B. Subramaniam, eds. ACS Symposium Series, Vol. 1006, pp. 274–289, 2009.
81. E. Reverchon, H. Kröber, and U. Teipel. Crystallization with compressed gases. In *Energetic materials: Particle processing and characterization*, U. Teipel, ed. Wiley-VCH Verlag GmbH & Co. KGaA, Weinheim, Germany, pp. 171–178, 2005.
82. E. Weidner, Z. Knez, and Z. Novak. Process for preparing particles or powders. WO Patent 9521688, 1995.
83. E. Lack, E. Weidner, Z. Knez, S. Grüner, B. Weinreich, and H. Seidlitz. Particle generation with supercritical CO_2. In *Proceedings of the 1st Vienna International conference: Micro- and nano-technologies*, Vienna, Austria, 2005.
84. P. Senčar-Božič, S. Srčič, Ž. Knez, and J. Kerč. *International J. of Pharmaceutics* Vol. 148, pp. 123–130, 1997.
85. T. Wendt, G. Brandin, E. Weidner, and M. Petermann. PGSS - The innovative production of fluid-filled microcapsules for the food industry. In *Proceedings of the 6th European Congress of chemical engineering*, Copenhagen, Denmark, 2007.
86. A.R. Sampaio de Sousa, M. Calderone, E. Rodier, J. Fages, and C.M.M. Duarte. *J. of Supercritical Fluids* Vol. 39, pp. 13–19, 2006.
87. A.V.M. Nunes, A.P.C. Almeida, S.R. Marques, A.R. Sampaio de Sousa, T. Casimiro, and C.M.M. Duarte. *J. of Supercritical Fluids* Vol. 54, pp. 357–361, 2010.
88. P. Kappler, W. Leiner, M. Petermann, and E. Weidner. Size and morphology of particles generated by spraying polymer-melts with carbon dioxide. In *Proceedings of the 6th international symposium on supercritical fluids*, Versailles, France, 2003.
89. J. Hao, M.J. Whitaker, B. Wong, G. Serhatkulu, K.M. Shakesheff, and S.M. Howdle. *J. of Pharmaceutical Sciences* Vol. 93, pp. 1083–1090, 2004.
90. S. Varona, S. Kareth, Á. Martín, and M.J. Cocero. *J. of Supercritical Fluids* Vol. 54, pp. 369–377, 2010.
91. R.E. Sievers and U. Karst. Methods for fine particle formation. US Patent 5639441, assigned to University Technology Corporation, Boulder, CO, U.S.A., June 17, 1997.
92. E. Reverchon. *Industrial and Engineering Chemistry Research* Vol. 41, pp. 2405–2411, 2002.
93. E. Reverchon, and A. Antonacci. *Biotechnology and Bioengineering* Vol. 97, pp. 1626–1637, 2007.
94. E. Reverchon, and A. Antonacci. *J. of Supercritical Fluids* Vol. 39, pp. 444–452, 2007.
95. D. Meterc, M. Petermann, and E. Weidner. *J. of Supercritical Fluids* Vol. 45, pp. 253–259, 2008.

96. S. Varona, Á. Martín, and M.J. Cocero. *Industrial and Engineering Chemistry Research* Vol. 50, pp. 2088–2097, 2011.
97. E. de Paz, Á. Martín, and M.J. Cocero. *J. of Supercritical Fluids* Vol. 72, pp. 125–133, 2012.
98. E. Alonso, I. Montequi, S. Lucas, and M.J. Cocero. *J. of Supercritical Fluids* Vol. 39, pp. 453–461, 2007.
99. V. Pessey, D. Mateos, F. Weill, F. Cansell, J. Etourneau, and B. Chevalier. *J. of Alloys and Compounds* Vol. 323–324, pp. 412–416, 2001.
100. E. Loste, J. Fraile, M.A. Fanovich, G.F.Woerlee, and C. Domingo. *Advanced Materials* Vol. 16, pp. 739–744, 2004.
101. S.G. Aspromonte, Á. Sastre, A.V. Boix, M.J. Cocero, and E. Alonso. *Microporous and Mesoporous Materials* Vol. 148, pp. 53–61, 2012.
102. S.P. Nalawade, F. Picchioni, and L.P.B.M. Janssen. *Progress in Polymer Science* Vol. 31, pp. 19–43, 2006.

Index

Also of Interest

Check out these published and forthcoming related titles from Scrivener Publishing

Atmospheric Pressure Plasma Treatment of Polymers
Edited by Michael Thomas and K.L. Mittal
Published 2013. ISBN 978-1-118-59621-0

Polymers for Energy Storage and Conversion
Edited by Vikas Mittal
Published 2013. ISBN 978-1-118-34454-5

Encapsulation Nanotechnologies
Edited by Vikas Mittal
Published 2013. ISBN 978-1-118-34455-2

Plastics Additives and Testing
By Muralisrinivasan Subramanian
Published 2013. ISBN 978-1-118-11890-0

Atmospheric Pressure Plasma for Surface Modification
By Rory A. Wolf
Published 2012. ISBN 9781118016237

Polymeric Sensors and Actuators
by Johannes Karl Fink
Published 2012. ISBN 978-1-118-41408-8

Handbook of Troubleshooting Plastics Processes A Practical Guide
Edited by John R. Wagner, Jr
Published 2012. ISBN 978-0-470-63922-1

Introduction to Industrial Polypropylene: Properties, Catalysts, Processes
By Dennis P. Malpass and Elliot Band.
Published 2012. ISBN 978-1-118-06276-0

Antioxidant Polymers: Synthesis, Properties and Applications
Edited by Giuseppe Cirillo and Francesca Iemma
Published 2012. ISBN 978-1-118-20854-0

Handbook of Bioplastics and Biocomposites Engineering Applications
Edited by Srikanth Pilla
Published 2011. ISBN 978-0-470-62607-8

Biopolymers Biomedical and Environmental Applications
Edited by Susheel Kalia and Luc Avérous
Published 2011. ISBN 978-0-470-63923-8

Renewable Polymers: Synthesis, Processing, and Technology
Edited by Vikas Mittal
Published 2011. ISBN 978-0-470-93877-5

Plastics Sustainability Towards a Peaceful Coexistence between Bio-based and Fossil fuel-based Plastics
Michael Tolinski
Published 2011. ISBN 978-0-470-93878-2

Green Chemistry for Environmental Remediation
Edited by Rashmi Sanghi and Vandana Singh
Published 2011 ISBN 978-0-470-94308-3

High Performance Polymers and Engineering Plastics
Edited by Vikas Mittal
Published 2011. ISBN 978-1-1180-1669-5

Handbook of Engineering and Specialty Thermoplastics
Part 1: Polyolefins and Styrenics
By Johannes Karl Fink
Published 2010. ISBN 978-0-470-62483-5

Part 2: Water Soluble Polymers
By Johannes Karl Fink
Published 2011. ISBN 978-1-118-06275-3
Part 3: Polyethers and Polyesters
Edited by Sabu Thomas and Visakh P.M.
Published 2011. ISBN 978-0-470-63926-9
Part 4: Nylons
Edited by Sabu Thomas and Visakh P.M.
Published 2011. ISBN 978-0-470-63925-2

The Basics of Troubleshooting in Plastics Processing
By Muralisrinivasan Subramanian
Published 2011. ISBN 978-0-470-62606-1

A Concise Introduction to Additives for Thermoplastic Polymers
By Johannes Karl Fink.
Published 2010. ISBN 978-0-470-60955-2

Introduction to Industrial Polyethylene: Properties, Catalysts,
Processes by Dennis P. Malpass.
Published 2010. ISBN 978-0-470-62598-9

Polymer Nanotube Nanocomposites: Synthesis, Properties, and Applications
Edited by Vikas Mittal.
Published 2010. ISBN 978-0-470-62592-7

Rubber as a Construction Material for Corrosion Protection
A Comprehensive Guide for Process Equipment Designers
2010. ISBN 978-0-470-62594-1

Miniemulsion Polymerization Technology
Edited by Vikas Mittal
Published 2010. ISBN 978-0-470-62596-5